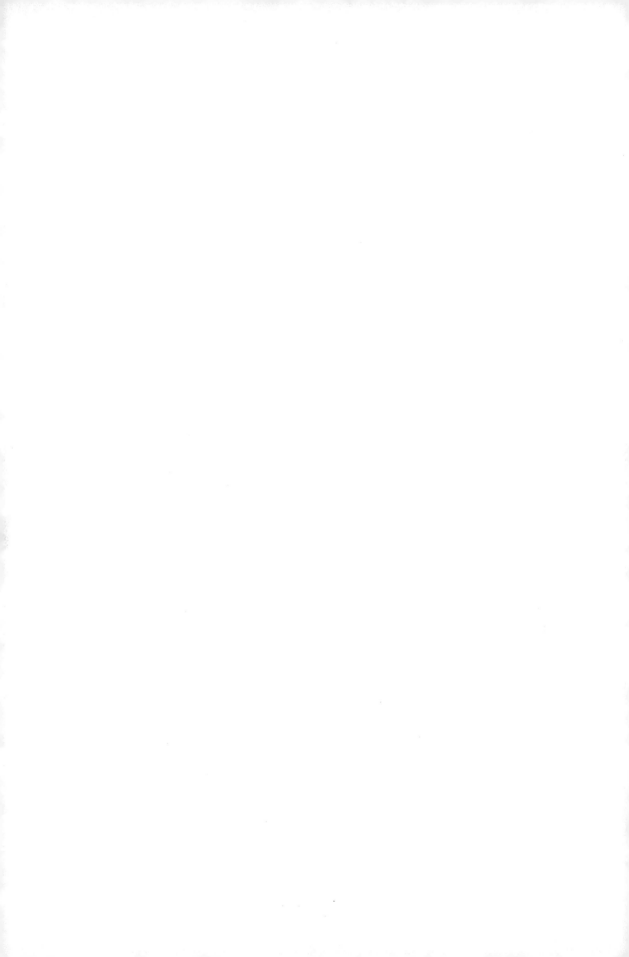

# FDG-PET/CT vs. Non-FDG Tracers in Less Explored Domains

*Editors*

SANDIP BASU
RAKESH KUMAR
ABASS ALAVI

# PET CLINICS

www.pet.theclinics.com

*Consulting Editor*
ABASS ALAVI

July 2022 • Volume 17 • Number 3

**ELSEVIER**

1600 John F. Kennedy Boulevard • Suite 1800 • Philadelphia, Pennsylvania, 19103-2899

http://www.pet.theclinics.com

**PET CLINICS Volume 17, Number 3**
**July 2022 ISSN 1556-8598, ISBN-13: 978-0-323-89718-1**

Editor: John Vassallo (j.vassallo@elsevier.com)
Developmental Editor: Karen Solomon

*PET Clinics* (ISSN 1556-8598) is published quarterly by Elsevier Inc., 360 Park Avenue South, New York, NY 10010-1710. Months of issue are January, April, July, and October. Periodicals postage paid at New York, NY, and additional mailing offices. Subscription prices per year are $262.00 (US individuals), $526.00 (US institutions), $100.00 (US students), $290.00 (Canadian individuals), $552.00 (Canadian institutions), $100.00 (Canadian students), $283.00 (foreign individuals), $552.00 (foreign institutions), and $140.00 (foreign students). To receive student and resident rate, orders must be accompanied by name of affiliated institution, date of term, and the signature of program/residency coordinator on institution letterhead. Orders will be billed at individual rate until proof of status is received. Foreign air speed delivery is included in all Clinics subscription prices. All prices are subject to change without notice. POSTMASTER: Send address changes to PET Clinics, Elsevier Health Sciences Division, Subscription Customer Service, 3251 Riverport Lane, Maryland Heights, MO 63043. **Customer Service: 1-800-654-2452 (U.S. and Canada); 314-447-8871 (outside U.S. and Canada). Fax: 314-447-8029. E-mail: journalscustomerservice-usa@elsevier.com (for print support); journalsonlinesupport-usa@elsevier.com (for online support).**

*Reprints.* For copies of 100 or more of articles in this publication, please contact the Commercial Reprints Department, Elsevier Inc., 360 Park Avenue South, New York, NY 10010-1710. Tel.: 212-633-3874; Fax: 212-633-3820; E-mail: reprints@elsevier.com.

PET Clinics is covered in MEDLINE/PubMed (Index Medicus).

# Contributors

## CONSULTING EDITOR

**ABASS ALAVI, MD, MD (Hon), PhD (Hon), DSc (Hon)**
Professor of Radiology and Neurology, Director of Research Education, Division of Nuclear Medicine, Department of Radiology, Hospital of the University of Pennsylvania, University of Pennsylvania Perelman School of Medicine, Philadelphia, Pennsylvania, USA

## EDITORS

**SANDIP BASU, MBBS, MD, DRM, DNB, MNAMS**
Radiation Medicine Centre (BARC), Tata Memorial Centre Annexe, Parel, Mumbai, India; Homi Bhabha National Institute, Mumbai, India; Department of Nuclear Medicine, All India Institute of Medical Sciences, New Delhi, India

**RAKESH KUMAR, MBBS, DRM, DNB, MNAMS, PhD**
Professor and Head, Division of Diagnostic Nuclear Medicine, Department of Nuclear Medicine, All India Institute of Medical Sciences, New Delhi, India; Homi Bhabha National Institute, Mumbai, India

**ABASS ALAVI, MD, MD (Hon), PhD (Hon), DSc (Hon)**
Professor of Radiology and Neurology, Director of Research Education, Division of Nuclear Medicine, Department of Radiology, Hospital of the University of Pennsylvania, University of Pennsylvania Perelman School of Medicine, Philadelphia, Pennsylvania, USA

## AUTHORS

**AADIL ADNAN, MBBS, MD**
Radiation Medicine Centre (BARC), Tata Memorial Centre Annexe, Parel, Mumbai, India; Homi Bhabha National Institute, Mumbai, India

**KANHAIYALAL AGRAWAL, MD**
Associate Professor, All India Institute of Medical Sciences, Bhubaneswar, India

**ABASS ALAVI, MD, MD (Hon), PhD (Hon), DSc (Hon)**
Professor of Radiology and Neurology, Director of Research Education, Division of Nuclear Medicine, Department of Radiology, Hospital of the University of Pennsylvania, University of Pennsylvania Perelman School of Medicine, Philadelphia, Pennsylvania, USA

**CYRUS AYUBCHA, MSc**
Harvard Medical School, Boston, Massachusetts, USA

**SANDIP BASU, MBBS, MD, DRM, DNB, MNAMS**
Radiation Medicine Centre (BARC), Tata Memorial Centre Annexe, Parel, Mumbai, India; Homi Bhabha National Institute, Mumbai, India; Department of Nuclear Medicine, All India Institute of Medical Sciences, New Delhi, India

**AUSTIN J. BORJA, BA**
Department of Radiology, Hospital of the University of Pennsylvania, Philadelphia, Pennsylvania, USA

**ROGER COBLE, BA**
University of California Berkeley, Berkeley, California, USA; Marcus Institute of Integrative Health, Thomas Jefferson University, Philadelphia, Pennsylvania, USA

**PATRICK M. COLLETTI, MD**
Professor of Radiology, Division of Nuclear Medicine, Department of Radiology, Keck School of Medicine of USC, University of Southern California, Los Angeles, California, USA

**VANDANA KUMAR DHINGRA, DNB**
Department of Nuclear Medicine, All India Institute of Medical Sciences, Rishikesh, India

**GOPINATH GNANASEGARAN, MSc, MD, FRCP**
Consultant in Nuclear Medicine, Royal Free London NHS Foundation Trust, London, United Kingdom

**ANGEL HEMROM, MD**
Department of Nuclear Medicine, All India Institute of Medical Sciences, New Delhi, India

**STEPHEN J. HUNT, MD, PhD**
Department of Radiology, Perelman School of Medicine, Penn Image-Guided Interventions Lab, University of Pennsylvania, Philadelphia, Pennsylvania, USA

**ROLAND HUSTINX, MD, PhD**
Division of Nuclear Medicine and Oncological Imaging, Department of Medical Physics CHU of Liege, Quartier Hopital, Liege 1, Belgium; GIGA-CRC in vivo imaging, University of Liege, Belgium

**HOSSEIN JADVAR, MD, PhD, MPH, MBA**
Professor of Radiology, Urology, and Biomedical Engineering, Division of Nuclear Medicine, Department of Radiology, Keck School of Medicine of USC, Kenneth Norris Jr. Comprehensive Cancer Center, University of Southern California, Los Angeles, California, USA

**JASIM JALEEL, MD**
Department of Nuclear Medicine, All India Institute of Medical Sciences, New Delhi, India

**DIKHRA KHAN, MD**
Department of Nuclear Medicine, All India Institute of Medical Sciences, New Delhi, India

**MOHSEN KHOSRAVI, MD**
Marcus Institute of Integrative Health, Thomas Jefferson University, Philadelphia, Pennsylvania, USA

**RAKESH KUMAR, MBBS, DRM, DNB, MNAMS, PhD**
Professor and Head, Division of Diagnostic Nuclear Medicine, Department of Nuclear Medicine, All India Institute of Medical Sciences, New Delhi, India; Homi Bhabha National Institute, Mumbai, India

**CHANDANA NAGARAJ, DNB**
Department of Neuro Imaging and Interventional Radiology, National Institute of Mental Health and Neurosciences, Bengaluru, Karnataka, India

**ANDREW B. NEWBERG, MD**
Marcus Institute of Integrative Health, Thomas Jefferson University, Philadelphia, Pennsylvania, USA; Department of Radiology, Thomas Jefferson University

**RAHUL V. PARGHANE, MBBS, MD**
Radiation Medicine Centre (BARC), Tata Memorial Hospital Annexe, Parel, Mumbai, India; Homi Bhabha National Institute, Mumbai, India

**ANKITA PHULIA, MBBS**
Maulana Azad Medical College, New Delhi, India

**SWATI SODAGAR RACHH, MBBS, DRM, DNB, MNAMS**
Department of Nuclear Medicine, Gujarat Cancer & Research Institute, Ahmedabad, India; Radiation Medicine Centre (BARC), Tata Memorial Centre Annexe, Parel, Mumbai, India

**SHOBHANA RAJU, MBBS, MD**
Homi Bhabha National Institute, Mumbai, India; Department of Nuclear Medicine, All India Institute of Medical Sciences, New Delhi, India

**WILLIAM Y. RAYNOR, MD**
Department of Radiology, Hospital of the
University of Pennsylvania, Philadelphia,
Pennsylvania, USA

**MONA-ELISABETH REVHEIM, MD, PhD, MHA**
Division of Radiology and Nuclear Medicine,
Oslo University Hospital, Institute of Clinical
Medicine, Faculty of Medicine, University of
Oslo, Oslo, Norway

**SAMBIT SAGAR, MD**
Department of Nuclear Medicine, All India
Institute of Medical Sciences, New Delhi, India

**JITENDER SAINI, DM**
Department of Neuro Imaging and
Interventional Radiology, National Institute of
Mental Health and Neurosciences, Bengaluru,
Karnataka, India

**JOEY SAUCEDO, BS**
Department of Radiology, Perelman School of
Medicine, University of Pennsylvania,
Philadelphia, Pennsylvania, USA

**JAYA SHUKLA, MSc, PhD**
Additional Professor, Department of Nuclear
Medicine and PET, PGIMER, Chandigarh, India

**AVINASH TUPALLI, MD, DM**
Department of Nuclear Medicine, All India
Institute of Medical Sciences, New Delhi, India

**ARASTOO VOSSOUGH, MD, PhD**
Department of Radiology, Division of
Neuroradiology, The Children's Hospital of
Philadelphia, Department of Radiology,
Perelman School of Medicine, University of
Pennsylvania, Philadelphia, Pennsylvania,
USA

**SIMON WAN, FRCR**
Consultant in Radionuclide Radiologist,
University College London Hospitals, NHS
Foundation Trust, London, United Kingdom

**THOMAS J. WERNER, MS**
Department of Radiology, Hospital of the
University of Pennsylvania, Philadelphia,
Pennsylvania, USA

**NADIA WITHOFS, MD, PhD**
Division of Nuclear Medicine and Oncological
Imaging, Department of Medical Physics CHU
of Liege, Quartier Hopital, Liege 1, Belgium;
GIGA-CRC in vivo imaging, University of Liege,
Belgium

**DIVYA YADAV, MD**
The University of Texas MD Anderson Cancer
Center, Houston, Texas, USA

**ALIREZA ZANDIFAR, MD**
Department of Radiology, Division of
Neuroradiology, The Children's Hospital of
Philadelphia, Philadelphia, Pennsylvania,
USA

# Contents

MRI is the first-choice imaging technique for brain tumors. Positron emission tomography can be combined together with multiparametric MRI to increase diagnostic confidence. Radiolabeled amino acids have gained wide clinical acceptance. The reported pooled specificity of [18F]FDG positron emission tomography is high and [18F]FDG might still be the first-choice positron emission tomography tracer in cases of World Health Organization grade 3 to 4 gliomas or [18F]FDG-avid tumors, avoiding the use of more expensive and less available radiolabeled amino acids. The present review discusses the additional value of positron emission tomography with a focus on [18F]FDG and radiolabeled amino acids.

Endocrine neoplasms and malignancies are a group of tumors with varied clinical, histopathologic, and functional features. These tumors may vary from sporadic to hereditary, isolated entities to multiple neoplastic syndromes, unifocal locally invasive, and advanced to multifocal tumors with disseminated distant metastases. The presence of various specific biomarkers and specific receptor targets serves as a valuable tool for diagnosis, prognosis, and management. Nuclear medicine techniques using the historical rectilinear scanners and planner gamma camera imaging for a long time have been incorporated in the management of endocrine neoplasms.

Molecular imaging with PET-computerized tomography (PET-CT) plays an important role in oncology. There is current and evolving evidence supporting the use of fluorodeoxyglucose (FDG) and non-FDG tracers in assessment patients with hepatobiliary and pancreatic cancers in various clinical scenarios. In this chapter, we discuss the advantages and limitations of FDG and non-FDG PET-CT in the management of patients with hepatobiliary and pancreatic cancers.

Hormonal therapy has long been recognized as a mainstay treatment for prostate cancer. New generation imaging agents have provided unprecedented opportunities at all phases along the natural history of prostate cancer. We review the literature on the effect of androgens and androgen deprivation therapy on prostate tumor at its various biological phases using the new generation molecular imaging agents in conjunction with positron emission tomography.

Divya Yadav, Rakesh Kumar, Ankita Phulia, Sandip Basu, and Abass Alavi

Hormone-sensitive breast cancer, which demonstrates hormone receptor positivity, accounts for approximately 75% of newly diagnosed breast cancer. 2-[18F]-Fluoro-2-deoxy-glucose is the nonspecific radiotracer of glucose metabolism as opposed to specific receptor based tracers like 16α-[18F]-fluoro-17β-estradiol and [18F]-fluoro-furanyl-norprogesterone, which provide essential information about receptor status in the management of hormonally active malignancies. The complementary information provided by (a) 2-[18F]-fluoro-2-deoxy-glucose imaging for staging and prognostication along with (b) analyzing the hormonal receptor status with receptor-based PET imaging in breast cancer can optimize tumor characterization and influence patient management.

Angel Hemrom, Avinash Tupalli, Abass Alavi, and Rakesh Kumar

Multiple myeloma (MM) accounts for 0.9% of cancer diagnoses, and incidence and mortality rate have increased in previous years. 18F-fluorodeoxyglucose (FDG) PET–computed tomography (CT) is an established modality for MM evaluation. MR imaging is helpful where 18F-FDG PET-CT is lacking. To standardize PET reporting, methods like Italian Myeloma Criteria for PET Use and Deauville criteria have been studied. Tracers like 11C-acetate and 11C-choline/18F-fluoromethylcholine (FCH) have shown higher sensitivity and detected more focal lesions and diffuse involvement than 18F-FDG PET-CT. 18F-FCH showed higher maximum standardized uptake value than 18FDG. 11C-methionine appears to be the best radiopharmaceutical, apart from 18F-FDG, for evaluating MM.

Austin J. Borja, Jitender Saini, William Y. Raynor, Cyrus Ayubcha, Thomas J. Werner, Abass Alavi, Mona-Elisabeth Revheim, and Chandana Nagaraj

Gliomas are the most common primary brain tumors. Hybrid PET/MR imaging has revolutionized brain tumor imaging, allowing for noninvasive, simultaneous assessment of morphologic, functional, metabolic, and molecular parameters within the brain. Molecular information obtained from PET imaging may aid in the detection, classification, prognostication, and therapeutic decision making for gliomas. $^{18}$F-fluorodeoxyglucose (FDG) has been widely used in the setting of brain tumor imaging, and multiple techniques may be employed to optimize this methodology. More recently, a number of non–$^{18}$F-FDG–PET radiotracers have been applied toward brain tumor imaging and are used in clinical practice.

The evolution of the fibroblast activation protein inhibitor molecules over the past decade has brought into the forefront a novel theranostic agent that has the potential of matching the workhorse of PET/computed tomography, [fluorine-18] fluoro-2-deoxy-d-glucose (18F-FDG). It is hoped that in the next decade it can act as a complementary tracer to 18F-FDG, in providing phenotypic and biomarker information and also in directing fibroblast activation protein–targeted therapies.

The various semiquantitative and quantitative PET-CT parameters provide measurement of disease activity and assessment of treatment response in the PET-CT studies. These include standardized uptake value (SUV), metabolic tumor volume (MTV) and total lesion glycolysis (TLG), and total metabolic tumor volume (TMTV). Thresholding and adaptive thresholding methods are commonly used algorithms for the evaluation of global disease activity. Readily available commercial software frequently in-built with the current generation PET-CT scanners for providing easy, less time consuming, highly reproducible, and more accurate measurement of global disease activity on PET-CT imaging in evaluation of malignant as well as benign disorders.

Positron emission tomography (PET) has been a key component in the diagnostic armamentarium for assessing neurodegenerative diseases such as Alzheimer or Parkinson disease. PET imaging has been useful for diagnosing these disorders, identifying their pathophysiology, and following their treatment. Further, PET imaging has been extensively used for both clinical and research purposes, particularly for helping with potential therapeutic approaches for managing neurodegenerative diseases. This article will review the current literature regarding PET imaging in patients with neurodegenerative disorders. This includes an evaluation of the most commonly used tracer fluorodeoxyglucose that measures cerebral glucose metabolism, tracers that assess neurotransmitter systems, and tracers designed to reveal disease-specific pathophysiological processes. With the continuing development of an expanding variety of radiopharmaceuticals, PET imaging will likely play a prominent role in future research and clinical applications for neurodegenerative diseases.

PET/computed tomography (CT) with fluorodeoxyglucose and nonfluorodeoxyglucose PET tracers has established itself in the management of malignant disorders. Its role in the assessment of nonmalignant conditions, such as infectious and noninfectious inflammatory diseases and other benign conditions, has emerged independently and alongside its role being evaluated in malignancy and continues to evolve.

It is evident that PET/CT has the potential to play a significant role in various nonmalignant disorders of the thorax. This review highlights current developments and areas where PET/CT has a potential to impact the clinical management of nonmalignant thoracic conditions with special focus on nonfluorodeoxyglucose tracers.

Infection imaging has been an important part of nuclear medicine practice. Infections in prosthetic joints and diabetic foot are associated with devastating complications, posing substantial challenge for both diagnosis and overall management. For many years, conventional nuclear medicine techniques have been used to frame a painful joint arthroplasty or diabetic foot infection. The various functional nuclear imaging modalities used include labeled leukocyte imaging, combined leukocyte-marrow scintigraphy, antigranulocyte antibody scintigraphy, 3-phase bone scintigraphy, and fluorodeoxyglucose PET/computed tomography, yet no single method has proved to be highly sensitive and specific and at the same time safe, simple, and time-effective.

The role of nuclear medicine for noninvasive assessment of infection and inflammation is well established. The role of nuclear medicine is limited to initial diagnosis, recurrence, and response assessment of infections and inflammations such as tuberculosis, sarcoidosis, vasculitis, osteomyelitis, immunoglobulin G4–related diseases, and coronavirus disease 2019, as the specificity is affected by false positivity due to physiologic fluorodeoxyglucose uptake in specific organ and nonspecific uptake in postoperative cases. PET with fludeoxyglucose F 18/CT is a well-established modality for diagnosis of fever of unknown origin helping in optimized management of the patient.

Fluorodeoxyglucose (FDG)-PET has expanding applications in the field of interventional radiology. FDG-PET provides both qualitative and quantitative assessments of malignancy, infection, and inflammation. These assessments can assist interventional radiologists in selecting the most appropriate treatment options for their oncology patients. FDG-PET is also useful for evaluating the response to interventional treatments and in predicting the prognosis of oncology patients. Finally, FDG-PET can assist the interventional radiologist in diagnosing and monitoring response to treatment of infection and inflammation. Nevertheless, there is a need for additional prospective studies to further establish the role of FDG-PET in these applications.

# PET CLINICS

**THE CLINICS ARE AVAILABLE ONLINE!**
Access your subscription at:
www.theclinics.com

## PROGRAM OBJECTIVE

The goal of the *PET Clinics* is to keep practicing radiologists and radiology residents up to date with current clinical practice in positron emission tomography by providing timely articles reviewing the state of the art in patient care.

## TARGET AUDIENCE

Practicing radiologists, radiology residents, and other health care professionals who provide patient care utilizing radiologic findings.

## LEARNING OBJECTIVES

Upon completion of this activity, participants will be able to:

1. Review the purpose of FDG and non-FDG PET tracers as the standard of care for diagnosing, staging, assessing, and treatment planning in malignancies, non-malignant conditions, infectious disease, and inflammatory disorders.
2. Discuss the role, response, and benefits of using FDG and non-FDG PET tracers, both traditional and novel, in accurately assessing, diagnosing, and treatment planning and prediction in malignancies, non-malignant conditions, infectious disease, and inflammatory disorders.
3. Recognize the importance of FDG and non-FDG PET tracers for diagnosing, staging, treatment response, early detection of recurrence, and prognostication of malignancies, infectious disease, and inflammatory disorders.

## ACCREDITATION

The Elsevier Office of Continuing Medical Education (EOCME) is accredited by the Accreditation Council for Continuing Medical Education (ACCME) to provide continuing medical education for physicians.

The EOCME designates this journal-based CME activity for a maximum of 14 *AMA PRA Category 1 Credit*(s)™. Physicians should claim only the credit commensurate with the extent of their participation in the activity.

All other health care professionals requesting continuing education credit for this enduring material will be issued a certificate of participation.

## DISCLOSURE OF CONFLICTS OF INTEREST

The EOCME assesses conflict of interest with its instructors, faculty, planners, and other individuals who are in a position to control the content of CME activities. All relevant conflicts of interest that are identified are thoroughly vetted by EOCME for fair balance, scientific objectivity, and patient care recommendations. EOCME is committed to providing its learners with CME activities that promote improvements or quality in healthcare and not a specific proprietary business or a commercial interest.

**The planning committee, staff, authors, and editors listed below have identified no financial relationships or relationships to products or devices they or their spouse/life partner have with commercial interest related to the content of this CME activity:**

Aadil Adnan, MBBS, MD; Kanhaiyalal Agrawal, MD; Abass Alavi, MD, MD (Hon), PhD (Hon), DSc (Hon); Cyrus Ayubcha, MSc; Sandip Basu, MBBS, MD, DRM, DNB, MNAMS; Austin J. Borja, BA; Roger Coble, BA; Patrick M. Colletti, MD; Vandana Kumar Dhingra, DNB; Gopinath Gnanasegaran, MSc, MD, FRCP; Angel Hemrom, MD; Stephen J. Hunt, MD, PhD; Roland Hustinx, MD, PhD; Hossein Jadvar, MD, PhD, MPH, MBA; Jasim Jaleel, MD; Dikhra Khan, MD; Mohsen Khosravi, MD; Manoj Krishnamoorthy; Rakesh Kumar, MBBS, DRM, DNB, MNAMS, PhD; Chandana Nagaraj, DNB; Andrew B. Newberg, MD; Rahul V. Parghane, MBBS, MD; Ankita Phulia, MBBS; Swati Sodagar Rachh, MBBS, DRM, DNB, MNAMS; Shobhana Raju, MBBS, MD; William Y. Raynor, MD; Mona-Elisabeth Revheim, MD, PhD, MHA; Sambit Sagar, MD; Jitender Saini, DM; Joey Saucedo, BS; Jaya Shukla, MSc, PhD; Doreen Thomas-Payne, MSN, BSN, RN, PMHNP-BC; Avinash Tupalli, MD, DM; Arastoo Vossough, MD, PhD; Simon Wan, FRCR; Thomas J. Werner, MS; Nadia Withofs, MD, PhD; Divya Yadav, MD; Alireza Zandifar, MD

## UNAPPROVED/OFF-LABEL USE DISCLOSURE

The EOCME requires CME faculty to disclose to the participants:

1. When products or procedures being discussed are off-label, unlabelled, experimental, and/or investigational (not US Food and Drug Administration [FDA] approved); and
2. Any limitations on the information presented, such as data that are preliminary or that represent ongoing research, interim analyses, and/or unsupported opinions. Faculty may discuss information about pharmaceutical agents that is outside of FDA-approved labelling. This information is intended solely for CME and is not intended to promote off-label use of these medications. If you have any questions, contact the medical affairs department of the manufacturer for the most recent prescribing information.

## TO ENROLL

To enroll in the *PET Clinics* Continuing Medical Education program, call customer service at 1-800-654-2452 or sign up online at http://www.theclinics.com/home/cme. The CME program is available to subscribers for an additional annual fee of USD 254.00

## METHOD OF PARTICIPATION

In order to claim credit, participants must complete the following:

1. Complete enrolment as indicated above.

2. Read the activity.
3. Complete the CME Test and Evaluation. Participants must achieve a score of 70% on the test. All CME Tests and Evaluations must be completed online.

## CME INQUIRIES/SPECIAL NEEDS

For all CME inquiries or special needs, please contact elsevierCME@elsevier.com.

# Preface

# Fluorodeoxyglucose versus Non-Fluorodeoxyglucose PET-Computed Tomography in Less-Explored Domains: An Appraisal

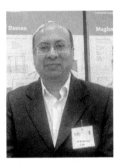

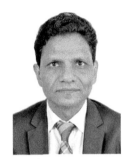

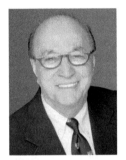

Sandip Basu, MBBS, DRM, DNB, MNAMS

Rakesh Kumar, MBBS, DRM, DNB, MNAMS, PhD

Abass Alavi, MD, MD (Hon), PhD (Hon), DSc (Hon)

*Editors*

The past two decades have witnessed remarkable growth of molecular PET imaging in cancer and other noncancerous disorders. The combined structure-function approach based on metabolic/anatomic information through integrated PET and computed tomographic (CT) scanners (PET-CT) was a milestone development in the field that led to its widespread application in the clinical workup of patients with cancer. Among the different PET tracers in the clinical arena, fluorodeoxyglucose (FDG) has been at the forefront and dominated the clinical practice, with FDG-PET-CT becoming an integral part of routine patient care in a plethora of clinical conditions. The metrics and change in glucose consumption by the tumor cells were found useful in a number of applications of FDG-PET beyond diagnostic staging, which includes treatment response monitoring early in the course of treatment, aiding in assessing and predicting treatment outcome, treatment planning including radiation therapy, and so on. New drug development is one area that has immensely benefited through the effective evaluation of new therapeutic modalities made possible through molecular PET.

Over time, a number of non-FDG-PET tracers have also been developed and employed clinically, that explored tumor cell proliferation and angiogenesis, certain specific metabolic characteristics of tumor cells, such as amino acid metabolism, radiolabeled receptor ligands for assessing specific receptor-protein overexpression on tumor cells (somatostatin receptors and Prostate Specific Membrane Antigen are some notable examples that provided boost to the development of clinical theranostics), and more recently, tracers targeting stromal cells of the tumor microenvironment by small molecule inhibitors of fibroblast activation protein (FAPI). The non-FDG-PET tracers have been of particular interest and have been examined more where FDG demonstrates limitations, either due to the physiologic distribution of the radiotracer (such as brain, liver, renal system) or due to tumors exhibiting low-glycolytic activity and hence low [18]F-FDG avidity and uptake (such as mucin-producing low-grade carcinomas, such as ovarian and gastric malignancies, grade 1 and grade 2 neuroendocrine tumors, endocrine malignancies, such as thyroid carcinoma, hormonally sensitive malignancies, such as prostate carcinoma and breast carcinoma).

This issue of *PET Clinics* endeavors to provide an update and a comparative appraisal of FDG and non-FDG-PET tracers, in areas where the

PET Clin 17 (2022) xv–xvi
https://doi.org/10.1016/j.cpet.2022.05.001
1556-8598/22/© 2022 Published by Elsevier Inc.

use of FDG has been relatively limited and critically examined for its feasibility on a routine clinical basis. In these relatively less-employed clinical domains, the recent advances and development of newer PET radiotracers for imaging have been discussed vis-à-vis FDG with regard to the current status and place in assessment of different aspects of tumor biology, and molecular targets, and also in nonmalignant conditions, including nonmalignant thoracic disorders, infectious and inflammatory conditions, and certain benign conditions within the central nervous system. The reviews have been sequenced in a similar order, such as cancerous conditions first, followed by the nonmalignant conditions. Three related and relevant articles have been interposed in between that describe (a) current status of FAPI-based PET imaging and its potential future applications, (b) PET-CT-based quantitative parameters for assessment of treatment response and disease activity in cancer and noncancerous disorders, along with two articles that describe current and (c) future state of FDG-PET applications in the field of interventional radiology.

We hope the collection of articles provide the readers a balanced view of the value and limitations of the different PET tracers in the enlisted domains and also sustain insight regarding their potential future applications. Finally, the editors would like to extend thanks to all contributors of this issue of *PET Clinics* for their sincere commitments and support.

Sandip Basu, MBBS, DRM, DNB, MNAMS
Radiation Medicine Centre (B.A.R.C.)
Tata Memorial Hospital Annexe
Jerbai Wadia Road, Parel
Mumbai 400012, India

Homi Bhabha National Institute
Mumbai, Maharashtra, India

Rakesh Kumar, MBBS, DRM, DNB, MNAMS, PhD
Division of Diagnostic Nuclear Medicine
Department of Nuclear Medicine
All India Institute of Medical Sciences
New Delhi 110029, India

Abass Alavi, MD, MD (Hon), PhD (Hon), DSc
(Hon)
Division of Nuclear Medicine
Department of Radiology
University of Pennsylvania School of Medicine
Hospital of the University of Pennsylvania
3400 Spruce Street
Philadelphia, PA 19104, USA

*E-mail addresses:*
drsanb@yahoo.com (S. Basu)
rkphulia@yahoo.com (R. Kumar)
Abass.Alavi@pennmedicine.upenn.edu (A. Alavi)

# Facts and Fictions About [18F]FDG versus Other Tracers in Managing Patients with Brain Tumors
## It Is Time to Rectify the Ongoing Misconceptions

Nadia Withofs, MD, PhD[a,b,*], Rakesh Kumar, MBBS, DRM, DNB, MNAMS, PhD[c],
Abass Alavi, MD[d], Roland Hustinx, MD, PhD[a,b]

## KEYWORDS

- Brain tumor • Neuro-oncology • FDG • FDOPA • FET • PET

## KEY POINTS

- [18F]FDG positron emission tomography/computed tomography scanning is a valuable tool for characterizing suspicious MRI lesions, and identifying recurrence/persistence of high-grade gliomas.
- [18F]FET better defines gliomas boundaries within the normal brain than with [18F]FDG, including low-grade gliomas, although it can be falsely negative in up to 30% of World Health Organization grade 2 gliomas.
- The specificity of amino acids positron emission tomography is not perfect. False- positive results occur in a wide variety of nontumor pathologic conditions.
- Both [18F]FDG and radiolabeled amino acids positron emission tomography performances should be further assessed, integrating gliomas molecular profile presented in the latest World Health Organization CNS5 classification.

## INTRODUCTION

Brain metastases are the most common malignant brain tumor in adults, most frequently related to lung cancer, breast cancer, and melanoma.[1] Brain metastases incidence is distinctly higher than that of primary malignant brain tumors. Overall, the latter account for less than 1% of all invasive cancer cases in the United States, but they are the second most common cancer in children and adolescents and the leading cause of cancer death among males aged less than 40 years and females aged less than 20 years.[2] The fifth edition of the World Health Organization (WHO) classification of tumors of the central nervous system (WHO CNS5) published in 2021 increasingly incorporates molecular diagnostic markers to histology and immunohistochemistry.[3] Such evolution complexifies the

[a] Division of Nuclear Medicine and Oncological Imaging, Department of Medical Physics, CHU of Liege, Quartier Hopital, Avenue de l'hopital, 1, Liege 1 4000, Belgium; [b] GIGA-CRC in vivo imaging, University of Liege, GIGA CHU - B34 Quartier Hôpital Avenue de l'Hôpital,11, 4000 Liège, Belgium; [c] Diagnostic Nuclear Medicine Division, All India Institute of Medical Sciences, New Delhi 110029, India; [d] Department of Radiology, Hospital of the University of Pennsylvania, 3400 Spruce Street, Philadelphia, PA 19104, USA
* Corresponding author: Nadia Withofs; email: nwithofs@chuliege.be; Division of Nuclear Medicine and Oncological Imaging, Department of Medical Physics, CHU of Liege, Quartier Hopital, Avenue de l'hopital, 1, Liege 1 4000, Belgium.
*E-mail address:* nwithofs@chuliege.be

PET Clin 17 (2022) 327–342
https://doi.org/10.1016/j.cpet.2022.03.004
1556-8598/22/© 2022 Elsevier Inc. All rights reserved.

distinction between low-grade and high-grade gliomas. For example, the presence of 1p/19q codeletion and *IDH* mutation in patients with WHO grade 2 diffuse gliomas is associated with a more favorable outcome. By contrast, patients with IDH–mutant astrocytoma and a CDKN2A/B homozygous deletion are doomed with a poor prognosis, regardless of the WHO glioma grade.[4,5] In the present review, we avoided using the terms low-grade and high-grade gliomas and replaced these terms by WHO grade 2 (and 1) versus WHO grade 3 and 4 gliomas, respectively, unless otherwise stated.

MRI is the first-choice imaging technique for brain tumors.[5–8] The T2-weighted and/or T2 fluid-attenuated inversion recovery is performed for tumor detection and delineation, but cannot reliably differentiate tumor from other conditions, such as demyelination, ischemic injury, and edema, especially once treatment, for example, radiation therapy and/or chemotherapy, has been initiated.[9] Moreover, inflammation induced by immunotherapies can alter T2 signal intensity.[6] Diffusion-weighted imaging sequence and apparent diffusion coefficient (ADC) measurements are used to characterize brain lesions and assess tumor response to treatments but similarly high ADC values can be observed in high-grade gliomas as well as in necrotic areas and abscesses.[9–11] Thin-section 3D T1-weighted sequences before and after injection of a gadolinium-based contrast agent identifies brain areas with blood–brain barrier (BBB) disruption. The latter is usually present in WHO grade 3 and 4 gliomas but also in WHO grade 2 oligodendrogliomas, lymphomas, and other non-neoplastic conditions.[6,12] Treatments, including radiation therapy, antiangiogenic therapies and immunotherapies can induce transient changes in contrast enhancement that can be misleading in assessing response to treatment.[6] The MR spectroscopy can contribute to lesion characterization, including distinction of tumor from non-neoplastic conditions, for example, post-therapy changes, but it lacks both sensitivity and specificity.[13] Perfusion MRI, dynamic contrast enhanced and dynamic susceptibility contrast MRI, allows distinction between WHO grade 3 and 4 gliomas and WHO grade 2 gliomas at diagnosis using relative cerebral blood volume (rCBV) values measured using dynamic susceptibility contrast MRI with high sensitivity (95%), but low specificity (57%), mainly due to WHO grade 2 oligodendrogliomas with elevated rCBV.[12–14] At diagnosis, perfusion MRI can guide biopsy to areas of higher WHO grade tumor. Within 24 to 48 hours after surgery, the extent of resection can be assessed by MRI. Advanced MRI techniques (eg, diffusion-weighted imaging

and ADC values; dynamic susceptibility contrast/dynamic contrast enhanced MRI and rCBV values; and MR spectroscopy) showed high diagnostic accuracy in the differentiation between treatment-induced changes (eg, pseudoprogression and radiation necrosis) and true progression, with both sensitivity and specificity of more than 85%.[6,15–17]

Even when multiple MRI sequences are performed, MRI still has limitations.[8,18] Positron emission tomography (PET) combined with computed tomography (CT) scan (or MRI) is not recommended routinely but contributes to the management of brain tumors from diagnosis to follow-up, in particular when recurrence is suspected.[19–21] Brain tumor cells metabolic adaptation is driven by tumor's phenotype (eg, mutation of the gene *IDH1* coding for isocitrate dehydrogenase 1, component involved in the tricarboxylic acid cycle) and microenvironment changes (eg, frequent hypoxic environment).[22] The brain is a special environment restricted by the BBB; gliomas and cancer cells take up nutrients from the extracellular environment, including glucose, acetate, glutamine and other amino acids (AAs) and fatty acids, to ensure tumor growth.[22]

Borja and colleagues[23] recently presented the use of PET tracers for brain tumor imaging for tumor grading, delineation, and treatment response assessment. The present work aims at further discussing the role of 2-[$^{18}$F]fluoro-2-deoxy-D-glucose ([$^{18}$F]FDG) and alternative PET tracers in the management of brain tumors.

## 2-[$^{18}$F]FLUORO-2-DEOXY-D-GLUCOSE

2-[$^{18}$F]fluoro-2-deoxy-D-glucose ([$^{18}$F]FDG) is transported across the intact BBB by glucose transporters (GLUT), mainly GLUT1 and GLUT3, and [$^{18}$F]FDG accumulation in brain tumors does not depend on BBB disruption.[24,25] Glucose is a major energy substrate of cancer cells in brain, even in the presence of oxygen (aerobic glycolysis; Warburg effect). GLUT1 and GLUT3 are upregulated in tumors, especially in aggressive tumors, and GLUT3 upregulation has been correlated with poor survival.[24,26] The glucose metabolic rate correlates with both GLUT expression and the cell proliferation rate.[26] Various methods have been used to quantify glucose metabolic rate of brain lesions using [$^{18}$F]FDG PET/CT scans, but none of them have been validated and there is no role for such measurements in routine clinical practice.[27] As a rule of thumb, the WHO grade 3 andand 4 gliomas are more likely to show high [$^{18}$F]FDG uptake, higher or similar to gray matter, whereas [$^{18}$F]FDG uptake of WHO grade 2 glioma tends to be similar

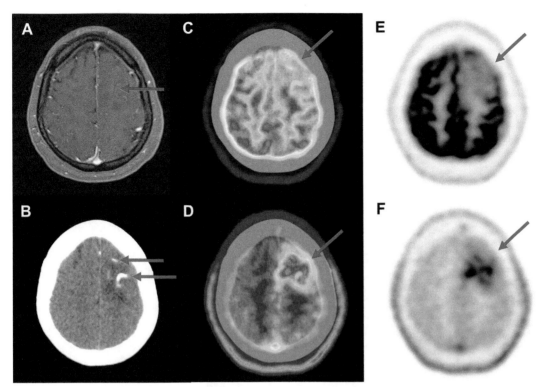

Fig. 1. Brain images of a 39-year-old patient with a left frontal lesion with mild enhancement after gadolinium injection in MR images (*A*, postgadolinium T1-weighted MRI; *red arrow*) and increased perfusion described by multiparametric MRI (not shown). The CT images of the PET/CT scans showed calcifications (*B*, CT scan of PET/CT scan; *red arrows*), characteristic of oligodendrioglial tumors. The lesion seemed to be hypometabolic in [$^{18}$F] FDG PET images (*C*, fused PET/CT scan; *E*, PET image, SUV scale of 0–8; *red arrows*) with [$^{18}$F]FDG uptake (maximum SUV 5.6) slightly higher than white matter and lower than gray matter. The [$^{18}$F]FDG TBR$_{max}$ (maximum tumoral SUV/maximum SUV in the contralateral healthy hemisphere) estimated at 0.5 suggested a WHO grade 2 glioma.[29] The [$^{18}$F]FET PET images (*D*, fused PET/CT scan; *F*, PET image, SUV scale 0–5; *red arrows*) allowed to better estimate the extent of the lesion; the [$^{18}$F]FET TBR$_{max}$ (maximum tumoral SUV/mean SUV in the contralateral healthy hemisphere), estimated at 4.5, suggested a WHO grade 3 andand 4 glioma.[75] The pathologic diagnosis was an oligodendroglioma WHO grade 2, IDH-mutant (IDH1 p.R132 mutation), and 1p/19q-codeleted. The [$^{18}$F]FDG TBR$_{max}$ correctly predicted the WHO grade 2 glioma whereas [$^{18}$F]FET TBR$_{max}$ overestimated it.

to white matter. As a result, they are most of the time not seen, or present as cortical hypometabolic areas. One method helpful to differentiate those lesions is to calculate the tumor to contralateral normal brain standardized uptake value (SUV) ratios (TBRs). TBR cutoff values help to differentiate WHO grade 3 and 4 from WHO grade 1 to 2 gliomas (eg, a TBR cutoff value of 0.6 for tumor-to-cortex maximum SUV ratio is often used).[27–29] Although the [$^{18}$F]FDG TBR is usually higher in WHO grade 3 andand 4 gliomas, it could also be similarly increased in WHO grade 1 pilocytic astrocytoma and WHO grade 2 gliomas with oligodendroglial component, which somehow limits the accuracy of [$^{18}$F]FDG PET/CT scans to predict glioma grade at diagnosis (**Fig. 1**).[30,31] Moreover, in the differential diagnosis between neoplastic and non-neoplastic lesions, [$^{18}$F]FDG PET/CT scans can be falsely negative in WHO grade 2 gliomas or metastases, and it can be falsely positive in inflammatory brain lesions.[19,32,33] Nonetheless, the combination of metabolic and MRI features is usually quite efficient for characterizing those lesions. Furthermore, [$^{18}$F]FDG uptake is an independent prognostic marker in primary central nervous system lymphoma and in WHO grade 4 gliomas at diagnosis and after treatment initiation.[28,34–36] Environmental conditions influence [$^{18}$F]FDG transport at the BBB and in brain tumors, for example, hyperglycemia associated with diabetes or hypoxia.[24] The major drawback of [$^{18}$F]FDG is the uptake in brain cells, including astrocytes, microglia and neurons, and hampering precise tumor delineation.[24]

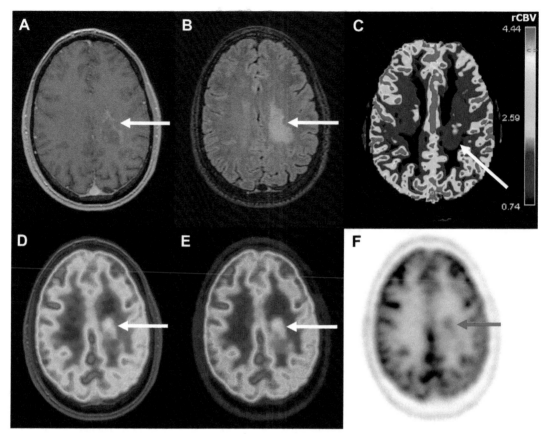

Fig. 2. [$^{18}$F]FDG PET and MR images of a 34-year-old patient who presented with neurologic deficits related to a left frontoparietal brain lesion. The postgadolinium T1-weighted MR images demonstrated peripheral contrast enhancement (A, white arrow), whereas the T2/fluid-attenuated inversion recovery (FLAIR) sequence allowed visualization of the lesion with better contrast (B, white arrow). The perfusion MR images showed increased rCBV (C, white arrow). The [$^{18}$F]FDG PET images highlighted a tumor area with high [$^{18}$F]FDG uptake in the most anterior part of the lesion (D, E, fused PET/MRI, white arrows; F, PET image, SUV scale 0–10; lesion maximum SUV, 6.1; TBR$_{max}$, 0.6; red arrow), which therefore was suggested as the best biopsy site to neurosurgeon. The pathologic diagnosis was a WHO grade 4 glioma.

Even though [$^{18}$F]FDG PET/CT alone has limited accuracy in the diagnosis of a suspected brain tumor, it can be a reliable imaging technique to guide stereotactic brain biopsy to tumor areas with the highest [$^{18}$F]FDG uptake, more likely to correspond with WHO grade 3 and 4 gliomas, avoiding sampling errors and undergrading gliomas based on MRI only (Fig. 2).[37–39] Pirotte and colleagues,[37,40] in a work published in 2004 when more advanced MRI techniques such as perfusion were in its infancy, were able to use [$^{18}$F]FDG PET for guiding stereotactic biopsy in almost one-half of patients (n = 14/32). The combination of [$^{18}$F]FDG PET and multiparametric MRI might significantly increase the performance of [$^{18}$F]FDG PET for stereotactic biopsy target definition but this has not been addressed in the era of multiparametric MRI.[13]Note that in case of suspected primary central nervous system lymphoma, additional whole-body [$^{18}$F]FDG PET/CT scanning is recommended for staging.[41]

[$^{18}$F]FDG PET/CT scanning can be considered in combination with multiparametric MRI for WHO grade 3 and 4 gliomas or [$^{18}$F]FDG-avid metastases for differentiating tumor recurrence from treatment-induced changes induced by BBB breakdown and edema, including pseudoprogression and radiation necrosis.[7,19,27,36,42] In the follow-up MRI, the extent of contrast enhancement in T1-weighted sequence or T2/fluid-attenuated inversion recovery–weighted MR signal can temporarily increase within the first 3 months after radiation therapy completion in up to two-third of patients with WHO grade 4 gliomas, mimicking progression. And, there is an increased likelihood of pseudoprogression in WHO grade 4 gliomas with O$^6$-methylguanine–DNA methyltransferase (MGMT) promoter methylation.[7,36,43]

Beyond 6 months and up to several years after radiation therapy for metastases or gliomas, radiation necrosis can occur within the irradiated field in up to one-quarter of cases, with the risk increasing with total radiation dose, irradiated volume, and additional chemotherapy.[7,36] [$^{18}$F]FDG PET/CT scanning can help to differentiate tumor progression or recurrence from tumor pseudoprogression or radiation injuries.[44] Meta-analyses showed that sensitivity and specificity of [$^{18}$F]FDG PET scans for distinction between WHO grade 3 and 4 gliomas progression versus treatment-related changes are 78% to 84% and 70% to 87%, respectively, with wide 95% confidence intervals (CI), especially in term of specificity.[44–46] The sensitivity of [$^{18}$F]FDG PET/CT scanning is limited by the high [$^{18}$F]FDG background uptake, especially when lesions are small (≤20 mm in diameter) and located in the gray matter.[47] The specificity might be limited by inflammation, especially early after surgery and/or radiation therapy. Again, the combined use of multiparametric MRI and [$^{18}$F]FDG provides higher accuracy, in particular when including information provided by perfusion MRI.[48,49]

## RADIOLABELED AMINO ACIDS

An alternate metabolic pathway was investigated when the radiolabeled AA, L-methyl-[$^{11}$C]methionine ([$^{11}$C]MET) was developed in the 1980s.[50] L-type AAs are actively transported from systemic circulation across the BBB into the brain by L-type AA transporter 1 (LAT1) expressed in luminal and abluminal sides of the BBB endothelial cells.[51] The L-type AAs are, therefore, transported in normal brain and brain lesions without BBB disruption such as WHO grade 2 gliomas.[52] By contrast with [$^{18}$F]FDG PET scans, the radiolabeled [$^{11}$C]MET PET images show a low background activity in normal brain, providing higher tumor-to-background contrast, even in low-grade gliomas.[53] LAT1 is expressed by endothelial cells and tumor cells, and the high AAs transport in higher grade gliomas and brain metastases might be related to increased microvessel density (angiogenesis) and/or increased tumor cell density and/or LAT1 overexpression and transport activity, ultimately reflecting tumor cells proliferation activity.[54–56] The sensitivity and specificity of [$^{11}$C]MET PET for the diagnosis of suspected glioma are variable, at 76% to 100% and 75% to 100%, respectively.[56] Some WHO grade 2 gliomas show no [$^{11}$C]MET uptake, resulting in false-negative results.[56,57] Similar to [$^{18}$F]FDG, false-positive cases have been reported using [$^{11}$C]MET PET due to uptake in inflammatory

processes and treatment-related changes owing to BBB disruption and vascular proliferation, including leucoencephalitis, brain abscesses, multiple sclerosis, hematoma, necrosis, acute demyelination, and ischemia.[56,58–61] The WHO grade 3 and 4 gliomas are more likely to show higher [$^{11}$C]MET uptake than WHO grade 2 gliomas.[56] Various TBR cutoff values, ranging from 1.3 to 2.05, have been used to predict glioma grade using [$^{11}$C]MET PET, providing limited accuracy as a consequence ofas large TBR values overlaps between WHO grade 2, 3, and 4 gliomas.[56] Similar to [$^{18}$F]FDG, high [$^{11}$C]MET TBR have been reported in oligodendrogliomas with 1p/19q codeletion, as high as in WHO grade 3 and 4 gliomas.[31,53] Overall, areas of highest [$^{18}$F]FDG uptake and [$^{11}$C]MET uptake are concordant in gliomas; however, owing to the low background activity using [$^{11}$C]MET PET scans, the latter is preferred for guiding biopsy, but also to better delineate tumor extent for radiation therapy planning.[37,62]

The drawbacks of PET imaging using [$^{11}$C]MET are many, including the short half-life of [$^{11}$C] (20 minutes) requiring on-site cyclotron, and the rapid incorporation after a few minutes of [$^{11}$C]MET into proteins and tracer metabolization into radiolabeled metabolites.[63] Therefore, in the 1990s, the [$^{18}$F]-labeled artificial AA, O-(2-[$^{18}$F]fluoroethyl)-L-tyrosine ([$^{18}$F]FET), was developed with the advantages of the longer half-life of [$^{18}$F] (110 minutes) and of not being incorporated into proteins, resulting in the absence of radiolabeled metabolites.[64,65] Owing to its low lipophilicity, brain [$^{18}$F]FET uptake by diffusion through the BBB is not significant.[64] Another advantage of [$^{18}$F]FET is its lower uptake in inflammatory cells compared with [$^{11}$C]MET.[58,59] Similar clinical performances are reported for [$^{11}$C]MET and [$^{18}$F]FET in the management of gliomas and metastases.[66] In a meta-analysis assessing the diagnostic performance of [$^{18}$F]FET and [$^{18}$F]FDG PET in suspected brain tumors, Dunet and colleagues[32] demonstrated a significantly higher sensitivity of [$^{18}$F]FET PET (0.94; 95% CI, 0.79–0.98) compared with [$^{18}$F]FDG (0.38; 95% CI, 0.27–0.50) for the diagnosis of brain tumor versus nontumoral lesions, with comparable specificity (0.88; 95% CI, 0.37–0.99, and 0.86; 95% CI, 0.31–0.99, respectively). Even though [$^{18}$F]FET is transported in gliomas irrespective of BBB disruption, passive tracer influx through disrupted BBB disruption, passive tracer influx through disrupted BBB and in nonneoplastic brain lesions limits the specificity of [$^{18}$F]FET.[67] As with [$^{18}$F]FDG and [$^{11}$C]MET PET, [$^{18}$F]FET PET can be falsely positive in brain abscesses, intracerebral acute hematomas, acute infarctions, demyelinating inflammatory central

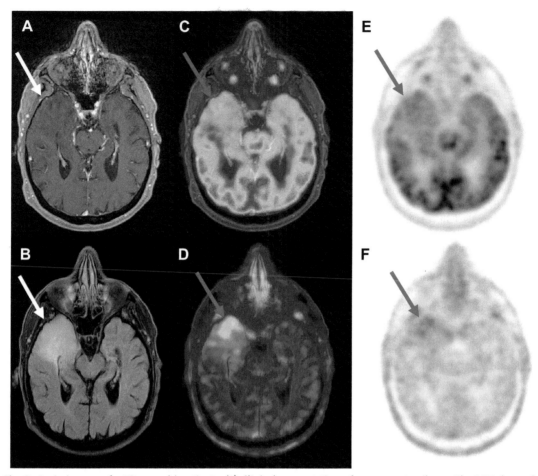

**Fig. 3.** Brain images of a 73-year-old patient with clinical presentation of new-onset epilepsy. The MRI showed a right temporal lesion with mild enhancement (*A*, postgadolinium T1-weighted sequence; *B*, T2-weighted/fluid-attenuated inversion recovery [FLAIR] MR image; *white arrows*). The [$^{18}$F]FDG PET scan showed tumoral uptake lower than gray matter (*C*, fused PET/MRI; *E*, PET image SUV scale 0–8; TBR$_{max}$ 0.7; *red arrows*). The [$^{18}$F]FET PET scan showed a heterogeneous lesion with foci of higher [$^{18}$F]FET uptake (*D*, fused PET/MRI; *F*, PET image SUV scale 0–5; TBR$_{max}$ 2.8; red *arrows*). The pathologic analyses showed a WHO grade 4 glioma, *IDH* wild type.

nervous system lesions (eg, multiple sclerosis), meningoencephalitis, and other conditions with acute inflammation and/or reactive astroglio-sis[33,59,67,68] Both [$^{18}$F]FDG and radiolabeled AAs PET can also be falsely positive in (neuro)sarcoid-osis.[67,69] In addition, high [$^{18}$F]FET activity can be observed in vascular malformations, including cavernoma.[67] [$^{11}$C]MET and [$^{18}$F]FET uptake mimicking tumor activity has been reported in (subclinical) epileptic activity associated with brain tumors, radiation necrosis, focal cortical dysplasia, or arteriovenous malformations.[70–73] In contrast, the negative predictive value of [$^{18}$F]FET PET to exclude gliomas is limited because [$^{18}$F]FET PET scans can be negative in about 30% of WHO grade 2 gliomas.[73–75] Nevertheless, a negative [$^{18}$F]FET PET scans excludes WHO grade 3 and 4 gliomas with a high probability

(with the exception for small lesions).[73,75] [$^{18}$F]FET PET scans actually identify WHO grade 3 and 4 gliomas in up to one-third of the patients whose preoperative MRI suspected WHO grade 2 glioma, with a sensitivity of 95%, specificity of 72%, positive predictive value of 74%, and nega-tive predictive value of 95%.[62,76,77] The radiola-beled AAs PET, thanks to the lower background activity compared with [$^{18}$F]FDG, can better iden-tify the most appropriate site of biopsy in hetero-geneous lesions, detecting foci of higher grade gliomas with no or mild contrast enhancement in MR images, avoiding biopsy undersampling (**Fig. 3**).[19] Similar to [$^{11}$C]MET, there are large over-laps in TBR values across WHO grade 2, 3, and 4 gliomas (see **Fig. 1**).[73] However, the accuracy to distinguish WHO grade 2 from WHO grade 3 and 4 gliomas is improved when evaluating the kinetics

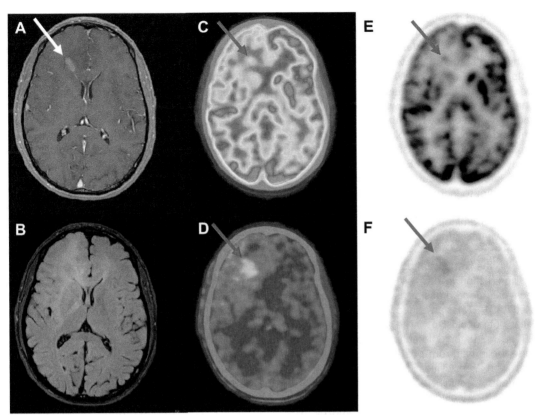

Fig. 4. Brain images of a 25-year-old patient with the initial diagnosis of WHO grade 2 diffuse astrocytoma located in the right frontal lobe, who underwent maximal surgical resection. Five years later, a follow-up MRI showed the appearance of a focal area of gadolinium enhancement in T1-weighted sequence (*A*, T1-weighted sequence, *white arrow*; *B*, T2/fluid-attenuated inversion recovery [FLAIR] sequence). The [$^{18}$F]FDG PET images (*C*, fused PET/MRI; *E*, PET image SUV scale 0–8; red *arrows*) showed a focal high uptake corresponding to the gadolinium enhancement with $TBR_{max}$ estimated at 0.6, suggesting malignant transformation. The [$^{18}$F]FET PET images (*D*, fused PET/MRI; *F*, PET image SUV scale 0–5; red *arrows*) showed larger extent of uptake and a slightly higher uptake in the same region as [$^{18}$F]FDG PET scan and MRI with a $TBR_{max}$ estimated at 2.6. Note that 2-[$^{18}$F]fluoro-L-tyrosine ([$^{18}$F]TYR) did not show tumoral uptake at diagnosis (image not showed). Pathology confirmed transformation into WHO grade 3 glioma.

of [$^{18}$F]FET uptake. Indeed, the time–activity curves increase for WHO grade 2 gliomas, and decrease for WHO grade 3 and 4 gliomas, with the early timeframe (5–15 minutes) showing the greater difference.[27,62,75,78,79] The biological processes underlying [$^{18}$F]FET time–activity curve patterns are not yet elucidated and the contribution of [$^{18}$F]FET transport activity, blood volume and perfusion (related to increased angiogenesis in WHO grade 4 gliomas), possible passive diffusion in disrupted BBB in WHO grade 3 and 4 gliomas and [$^{18}$F]FET efflux, respectively, is not known.[80,81] Even if the kinetic parameters are taken into account, [$^{18}$F]FET PET scanning has limited accuracy to predict glioma grade at diagnosis, as well as detecting malignant transformation of WHO grade 2 gliomas.[82,83] **Fig. 4** illustrates a case for which both [$^{18}$F]FET PET and [$^{18}$F]FDG PET scans were performed for a

suspected malignant transformation of a WHO grade 2 diffuse astrocytoma; the [$^{18}$F]FDG PET scan alone correctly detected malignant transformation to WHO grade 3 glioma. However, the [$^{18}$F]FET PET scan allowed better delineation of tumor recurrence extent, which might be a valuable complementary information for surgical planning.

The undisputed advantage of radiolabeled AAs over [$^{18}$F]FDG is the better contrast between tumor uptake and cortical background, making possible the delineation of tumor extent, helping radiation oncologist for tumor delineation, especially beyond contrast-enhanced areas for which MRI has a limited ability to differentiate nonenhancing infiltrating tumor from edema or treatment-related changes in cases of recurrence.[36,84–89] A large retrospective multicenter study showed an association between overall survival and maximal resection of both contrast-enhanced and non–contrast-enhanced tumor using MRI in patients with newly diagnosed WHO grade 4 glioma regardless of *IDH* status, and methylation status of the *MGMT* promoter in patients with *IDH* wild-type WHO grade 4 glioma.[90] Baseline tumor volume based on [18F]FET PET scans in patients with newly diagnosed WHO grade 4 glioma before radiotherapy plus concomitant and adjuvant temozolomide was inversely correlated with progression-free survival and overall survival.[91] [18F]FET PET scanning might be of interest for surgical resection planning with the aim to increase the chances of maximal resection, in combination with preoperative MRI and using 5-aminolevulinic acid for the intraoperative visualization of areas of tumor infiltration.[92–94]

During the first 3 months after chemoradiotherapy completion in case WHO grade 4 gliomas, when pseudoprogression is suspected, radiolabeled AAs PET has an added value when perfusion MRI is not conclusive.[36] The accuracy of [18F]FET PET scanning in differentiating recurrent WHO grade 4 gliomas from post-treatment changes is high, with sensitivities ranging from 82% to 100% and specificities from 86% to 94%.[95–99] In a recent study including patients with WHO grade 4 gliomas treated with lomustine–temozolomide chemoradiation and for which MRI was equivocal after radiotherapy inside the radiation field (median time interval, 10 weeks; range, 5–34 weeks), [18F]FET PET imaging proved highly performant using a $TBR_{mean}$ cutoff of less than 1.95 (sensitivity, 82%; specificity, 92%; positive predictive value, 90%; negative predictive value, 85%; accuracy, 87%; area under the curve ± standard error, 0.77 ± 0.12).[95] When radiation necrosis is suspected in case of gliomas or metastases, radiolabeled AAs PET may help when perfusion MRI is uncertain.[36,42] However, the accuracy varies across studies (sensitivity of 74%–90%; specificity of 73%–100%); false-positive and false-negative results can occur, depending on tumor cell type and LAT activity, tracer activity related to passive diffusion across disrupted BBB and vascular volume and density associated with angiogenesis (Fig. 5).[42,100]

The AA 3, 4-dihydroxy-6-[18F]-fluoro-L-phenylalanine ([18F]DOPA) has also been used for imaging brain tumors; it is also transported across the BBB and in tumor cells by LAT and [18F]DOPA PET showed comparable performances to [18F]FET and [11C]MET PET scanning.[45,4645] One limitation of [18F]DOPA is that it is rapidly metabolized in the periphery and in the striatum, and released [18F]-labeled metabolites can be transported again and cross the BBB.[101–103] Tatekawa and colleagues[104] recently showed a relationship between [18F]DOPA uptake and ADC and rCBV measurements, respectively, in different molecular subtypes of gliomas. The [18F]DOPA SUV normalized to the median uptake value of the striatum was positively correlated with rCBV and negatively correlated with ADC in *IDH* wild-type and *IDH* mutant 1p/19q noncodeleted gliomas, whereas a significant positive correlation was observed between the SUV normalized to the median uptake value of the striatum and the ADC only in the subgroup of oligodendrogliomas with *IDH* mutant and 1p/19q codeletion.[104]

For the distinction between true recurrence and radiation necrosis in a small patients sample, Jena and colleagues[105] recently showed that the combination [18F]DOPA PET imaging of multiparametric MRI (perfusion, diffusion, and spectroscopy) achieved 95% accuracy with greater than 95% sensitivity and specificity.

The non-natural AA anti–1-amino-3-[18F]fluoro-cyclobutane-1-carboxylic acid ([18F]FACBC), originally developed for brain tumor imaging has been less investigated.[106] By contrast with [11C]MET, [18F]FET, and [18F]DOPA, the transport of [18F]FACBC across the BBB and in tumor cells is mediated mainly by the alanine, serine, cysteine transporter 2 (ASCT2; SLC1A5).[107] Michaud and colleagues[107] showed lower and slower uptake of [18F]FACBC than [11C]MET in brain lesions suspected of glioma recurrence or progression, although the [18F]FACBC normal brain background was lower.

## NON–AMINO ACID POSITRON EMISSION TOMOGRAPHY RADIOTRACERS

Similar to AAs, non-AAs unconventional tracers providing low or no background activity in brain compared with [18F]FDG and better contrast, are being investigated for glioma imaging.[108] The delivery of an imaging agent into the brain is challenged by highly restricted BBB.[109] After intravenous injection, for the tracer to reach brain tumor cells, when the BBB is intact, it must first be recognized by a receptor on the BBB (the imaging agent should mimic the structure of transporter substrate), be transported in luminal and abluminal sides of the BBB endothelial cells and reach the tumor cell target after entering into the brain parenchyma, and, ultimately, in a sufficient amount to obtain a detectable imaging signal.[110] For example, the promising radiolabeled ligand targeting fibroblast activation protein [68Ga]FAPI, shows high accumulation in *IDH*-wildtype WHO 4 gliomas and WHO grade 3 and 4 gliomas, with a disrupted BBB, but not in WHO grade II gliomas. It is highly

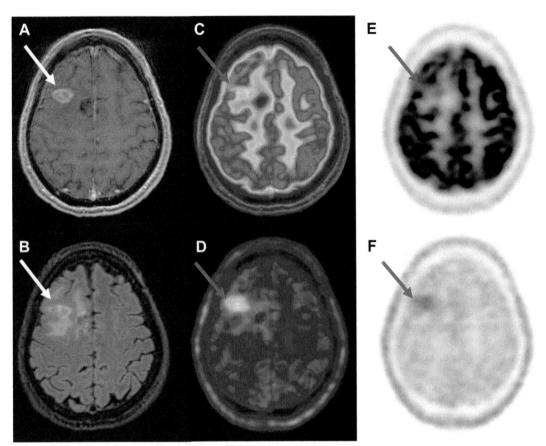

Fig. 5. Brain Images of a 65-year-old patient with a WHO grade 4 glioma with MGMT promotor methylation and suspected recurrence 4 months after the end of concomitant radiochemotherapy based on follow-up multiparametric MRI (*A*, postgadolinium T1-weighted sequence; *B*, T2/fluid-attenuated inversion recovery [FLAIR] MRI; *white arrows*) showing an area of gadolinium enhancement with increased rCBV (perfusion MRI not shown) next to surgical resection site in the right frontal lobe. The [$^{18}$F]FDG PET/CT scan did not show [$^{18}$F]FDG uptake higher than gray matter (*C*, fused PET/MR; *E*, PET image, SUV scale 0–8; *red arrows*). The [$^{18}$F]FET PET images (*D*, fused PET/MR; *F*, PET image, SUV scale 0–5; *red arrows*) showed [$^{18}$F]FET uptake with the TBR$_{max}$ estimated at 3.2 suggesting glioma recurrence. The lesion was resected, and the pathologic analyses showed radiation necrosis.

probable that it is not transported across an intact BBB, which in all likelihood will limit its clinical use for brain tumors.[111] Moreover, the BBB expresses efflux transporters, such as P-glycoprotein, to prevent drugs entering into the brain parenchyma, exporting them from endothelial cells back into circulating blood.[109] This efflux can occur with radiolabeled AAs such as [$^{18}$F]FET and [$^{11}$C]MET and [$^{11}$C]-labeled metabolites, being responsible for the decrease of PET signal with time.[80]

Many non-AAs PET tracers showed uptake in gliomas, but the PET signal is often not related solely to the glioma tumor cells. The mitochondrial translocator protein 18 kDa (TSPO) is upregulated in glioma cells and might be a target of interest for gliomas imaging; however, radiolabeled ligands of TSPO were originally developed for neuroinflammation imaging, because TSPO is upregulated in activated microglia and macrophages, thereby limiting the specificity of PET signal in glioma imaging.[112] Radiolabeled ligands of the prostate-specific membrane antigen PET/CT scans showed a high uptake in WHO grade 3 and 4 gliomas and might be used to differentiate WHO grade 3 and 4 from grade 2 gliomas, but the signal is mainly related to prostate-specific membrane antigen overexpression by activated endothelial cells of angiogenesis.[113–116] Similarly, WHO grade 4 gliomas showed uptake of the radiolabeled glycine–aspartic acid peptide [$^{18}$F]FPPRGD$_2$ targeting integrin $\alpha_v\beta_3$, not only owing to overexpression by glioma cells, but mainly related to integrin $\alpha_v\beta_3$ upregulation in activated endothelial cells of glioma neovasculature.[117] The radiolabeled ligands of the chemokine receptor 4 allows for imaging of glioma cells as well as-tumor associated neovasculature and immune cells of tumor microenvironment.[118]

Even though non-AA tracers are not specific for tumor cells imaging, they might still be used to better delineate tumor extent and, more importantly, being used as radiotheranostic agents.[119]

## DISCUSSION

Radiolabeled AAs and singularly [$^{18}$F]FET, developed more recently than [$^{18}$F]FDG, have gained wider clinical acceptance, and this was translated into official recommendations by the Response Assessment in Neuro-Oncology working group and European Association for Neuro-Oncology, who concluded in 2016 regarding the "superiority of AA PET over glucose PET."[19] It is obvious that [$^{18}$F]FET brings highly valuable information in several indications, but, in our opinion, it is more a matter of when to combine [$^{18}$F]FET with [$^{18}$F]FDG, rather than replacing one with another.

When it comes to distinguish neoplastic from non-neoplastic brain lesions, as well as predict glioma WHO grade, both [$^{18}$F]FDG and radiolabeled AAs present clinical limitations. In both cases, there are overlaps in the tracer uptake intensity across WHO grades 2, 3 and 4, especially in gliomas with an oligodendroglial component.[31,32,61,67,73] A shift toward using AAs has been advocated, notably based on a meta-analysis performed by Dunet and colleagues[32] in 2016. It compared the diagnostic performances of [$^{18}$F]FDG and [$^{18}$F]FET, based on a direct comparison of both tracers in the all patients and with histology as reference standard.[32] The performance of [$^{18}$F]FDG PET scanning for the diagnosis of brain tumor was significantly lower than [$^{18}$F]FET PET scanning (area under the curve, 0.56 [95% CI, 0.47–0.66] and 0.85 [95% CI, 0.77–0.93], respectively; $P<.0001$). Concluding to the definite superiority of [$^{18}$F]FET over [$^{18}$F]FDG in this setting would be misleading, however, considering the small number of studies (5 papers published between 2006 and 2010) and patients (n = 119 patients: n = 82 gliomas; n = 8 nonglioma tumors, and n = 29 nontumoral lesions). In addition to the sample size, variations in patient selection and imaging procedures are such as it would not be reasonable to generalize the conclusions.[32,120]

Several meta-analyses looked at the performances of the various radiotracers to assess tumor recurrence and progression after treatment, including radiation therapy. Nihashi and colleagues[44] showed in 2013 for [$^{18}$F]FDG and [$^{11}$C]MET a pooled sensitivity of 0.79 (0.67–0.88) and 0.70 (0.50–0.84), respectively, and a specificity of 0.70 (0.50–0.84) and 0.93 (0.44–1.0), respectively. More recently, de Zwart and colleagues[45] showed for [$^{18}$F]FDG, [$^{18}$F]FET, and [$^{11}$C]MET sensitivities of 0.82 (0.64–0.92), 0.90 (0.81–0.95), and 0.91 (0.78–0.97), respectively, and specificities of 0.79 (0.61–0.90), 0.85 (0.71–0.93), and 0.83 (0.68–0.92), respectively. Cui and colleagues, evaluated all 4 available tracers in 2021, and found a somewhat lower sensitivity of [$^{18}$F]FDG PET scanning with a pooled value of 0.76 (0.68–0.83) compared with radiolabeled AAs ([$^{18}$F]FET: 0.88, [$^{18}$F]DOPA: 0.85, and [$^{11}$C]MET: 0.92). However, [$^{18}$F]FDG PET scanning recorded the highest specificity with a pooled value of 0.87 (0.70–0.90), compared with 0.78, 0.70, and 0.78 for the 3 AAs, respectively.[46] A systematic review by Furuse and colleagues[121] further suggests that [$^{18}$F]FDG PET provides higher accuracy to differentiate radiation necrosis from tumor progression in patients with metastatic brain tumors than in patients with gliomas.

In this indication, and similar to the initial diagnosis setting, the picture as to which radiotracer should be preferred as a first-line PET is not as clear cut as it may seem. At the very least, [$^{18}$F]FDG is not thoroughly outperformed and surely cannot be discarded altogether.

Prognostic factors associated with progression-free survival and overall survival of patients with gliomas include age, tumor diameter, tumor crossing midline, performance status, and the molecular subgroup (eg, among patients with WHO grade 2 and 3 gliomas, IDH wild-type group is associated with the worst prognosis), and the extent of tumor debulking when maximal resection is possible.[7] Both [$^{18}$F]FDG and radiolabeled AA PET scans might provide independent prognostic information, such as the baseline metabolic tumor volume assessed using AAs PET scans and the extent of residual tumor early after surgery before radiation therapy.[35,88,91,122–126]

Despite the vastness of the available literature dealing with PET/CT scans or PET/MRI in brain tumors, these studies are often limited by the retrospective design and/or the small patient sample. Moreover, patients' selection criteria including the acquired sequences and results of multiparametric MRI may vary; the population of interest might also be heterogeneous as studies were performed before the latest updates of WHO CNS5 molecular classification published in 2021.[3] Eventually, the reference standard is most of the time based on imaging follow-up. Furthermore, despite valuable attempts by the European Association of Nuclear Medicine, the Society of Nuclear Medicine and Molecular Imaging, the European Association of Neuro-oncology, and the working group for

Response Assessment in Neuro-oncology with PET (PET-Response Assessment in Neuro-Oncology working group), there is not a single well-defined method that would consistently provide high diagnostic accuracy in the clinical setting (eg, various TBR$_{max}$ and TBR$_{mean}$ cutoff values based on early static vs kinetic parameters are proposed for [$^{18}$F]FET PET depending on clinical question).[27] Harmonization and prospective validation of PET image interpretation criteria should improve the interobserver agreement and facilitate comparison of studies results in literature. Future prospective studies should clarify the performance of [$^{18}$F]FDG PET scans and radiolabeled AA PET scans (and the combination) not in abstracto, but as a complementary tool to brain multiparametric MRI, taking into account the molecular profile of gliomas presented in the WHO CNS5 classification.[3] The past few years have witnessed major improvements in PET/CT detectors and reconstruction algorithms, which have further improved image resolution and lesion detectability with reduced image noise. This should positively impact the diagnostic performances of PET scanning, especially using [$^{18}$F]FDG as those images in which normal background is high.[127] Radiomics and artificial intelligence will certainly further enhance multimodality imaging performances; a recent review by Lohmann and colleagues[128] gives an overview of feature-based radiomics in neuro-oncology and examples of clinical applications.

The advantage of [$^{18}$F]FDG over radiolabeled AAs is its wide availability and low cost. Therefore, when multiparametric MRI is not conclusive, [$^{18}$F]FDG might be the first-choice PET tracer in cases of WHO grade 3 and 4 gliomas or [$^{18}$F]FDG-avid tumors, avoiding the use of more expensive and less available radiolabeled AAs (eg, [$^{11}$C]MET, [$^{18}$F]FET, or [$^{18}$F]DOPA). Radiolabeled AAs PET scans should be preferred in cases of WHO grade 2 gliomas or non [$^{18}$F]FDG-avid tumors. Ultimately, [$^{18}$F]FDG PET scans and radiolabeled AA PET scans can be combined together with multiparametric MRI to increase diagnostic confidence.[13,129]

## CLINICS CARE POINTS

- [$^{18}$F]FDG PET/CT scanning is a widely accessible imaging method that may be helpful for characterizing suspicious MRI lesions.
- [$^{18}$F]FDG PET/CT scanning performs fairly well for assessing the recurrence or persistence of high-grade gliomas.

- Tumor limits are more precisely delineated with [$^{18}$F]FET and [$^{18}$F]FDOPA than with [$^{18}$F]FDG, including low-grade gliomas.
- [$^{18}$F]FET PET scans can be falsely negative in up to 30% of WHO grade 2 gliomas.
- The specificity of AA PET scans is not perfect. Non-neoplastic brain conditions with increased blood flow and/or microvessel density, (sub-)acute inflammation or BBB disruption may all lead to false-positive results.
- Both [$^{18}$F]FDG and radiolabeled AA PET scan performances should be further assessed, integrating gliomas molecular profile presented in the latest WHO CNS5 classification.

## DISCLOSURE

The authors received no financial support for the work, authorship, and/or publication of this article.

## REFERENCES

1. Ostrom QT, Wright CH, Barnholtz-Sloan JS. Brain metastases: epidemiology. Handb Clin Neurol 2018;149:27–42.
2. Miller KD, Ostrom QT, Kruchko C, et al. Brain and other central nervous system tumor statistics. CA Cancer J Clin 2021;71(5):381–406.
3. Louis DN, Perry A, Wesseling P, et al. The 2021 WHO classification of tumors of the central nervous system: a summary. Neuro Oncol 2021;23(8):1231–51.
4. Leeper HE, Caron AA, Decker PA, et al. IDH mutation, 1p19q codeletion and ATRX loss in WHO grade II gliomas. Oncotarget 2015;6(30):30295–305.
5. Weller M, van den Bent M, Preusser M, et al. EANO guidelines on the diagnosis and treatment of diffuse gliomas of adulthood. Nat Rev Clin Oncol 2021;18(3):170–86.
6. Ellingson BM, Wen PY, Cloughesy TF. Modified criteria for radiographic response assessment in glioblastoma clinical trials. Neurotherapeutics 2017;14(2):307–20.
7. Nabors LB, Portnow J, Ahluwalia M, et al. Central nervous System Cancers, Version 3.2020, NCCN Clinical Practice Guidelines in Oncology. J Natl Compr Canc Netw 2020;18(11):1537–70.
8. Le Rhun E, Guckenberger M, Smits M, et al. EANO-ESMO Clinical Practice Guidelines for diagnosis, treatment and follow-up of patients with brain metastasis from solid tumours. Ann Oncol 2021;32(11):1332–47.
9. Wen PYC SM, Van den Bent MJ, Vogelbaum MA, et al. Response assessment in neuro-oncology clinical trials. J Clin Oncol 2017;35(21):2439–49.

10. Krabbe KG P, Wagn P, Hansen U, et al. MR diffusion imaging of human intracranial tumours. Neuroradiology 1997;39(7):483–9.

11. Hu R, Hoch MJ. Application of diffusion weighted imaging and diffusion tensor imaging in the pre-treatment and post-treatment of brain tumor. Radiol Clin North Am 2021;59(3):335–47.

12. Smits M. Imaging of oligodendroglioma. Br J Radiol 2016;89(1060):20150857.

13. Overcast WB, Davis KM, Ho CY, et al. Advanced imaging techniques for neuro-oncologic tumor diagnosis, with an emphasis on PET-MRI imaging of malignant brain tumors. Curr Oncol Rep 2021; 23(3):34.

14. Law M, Yang S, Wang H, et al. Glioma grading: sensitivity, specificity, and predictive values of perfusion MR imaging and proton MR spectroscopic imaging compared with conventional MR imaging. AJNR Am J Neuroradiol 2003;24(10): 1989–98.

15. van Dijken BRJ, van Laar PJ, Holtman GA, et al. Diagnostic accuracy of magnetic resonance imaging techniques for treatment response evaluation in patients with high-grade glioma, a systematic review and meta-analysis. Eur Radiol 2017;27(10): 4129–44.

16. Kaufmann TJ, Smits M, Boxerman J, et al. Consensus recommendations for a standardized brain tumor imaging protocol for clinical trials in brain metastases. Neuro Oncol 2020;22(6):757–72.

17. van Dijken BRJ, van Laar PJ, Smits M, et al. Perfusion MRI in treatment evaluation of glioblastomas: clinical relevance of current and future techniques. J Magn Reson Imaging 2019;49(1):11–22.

18. Thust SC, Heiland S, Falini A, et al. Glioma imaging in Europe: a survey of 220 centres and recommendations for best clinical practice. Eur Radiol 2018; 28(8):3306–17.

19. Albert NL, Weller M, Suchorska B, et al. Response Assessment in Neuro-Oncology working group and European Association for Neuro-Oncology recommendations for the clinical use of PET imaging in gliomas. Neuro Oncol 2016;18(9):1199–208.

20. Cooney TM, Cohen KJ, Guimaraes CV, et al. Response assessment in diffuse intrinsic pontine glioma: recommendations from the Response Assessment in Pediatric Neuro-Oncology (RAPNO) working group. The Lancet Oncol 2020;21(6): e330–6.

21. Fangusaro J, Witt O, Hernáiz Driever P, et al. Response assessment in paediatric low-grade glioma: recommendations from the Response Assessment in Pediatric Neuro-Oncology (RAPNO) working group. The Lancet Oncol 2020;21(6): e305–16.

22. Bi J, Chowdhry S, Wu S, et al. Altered cellular metabolism in gliomas - an emerging landscape of actionable co-dependency targets. Nat Rev Cancer 2020;20(1):57–70.

23. Borja AJ, Hancin EC, Raynor WY, et al. A critical review of PET tracers used for brain tumor imaging. PET Clin 2021;16(2):219–31.

24. Patching SG. Glucose transporters at the blood-brain barrier: function, regulation and gateways for drug delivery. Mol Neurobiol 2017;54(2): 1046–77.

25. Herholz K. Brain tumors: an update on clinical PET research in gliomas. Semin Nucl Med 2017;47(1): 5–17.

26. Flavahan WA, Wu Q, Hitomi M, et al. Brain tumor initiating cells adapt to restricted nutrition through preferential glucose uptake. Nat Neurosci 2013; 16(10):1373–82.

27. Law I, Albert NL, Arbizu J, et al. Joint EANM/EANO/RANO practice guidelines/SNMMI procedure standards for imaging of gliomas using PET with radiolabelled amino acids and [$^{18}$F]FDG: version 1.0. Eur J Nucl Med Mol Imaging 2019;46(3):540–57.

28. Toyonaga T, Yamaguchi S, Hirata K, et al. Hypoxic glucose metabolism in glioblastoma as a potential prognostic factor. Eur J Nucl Med Mol Imaging 2017;44(4):611–9.

29. Delbeke D, Meyerowitz C, Lapidus RL, et al. Optimal cutoff levels of F-18 fluorodeoxyglucose uptake in the differentiation of low-grade from high-grade brain tumors with PET. Radiology 1995;195(1):47–52.

30. Borgwardt L, Hojgaard L, Carstensen H, et al. Increased fluorine-18 2-fluoro-2-deoxy-D-glucose (FDG) uptake in childhood CNS tumors is correlated with malignancy grade: a study with FDG positron emission tomography/magnetic resonance imaging coregistration and image fusion. J Clin Oncol 2005;23(13):3030–7.

31. Manabe O, Hattori N, Yamaguchi S, et al. Oligodendroglial component complicates the prediction of tumour grading with metabolic imaging. Eur J Nucl Med Mol Imaging 2015;42(6):896–904.

32. Dunet V, Pomoni A, Hottinger A, et al. Performance of 18F-FET versus 18F-FDG-PET for the diagnosis and grading of brain tumors: systematic review and meta-analysis. Neuro Oncol 2016;18(3): 426–34.

33. Cecchin D, Garibotto V, Law I, et al. PET imaging in neurodegeneration and neuro-oncology: variants and pitfalls. Semin Nucl Med 2021;51(5):408–18.

34. Krebs S, Mauguen A, Yildirim O, et al. Prognostic value of [$^{18}$F]FDG PET/CT in patients with CNS lymphoma receiving ibrutinib-based therapies. Eur J Nucl Med Mol Imaging 2021;48(12):3940–50.

35. Chiang GC, Galla N, Ferraro R, et al. The added prognostic value of metabolic tumor size on FDG-PET at first suspected recurrence of glioblastoma multiforme. J Neuroimaging 2017;27(2):243–7.

36. Galldiks N, Niyazi M, Grosu AL, et al. Contribution of PET imaging to radiotherapy planning and monitoring in glioma patients - a report of the PET/RANO group. Neuro Oncol 2021;23(6):881–93.

37. Pirotte B, Goldman S, Massager N, et al. Comparison of 18F-FDG and 11C-methionine for PET-guided stereotactic brain biopsy of gliomas. J Nucl Med 2004;45(8):1293–8.

38. Pirotte BJ, Lubansu A, Massager N, et al. Clinical impact of integrating positron emission tomography during surgery in 85 children with brain tumors. J Neurosurg Pediatr 2010;5(5):486–99.

39. McCullough BJ, Ader V, Aguedan B, et al. Preoperative relative cerebral blood volume analysis in gliomas predicts survival and mitigates risk of biopsy sampling error. J Neurooncol 2018;136(1):181–8.

40. Petrella JR, Provenzale JM. MR perfusion imaging of the brain: techniques and applications. AJR Am J Roentgenol 2000;175(1):207–19.

41. Malani R, Bhatia A, Wolfe J, et al. Staging identifies non-CNS malignancies in a large cohort with newly diagnosed lymphomatous brain lesions. Leuk Lymphoma 2019;60(9):2278–82.

42. Galldiks N, Langen KJ, Albert NL, et al. PET imaging in patients with brain metastasis-report of the RANO/PET group. Neuro Oncol 2019;21(5):585–95.

43. Brandes AA, Franceschi E, Tosoni A, et al. MGMT promoter methylation status can predict the incidence and outcome of pseudoprogression after concomitant radiochemotherapy in newly diagnosed glioblastoma patients. J Clin Oncol 2008;26(13):2192–7.

44. Nihashi T, Dahabreh IJ, Terasawa T. Diagnostic accuracy of PET for recurrent glioma diagnosis: a meta-analysis. AJNR Am J Neuroradiol 2013;34(5):944–50. S941-S911.

45. de Zwart PL, van Dijken BRJ, Holtman GA, et al. Diagnostic Accuracy of PET tracers for the differentiation of tumor progression from treatment-related changes in high-grade glioma: a systematic review and metaanalysis. J Nucl Med 2020;61(4):498–504.

46. Cui M, Zorrilla-Veloz RI, Hu J, et al. Diagnostic accuracy of pet for differentiating true glioma progression from post treatment-related changes: a systematic review and meta-analysis. Front Neurol 2021;12:671867.

47. Dankbaar JW, Snijders TJ, Robe PA, et al. The use of (18)F-FDG PET to differentiate progressive disease from treatment induced necrosis in high grade glioma. J Neurooncol 2015;125(1):167–75.

48. Jena A, Taneja S, Jha A, et al. Multiparametric evaluation in differentiating glioma recurrence from treatment-induced necrosis using simultaneous (18)

F-FDG-PET/MRI: a single-institution retrospective study. AJNR Am J Neuroradiol 2017;38(5):899–907.

49. Hojjati M, Badve C, Garg V, et al. Role of FDG-PET/MRI, FDG-PET/CT, and dynamic susceptibility contrast perfusion MRI in differentiating radiation necrosis from tumor recurrence in glioblastomas. J Neuroimaging 2018;28(1):118–25.

50. Lilja A, Bergstrom K, Hartvig P, et al. Dynamic study of supratentorial gliomas with L-methyl-11C-methionine and positron emission tomography. AJNR Am J Neuroradiol 1985;6(4):505–14.

51. Huttunen J, Peltokangas S, Gynther M, et al. L-Type Amino Acid Transporter 1 (LAT1/Lat1)-utilizing prodrugs can improve the delivery of drugs into neurons, astrocytes and microglia. Sci Rep 2019;9(1):12860.

52. Meyer GJ, Schober O, Hundeshagen H. Uptake of 11C-L- and D-methionine in brain tumors. Eur J Nucl Med 1985;10(7–8):373–6.

53. Kim D, Chun JH, Kim SH, et al. Re-evaluation of the diagnostic performance of (11)C-methionine PET/CT according to the 2016 WHO classification of cerebral gliomas. Eur J Nucl Med Mol Imaging 2019;46(8):1678–84.

54. Okubo S, Zhen HN, Kawai N, et al. Correlation of L-methyl-11C-methionine (MET) uptake with L-type amino acid transporter 1 in human gliomas. J Neurooncol 2010;99(2):217–25.

55. Kracht LW, Friese M, Herholz K, et al. Methyl-[11C]-l-methionine uptake as measured by positron emission tomography correlates to microvessel density in patients with glioma. Eur J Nucl Med Mol Imaging 2003;30(6):868–73.

56. Glaudemans AW, Enting RH, Heesters MA, et al. Value of 11C-methionine PET in imaging brain tumours and metastases. Eur J Nucl Med Mol Imaging 2013;40(4):615–35.

57. Herholz K, Holzer T, Bauer B, et al. 11C-methionine PET for differential diagnosis of low-grade gliomas. Neurology 1998;50(5):1316–22.

58. Stober B, Tanase U, Herz M, et al. Differentiation of tumour and inflammation: characterisation of [methyl-3H]methionine (MET) and O-(2-[18F]fluoroethyl)-L-tyrosine (FET) uptake in human tumour and inflammatory cells. Eur J Nucl Med Mol Imaging 2006;33(8):932–9.

59. Salber D, Stoffels G, Oros-Peusquens AM, et al. Comparison of O-(2-18F-fluoroethyl)-L-tyrosine and L-3H-methionine uptake in cerebral hematomas. J Nucl Med 2010;51(5):790–7.

60. Nakajima R, Kimura K, Abe K, et al. 11)C-methionine PET/CT findings in benign brain disease. Jpn J Radiol 2017;35(6):279–88.

61. Van Laere K, Ceyssens S, Van Calenbergh F, et al. Direct comparison of 18F-FDG and 11C-methionine PET in suspected recurrence of glioma: sensitivity, inter-observer variability and prognostic

value. Eur J Nucl Med Mol Imaging 2005;32(1):
39–51.

62. Jansen NL, Graute V, Armbruster L, et al. MRI-suspected low-grade glioma: is there a need to perform dynamic FET PET? Eur J Nucl Med Mol Imaging 2012;39(6):1021–9.

63. Ishiwata K, Vaalburg W, Elsinga PH, et al. Comparison of L-[1-11C]methionine and L-methyl-[11C] methionine for measuring in vivo protein synthesis rates with PET. J Nucl Med 1988;29(8):1419–27.

64. Wester HJ, Herz M, Weber W, et al. Synthesis and radiopharmacology of O-(2-[18F]fluoroethyl)-L-tyrosine for tumor imaging. J Nucl Med 1999; 40(1):205–12.

65. Heiss P, Mayer S, Herz M, et al. Investigation of transport mechanism and uptake kinetics of O-(2-[18F]fluoroethyl)-L-tyrosine in vitro and in vivo. J Nucl Med 1999;40(8):1367–73.

66. Grosu AL, Astner ST, Riedel E, et al. An interindividual comparison of O-(2-[18F]fluoroethyl)-L-tyrosine (FET)- and L-[methyl-11C]methionine (MET)-PET in patients with brain gliomas and metastases. Int J Radiat Oncol Biol Phys 2011;81(4):1049–58.

67. Hutterer M, Nowosielski M, Putzer D, et al. [18F]-fluoro-ethyl-L-tyrosine PET: a valuable diagnostic tool in neuro-oncology, but not all that glitters is glioma. Neuro Oncol 2013;15(3):341–51.

68. Lohaus N, Mader C, Jelcic I, et al. Acute Disseminated Encephalomyelitis in FET PET/MR. Clin Nucl Med 2022;47(2):e137–9.

69. Yamada Y, Uchida Y, Tatsumi K, et al. Fluorine-18-fluorodeoxyglucose and carbon-11-methionine evaluation of lymphadenopathy in sarcoidosis. J Nucl Med 1998;39(7):1160–6.

70. Sasaki M, Ichiya Y, Kuwabara Y, et al. Hyperperfusion and hypermetabolism in brain radiation necrosis with epileptic activity. J Nucl Med 1996;37(7): 1174–6.

71. Sasaki M, Kuwabara Y, Yoshida T, et al. Carbon-11-methionine PET in focal cortical dysplasia: a comparison with fluorine-18-FDG PET and technetium-99m-ECD SPECT. J Nucl Med 1998;39(6):974–7.

72. Hutterer M, Ebner Y, Riemenschneider MJ, et al. Epileptic activity increases cerebral amino acid transport assessed by 18F-Fluoroethyl-l-Tyrosine amino acid PET: a potential brain tumor mimic. J Nucl Med 2017;58(1):129–37.

73. Rapp M, Heinzel A, Galldiks N, et al. Diagnostic performance of 18F-FET PET in newly diagnosed cerebral lesions suggestive of glioma. J Nucl Med 2013;54(2):229–35.

74. Floeth FW, Pauleit D, Sabel M, et al. Prognostic value of O-(2-18F-fluoroethyl)-L-tyrosine PET and MRI in low-grade glioma. J Nucl Med 2007;48(4): 519–27.

75. Albert NL, Winkelmann I, Suchorska B, et al. Early static (18)F-FET-PET scans have a higher accuracy for glioma grading than the standard 20-40 min scans. Eur J Nucl Med Mol Imaging 2016;43(6): 1105–14.

76. Ewelt C, Floeth FW, Felsberg J, et al. Finding the anaplastic focus in diffuse gliomas: the value of Gd-DTPA enhanced MRI, FET-PET, and intraoperative, ALA-derived tissue fluorescence. Clin Neurol Neurosurg 2011;113(7):541–7.

77. Scott JN, Brasher PM, Sevick RJ, et al. How often are nonenhancing supratentorial gliomas malignant? A population study. Neurology 2002;59(6): 947–9.

78. Popperl G, Kreth FW, Mehrkens JH, et al. FET PET for the evaluation of untreated gliomas: correlation of FET uptake and uptake kinetics with tumour grading. Eur J Nucl Med Mol Imaging 2007; 34(12):1933–42.

79. Langen KJ, Stoffels G, Filss C, et al. Imaging of amino acid transport in brain tumours: positron emission tomography with O-(2-[(18)F]fluoroethyl)-L-tyrosine (FET). Methods 2017;130: 124–34.

80. Richard MA, Fouquet JP, Lebel R, et al. Determination of an Optimal Pharmacokinetic Model of (18)F-FET for quantitative applications in rat brain tumors. J Nucl Med 2017;58(8):1278–84.

81. Gottler J, Lukas M, Kluge A, et al. Intra-lesional spatial correlation of static and dynamic FET-PET parameters with MRI-based cerebral blood volume in patients with untreated glioma. Eur J Nucl Med Mol Imaging 2017;44(3):392–7.

82. Bashir A, Brennum J, Broholm H, et al. The diagnostic accuracy of detecting malignant transformation of low-grade glioma using O-(2-[18F] fluoroethyl)-l-tyrosine positron emission tomography: a retrospective study. J Neurosurg 2018; 130(2):451–64.

83. Galldiks N, Stoffels G, Ruge MI, et al. Role of O-(2-18F-fluoroethyl)-L-tyrosine PET as a diagnostic tool for detection of malignant progression in patients with low-grade glioma. J Nucl Med 2013;54(12): 2046–54.

84. Lohmann P, Stavrinou P, Lipke K, et al. FET PET reveals considerable spatial differences in tumour burden compared to conventional MRI in newly diagnosed glioblastoma. Eur J Nucl Med Mol Imaging 2019;46(3):591–602.

85. Song S, Cheng Y, Ma J, et al. Simultaneous FET-PET and contrast-enhanced MRI based on hybrid PET/MR improves delineation of tumor spatial biodistribution in gliomas: a biopsy validation study. Eur J Nucl Med Mol Imaging 2020;47(6): 1458–67.

86. Verburg N, Koopman T, Yaqub MM, et al. Improved detection of diffuse glioma infiltration with imaging combinations: a diagnostic accuracy study. Neuro Oncol 2020;22(3):412–22.

87. Hirata T, Kinoshita M, Tamari K, et al. 11C-methio-nine-18F-FDG dual-PET-tracer-based target delineation of malignant glioma: evaluation of its geometrical and clinical features for planning radiation therapy. J Neurosurg 2019;131(3):676–86.

88. Poulsen SH, Urup T, Grunnet K, et al. The prognostic value of FET PET at radiotherapy planning in newly diagnosed glioblastoma. Eur J Nucl Med Mol Imaging 2017;44(3):373–81.

89. Kunz M, Albert NL, Unterrainer M, et al. Dynamic 18F-FET PET is a powerful imaging biomarker in gadolinium-negative gliomas. Neuro Oncol 2019; 21(2):274–84.

90. Molinaro AM, Hervey-Jumper S, Morshed RA, et al. Association of maximal extent of resection of contrast-enhanced and non-contrast-enhanced tumor with survival within molecular subgroups of patients with newly diagnosed glioblastoma. JAMA Oncol 2020;6(4):495–503.

91. Suchorska B, Jansen NL, Linn J, et al. Biological tumor volume in 18FET-PET before radiochemotherapy correlates with survival in GBM. Neurology 2015;84(7):710–9.

92. Bette S, Peschke P, Kaesmacher J, et al. Static FET-PET and MR imaging in anaplastic gliomas (WHO III). World Neurosurg 2016;91:524–531 e521.

93. Holzgreve A, Albert NL, Galldiks N, et al. Use of PET Imaging in neuro-oncological surgery. Cancers (Basel) 2021;13(9):2093.

94. Floeth FW, Sabel M, Ewelt C, et al. Comparison of (18)F-FET PET and 5-ALA fluorescence in cerebral gliomas. Eur J Nucl Med Mol Imaging 2011;38(4): 731–41.

95. Werner JM, Weller J, Ceccon G, et al. Diagnosis of pseudoprogression following lomustine-temozolomide chemoradiation in newly diagnosed glioblastoma patients using FET-PET. Clin Cancer Res 2021;27(13):3704–13.

96. Galldiks N, Dunkl V, Stoffels G, et al. Diagnosis of pseudoprogression in patients with glioblastoma using O-(2-[18F]fluoroethyl)-L-tyrosine PET. Eur J Nucl Med Mol Imaging 2015;42(5):685–95.

97. Werner JM, Stoffels G, Lichtenstein T, et al. Differentiation of treatment-related changes from tumour progression: a direct comparison between dynamic FET PET and ADC values obtained from DWI MRI. Eur J Nucl Med Mol Imaging 2019; 46(9):1889–901.

98. Kebir S, Fimmers R, Galldiks N, et al. Late pseudoprogression in glioblastoma: diagnostic value of dynamic O-(2-[18F]fluoroethyl)-L-Tyrosine PET. Clin Cancer Res 2016;22(9):2190–6.

99. Bashir A, Mathilde Jacobsen S, Molby Henriksen O, et al. Recurrent glioblastoma versus late posttreatment changes: diagnostic accuracy of O-(2-[18F]fluoroethyl)-L-tyrosine positron

emission tomography (18F-FET PET). Neuro Oncol 2019;21(12):1595–606.

100. Galldiks N, Stoffels G, Filss CP, et al. Role of O-(2-(18)F-fluoroethyl)-L-tyrosine PET for differentiation of local recurrent brain metastasis from radiation necrosis. J Nucl Med 2012;53(9):1367–74.

101. Heiss WD, Wienhard K, Wagner R, et al. F-Dopa as an amino acid tracer to detect brain tumors. J Nucl Med 1996;37(7):1180–2.

102. Chen W, Silverman DH, Delaloye S, et al. 18F-FDOPA PET imaging of brain tumors: comparison study with 18F-FDG PET and evaluation of diagnostic accuracy. J Nucl Med 2006;47(6): 904–11.

103. Huang SC, Yu DC, Barrio JR, et al. Kinetics and modeling of L-6-[18F]fluoro-dopa in human positron emission tomographic studies. J Cereb Blood Flow Metab 1991;11(6):898–913.

104. Tatekawa H, Hagiwara A, Yao J, et al. Voxelwise and patientwise correlation of (18)F-FDOPA PET, relative cerebral blood volume, and apparent diffusion coefficient in treatment-naive diffuse gliomas with different molecular subtypes. J Nucl Med 2021;62(3):319–25.

105. Jena A, Taneja S, Khan AA, et al. Recurrent glioma: does qualitative simultaneous 18F-DOPA PET/mp-MRI improve diagnostic workup? An initial Experience. Clin Nucl Med 2021;46(9):703–9.

106. Shoup TM, Olson J, Hoffman JM, et al. Synthesis and evaluation of [18F]1-amino-3-fluorocyclobutane-1-carboxylic acid to image brain tumors. J Nucl Med 1999;40(2):331–8.

107. Michaud L, Beattie BJ, Akhurst T, et al. 18)F-Fluciclovine ((18)F-FACBC) PET imaging of recurrent brain tumors. Eur J Nucl Med Mol Imaging 2020; 47(6):1353–67.

108. Laudicella R, Quartuccio N, Argiroffi G, et al. Unconventional non-amino acidic PET radiotracers for molecular imaging in gliomas. Eur J Nucl Med Mol Imaging 2021;48(12):3925–39.

109. Ruan S, Zhou Y, Jiang X, et al. Rethinking CRITID Procedure of Brain targeting drug delivery: circulation, blood brain barrier recognition, intracellular transport, diseased cell targeting, internalization, and drug release. Adv Sci (Weinh) 2021;8(9): 2004025.

110. Pike VW. PET radiotracers: crossing the blood-brain barrier and surviving metabolism. Trends Pharmacol Sci 2009;30(8):431–40.

111. Rohrich M, Loktev A, Wefers AK, et al. IDH-wild-type glioblastomas and grade III/IV IDH-mutant gliomas show elevated tracer uptake in fibroblast activation protein-specific PET/CT. Eur J Nucl Med Mol Imaging 2019;46(12):2569–80.

112. Vettermann FJ, Harris S, Schmitt J, et al. Impact of TSPO receptor Polymorphism on [(18)F]GE-180 binding in healthy brain and Pseudo-reference

regions of Neurooncological and Neurodegenerative Disorders. Life (Basel) 2021;11(6):484.

113. Salas Fragomeni RA, Menke JR, Holdhoff M, et al. Prostate-specific membrane antigen-targeted imaging with [18F]DCFPyL in high-grade gliomas. Clin Nucl Med 2017;42(10):e433–5.

114. Verma P, Malhotra G, Goel A, et al. Differential uptake of 68Ga-PSMA-HBED-CC (PSMA-11) in low-grade versus high-grade gliomas in treatment-Naive patients. Clin Nucl Med 2019;44(5):e318–22.

115. Liu D, Cheng G, Ma X, et al. PET/CT using (68) Ga-PSMA-617 versus (18) F-fluorodeoxyglucose to differentiate low- and high-grade gliomas. J Neuroimaging 2021;31(4):733–42.

116. Holzgreve A, Biczok A, Ruf VC, et al. PSMA Expression in Glioblastoma as a basis for theranostic approaches: a retrospective, correlational panel study including immunohistochemistry, clinical parameters and PET Imaging. Front Oncol 2021;11: 646387.

117. Andrei Iagaru M, Camila Mosci M, Erik Mittra M, et al. Glioblastoma multiforme recurrence: an Exploratory study of 18F FPPRGD2 PET/CT. Radiology 2015;277(2):497–506.

118. Santagata S, Ierano C, Trotta AM, et al. CXCR4 and CXCR7 signaling pathways: a focus on the crosstalk between cancer cells and tumor microenvironment. Front Oncol 2021;11:591386.

119. Shooli H, Nemati R, Ahmadzadehfar H, et al. Theranostics in brain tumors. PET Clin 2021;16(3): 397–418.

120. Huang X, Bai H, Zhou H, et al. Performance of 18F-FET-PET versus 18F-FDG-PET for the diagnosis and grading of brain tumors: inherent bias in meta-analysis not revealed by quality metrics. Neuro Oncol 2016;18(7):1028.

121. Furuse M, Nonoguchi N, Yamada K, et al. Radiological diagnosis of brain radiation necrosis after cranial irradiation for brain tumor: a systematic review. Radiat Oncol 2019;14(1):28.

122. Seidlitz A, Beuthien-Baumann B, Lock S, et al. Final results of the prospective biomarker trial PETra: [(11)C]-MET-Accumulation in Postoperative PET/MRI predicts outcome after radiochemotherapy in glioblastoma. Clin Cancer Res 2021;27(5): 1351–60.

123. Mittlmeier LM, Suchorska B, Ruf V, et al. (18)F-FET PET uptake characteristics of long-term IDH-wildtype diffuse glioma Survivors. Cancers (Basel) 2021;13(13).

124. Lundemann M, Munck Af, Rosenschold P, et al. Feasibility of multi-parametric PET and MRI for prediction of tumour recurrence in patients with glioblastoma. Eur J Nucl Med Mol Imaging 2019; 46(3):603–13.

125. Suchorska B, Giese A, Biczok A, et al. Identification of time-to-peak on dynamic 18F-FET-PET as a prognostic marker specifically in IDH1/2 mutant diffuse astrocytoma. Neuro Oncol 2018;20(2): 279–88.

126. Galldiks N, Dunkl V, Ceccon G, et al. Early treatment response evaluation using FET PET compared to MRI in glioblastoma patients at first progression treated with bevacizumab plus lomustine. Eur J Nucl Med Mol Imaging 2018;45(13): 2377–86.

127. Oen SK, Aasheim LB, Eikenes L, et al. Image quality and detectability in Siemens Biograph PET/MRI and PET/CT systems-a phantom study. EJNMMI Phys 2019;6(1):16.

128. Lohmann P, Galldiks N, Kocher M, et al. Radiomics in neuro-oncology: basics, workflow, and applications. Methods 2021;188:112–21.

129. Pirotte B, Goldman S, Massager N, et al. Combined use of 18F-fluorodeoxyglucose and 11C-methionine in 45 positron emission tomography-guided stereotactic brain biopsies. J Neurosurg 2004; 101(3):476–83.

# An Appraisal and Update of Fluorodeoxyglucose and Non-Fluorodeoxyglucose-PET Tracers in Thyroid and Non–Thyroid Endocrine Neoplasms

Aadil Adnan, MBBS, MD[a,b], Shobhana Raju, MBBS, MD[c],
Rakesh Kumar, MBBS, DRM, DNB, MNAMS, PhD[c],
Sandip Basu, MBBS, DRM, DNB, MNAMS[a,b,*]

## KEYWORDS

- Differentiated thyroid carcinoma • Aggressive variant of papillary thyroid carcinoma
- Thyroglobulin elevated negative iodine scintigraphy (TENIS)
- Anaplastic (undifferentiated) thyroid carcinoma • Medullary thyroid carcinoma
- Pheochromocytoma & Paraganglioma • Adrenocortical carcinoma • Parathyroid neoplasm

## KEY POINTS

- Endocrine malignancies are composed of a spectrum characterized by differentiated, hormone-producing tumors to poorly differentiated and nondifferentiated carcinomas. These neoplasms have a cellular population, which is actively involved in synthesis and packaging of bioactive hormones, their transport to target cells and tissues and receptor-mediated target cell activity.
- The fact that these cells synthesize hormones and are stimulated or inhibited through specific receptors is the core principle and can be exploited for various targeted approaches for diagnosis and treatment. Hence, functional molecular imaging provides opportunities for highly sensitive and specific targeted theranostic interventions.
- With increasing knowledge of pathogenesis, implicated genetic pathways, phenotypic expression, and overall tumor biology, demand for a specific target and corresponding radiotracers for better evaluation with potential for accurate clinical decision making is the need of the hour.
- The nuclear medicine fraternity has responded proportionately with many novel tracers evaluating various aspects of tumor biology, which are continuously being conceptualized and developed. Albeit the presence of several novel radiotracers and targets are on the horizon evaluating specific pathways in tumorigenesis, the importance of fluorodeoxyglucose as a prognostic marker cannot be undermined.
- The availability of a multitude of novel radiotracers and therapeutic targets mandates personalization of their use and is a significant challenge to the attending clinicians with respect to their deployment at different stages of disease course, so as to ensure maximum clinical benefit. In the present communication, therefore, on the basis of the authors' clinical experience and available literature, they have proposed recommendations for their appropriate use.

[a] Radiation Medicine Centre (B.A.R.C), Tata Memorial Centre Annexe, Parel, Mumbai, India; [b] Homi Bhabha National Institute, Mumbai, India; [c] Department of Nuclear Medicine, All India Institute of Medical Sciences, New Delhi, India
* Corresponding author. Radiation Medicine Centre (B.A.R.C.), Tata Memorial Hospital Annexe, Jerbai Wadia Road, Parel, Mumbai 400012, India.
E-mail address: drsanb@yahoo.com

PET Clin 17 (2022) 343–367
https://doi.org/10.1016/j.cpet.2022.03.010
1556-8598/22/© 2022 Elsevier Inc. All rights reserved.

# INTRODUCTION

Endocrine neoplasms and malignancies are a group of tumors with varied clinical, histopathologic, and functional features. These tumors may vary from sporadic to hereditary, isolated entities to multiple neoplastic syndromes, unifocal locally invasive, and advance to multifocal tumors with disseminated distant metastases. The presence of various specific biomarkers and specific receptor targets serves as a valuable tool for diagnosis, prognosis, and management. Nuclear medicine techniques using the historical rectilinear scanners and planner gamma camera imaging for a long time have been incorporated in the management of endocrine neoplasms. With technological advancements and development of novel radiotracers, PET-computed tomography (CT) has recently moved to the forefront of diagnosis, metastatic workup, treatment planning, response assessment, and prognostication of these malignancies.

This article enumerates the current uses and potential clinical scenarios where PET could have a role in disease management of thyroid, parathyroid, and adrenal neoplasms with particular emphasis on relative advantages of fluorod-eoxy-glucose (FDG) versus non-FDG-PET tracers. Furthermore, where applicable, a sequence of introducing these imaging modalities for better results and accuracy has been proposed.

# FLUORODEOXYGLUCOSE AND NON-FLUORODEOXYGLUCOSE-PET TRACERS IN THYROID NEOPLASMS

## Fluorodeoxyglucose-PET/Computed Tomography in Differentiated Thyroid Carcinoma

Differentiated thyroid carcinomas (DTCs) are indolent malignancies with a relatively better overall prognosis relative to anaplastic and medullary thyroid carcinomas (MTC) and other head and neck malignancies (Figs. 1 and 2).[1,2] The 10-year survival rates are 93% for papillary, 85% for follicular, and 76% for Hürthle cell carcinomas.[3] As such, there is no routine well-defined role of FDG or non-FDG-PET/CT in the initial diagnosis of DTCs, and no guidelines recommend the same. Soelberg and colleagues in their meta-analysis confirmed that approximately one-third (~35%) of all FDG-avid thyroid nodules proved to be cancerous. Various studies have reported a high negative predictive value (close to 90%) of FDG-PET-CT in preoperative evaluation of thyroid nodules and hence can effectively reduce unnecessary diagnostic surgeries in the presence of indeterminate cytology.[4–6] In recurrent DTCs, 2015 American Thyroid Association (ATA) guidelines recommend performing FDG-PET/CT for patients with suppressed thyroglobulin (Tg) levels greater than 10 ng/mL.

In Hürthle cell thyroid carcinoma (HTC or oncocytic thyroid carcinoma), a relatively rarer form of DTC characterized by poor prognosis owing to more aggressive tumor biology, there is a higher incidence of locoregional and distant metastases, and most patients show negative radio-iodine scan (~80%). FDG-PET is found to be an effective tool for both detection and prognostication.[7] Pryma and colleagues[8] recommended FDG-PET to be the imaging modality of choice in Hürthle cell carcinoma and reported a sensitivity of 95.8% and specificity of 95% for FDG-PET in 44 patients. They also reported a 6% increase in mortality with every 1-unit increase in maximum standardized uptake value ($SUV_{max}$) and showed that FDG $SUV_{max}$ less than 10 was associated with 5-year survival of 92%; FDG $SUV_{max}$ greater than 10 was associated with 5-year survival of just 64%.[8] Plotkin and colleagues[9] in a limited meta-analysis of 35 patients demonstrated a sensitivity of 92% and specificity of 80%. This increased FDG uptake in oncocytic tumors is attributed to inherent constitutive activation of glycolytic pathways rather than poorly differentiated phenotype and is because of mitochondrial dysfunction.[10]

Also, thyroid tumors are composed of both differentiated and undifferentiated cells; hence, FDG-PET and radio-iodine scans are complementary to each other and increase the accuracy. Furthermore, FDG-PET remains the only diagnostic tool in detecting persistent disease after thyroidectomy, where tumor cells do not secrete Tg. Nascimento and colleagues[11] in their study evaluating the potential role of FDG-PET/CT in DTC with aggressive histopathologies observed FDG-PET/CT to be more sensitive than radio-iodine scan for detection of individual lesions (69% vs 59%). They also inferred that both the imaging modalities are complementary, with 41% of lesions detected only by FDG-PET/CT and 32% detected only by radio-iodine scan. Hence, both of these scans should be routinely performed in such patients,[11] and tumor sites are missed in only 7% cases. [124]I PET/CT is used mainly for dosimetric studies, and its role in diagnosis and staging is limited.

## Recommendations

- There is no definitive role of FDG-PET/CT in DTC at baseline or at follow-up in

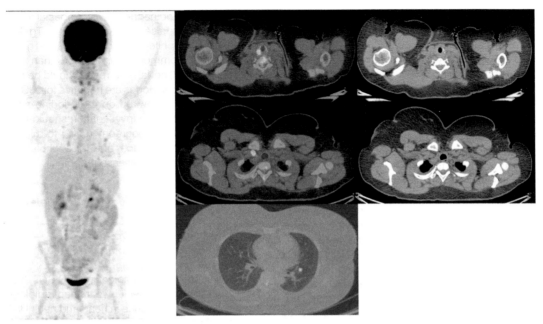

**Fig. 1.** In a 50-year-old patient with TENIS (diagnosed as papillary carcinoma thyroid 13 years previously and had undergone total thyroidectomy), the patient presented with recent radioiodine WBS-negative and an increase in serum Tg values of greater than 300 ng/dL. The $^{18}$F-FDG-PET/CT revealed metabolically active soft tissue lesion in the thyroid bed/cervical level VI lymph node and right supraclavicular lymph nodes and bilateral lung nodules suggestive of metastatic disease.

conventional case scenarios. However, FDG-PET/CT could be useful in certain situations.

- Patients with high risk of surgery or thyroid nodules with indeterminate cytology can be evaluated for metabolic activity.
- Planning completion surgery after hemithyroidectomy in very low to low-risk disease in patients not fit/not willing for surgery.

- Recurrent DTCs exist with high-serum Tg (cutoff >10 ng/mL); however, better yields are seen at still higher and stimulated Tg levels that can potentially direct/modify the plan of treatment.
- Persistent disease after thyroidectomy can be detected, in which tumor cells do not secrete Tg.

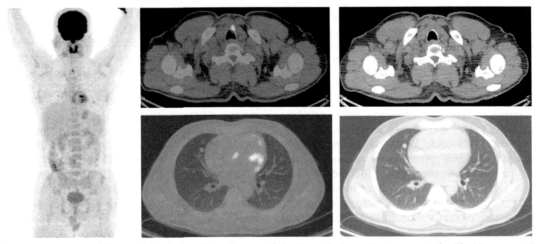

**Fig. 2.** In a 35-year-old man with Hürtle cell carcinoma of the thyroid, the patient presented with rising serum Tg values following total thyroidectomy and remnant ablation. $^{18}$F-FDG-PETPET/CT revealed soft tissue density lesion at the thyroid bed (suggestive of recurrent disease) with metastasis to the bilateral lungs.

- Hürthle cell carcinoma showing negative radio-iodine scan can be detected.
- Both radio-iodine scan and FDG-PET/CT are complementary to each other in aggressive histopathologies.

## Thyroglobulin Elevated Negative Iodine Scintigraphy

Thyroid tumor cells usually retain many of the characteristics of their normal progenitor cells, such as, capacity to concentrate iodine, capacity to synthesize thyroid hormone, and capacity to secrete Tg; hence, radio-iodine scan is well established in the management of thyroid malignancies, provided the original tumor cells are well differentiated and have the ability to concentrate radio-iodine. About one-third (30%) of DTC develop recurrent disease in the long run, and most of these recurrences are non-iodine-avid, as they tend to lose natrium-iodide (Na/I) symporter (NIS) owing to dedifferentiation of cells leading to decreased expression of NIS and increased GLUT1 expression, referred to as the "Flip-Flop" phenomenon, as defined by Feine and colleagues[12–15] in 1996. As a result, the whole-body scan shows no radio-iodine concentration despite high-serum Tg; this clinical situation was recently named thyroglobulin elevated negative iodine scintigraphy (TENIS) syndrome (ie, Tg elevated negative iodine scan) by Silberstein[15] in 2011.

TENIS is a rare entity, reported somewhere between 2% and 13% in available literature[15] and is challenging in terms of diagnosis and management. TENIS usually develops late in the course of disease in very few cases even after complete treatment, and 15% to 20% of recurrent DTC may become dedifferentiated, fail to concentrate radio-iodine, and is attributable mostly to mutation in the NIS gene.[16] The loss of iodine avidity is associated with aggressive disease pattern, and this dedifferentiation affects approximately one-third of patients with disseminated DTC.[14]

### Diagnostic approach for thyroglobulin elevated negative iodine scintigraphy

Diagnosis of TENIS is challenging, and certain factors need to be ruled out before a definitive diagnosis of TENIS could be made: (a) interference with stable iodine needs to be effectively ruled out (the most common reason behind negative iodine scintigraphy and proper preprocedure counseling and a thorough history taking just before the procedure could alleviate this); (b) poor imaging characteristics of [131]I as against [123]I, which could lead to radio-iodine uptake on posttherapy scan in cases with negative prethereapy (diagnostic) radio-iodine scan. Hence,

empirical radio-iodine therapy is of special importance here; (c) false-positive elevated Tg level owing to heterophile antibodies and anti-Tg antibodies (less common phenomenon than false negative); and (d) nodal recurrence should be ruled out (as these lymph nodes are negative for NIS and therefore do not show up on radio-iodine scan). Hence, the usual initial investigation should be (a) a reliable new ultrasonography (USG) to rule out/conform nodal recurrence, and (b) a whole-body FDG-PET/CT scan for disease mapping.

## Imaging in Thyroglobulin Elevated Negative Iodine Scintigraphy

### Fluorodeoxyglucose-PET/computed tomography in thyroglobulin elevated negative iodine scintigraphy

The initial imaging of choice in TENIS is high-resolution USG of the neck by a trained radiologist preferably with experience in head and neck USG, which is important in determining localized disease and which can be surgically treatable or amenable to external beam radiotherapy. However, in most cases, a whole-body FDG-PET/CT scan is required for metastatic workup and potentially can change the line of management. Furthermore, an FDG-PET/CT scan is the most important imaging/investigation in TENIS for disease mapping, prognostication, and response to systemic/localized therapy with the reported sensitivity ranging from 70% to 94% in the literature.[17] Özdemir and colleagues[18] demonstrated overall sensitivity, specificity, and diagnostic accuracy of 68.8%, 78.8%, and 71.9% respectively, of FDG-PET/CT in TENIS, and when analyzed according to stimulated Tg values, FDG-PET/CT was negative in those with stimulated Tg less than 5 ng/mL, whereas it was true positive in 70% of patients with stimulated Tg greater than 20 ng/mL. Sensitivity of FDG-PET/CT for detecting radio-iodine negative recurrent disease was reported to be 63% to 98%.[19–21] Sensitivity and accuracy increase with high-serum thyrotropin (TSH). Deichen and colleagues[22] demonstrated that TSH increases FDG uptake by thyrocytes in vitro, and Filetti and colleagues[23] demonstrated that TSH increases GLUT1 expression in cultured rat thyroid cells and hence increases FDG uptake.

The sensitivity of FDG-PET/CT scan improves with increasing values of Tg: Na and colleagues[21] in a series of 60 patients of TENIS inferred that sensitivity of FDG-PET/CT scan increases with an increase in stimulated Tg levels, 28.6% when stimulated Tg between 2 and 5 ng/mL, 57.1% when stimulated Tg between 5 and 10 ng/mL, 60% when stimulated Tg between 10 and 20 ng/

mL, and 85.7% when stimulated Tg greater than 20 ng/mL. Trybek and colleagues[24] reported 100% sensitivity and specificity for FDG-PET/CT to detect metastases at stimulated Tg cutoff value of 28.5 ng/mL in 19 patients of TENIS. Vural and colleagues in their study on 105 TENIS patients showed that highest accuracy of FDG-PET/CT was reached at suppressed Tg greater than 1.9 ng/mL and stimulated Tg greater than 38.2 ng/mL[25]. In a study on 40 patients with undetected Tg and high anti-Tg antibodies (>40 IU/mL), Asa and colleagues demonstrated the value of FDG-PET/CT in detecting recurrent/metastatic disease in this group of patients.

## Non-Fluorodeoxyglucose-PET Tracers in Differentiated Thyroid Carcinoma

### Somatostatin receptor analogue
Pazaitou-Panayiotou and colleagues[26] in their study demonstrated increased expression of all types of somatostatin receptor subtypes (SSTRs) in human nonmedullary thyroid carcinoma tissues, whereas the expression of SSTRs was low in non-neoplastic thyroid tissues obtained from the same operation material, and SSTR subtypes 2, 3, and 5 appeared to be most abundantly expressed and were located both in the cytoplasm and at plasma membrane of thyroid cells. Pisarek and colleagues[27] demonstrated that in TENIS syndrome, SSTR1 is the most commonly expressed subtype (88.8% of patients) followed by SSTR 3, 2, 5, and 4 in 55.5%, 44.4%, 33.3%, and 11.2% of patients, respectively. Of all the DOTA conjugates, DOTA-NOC PET/CT identified most lesions, as DOTA-NOC is the only radio-tracer having affinity for SSTR 2, 3, and 5 and moderate affinity for SSTR4.[28] Mourato and colleagues[29] demonstrated that SSTR-based PET/CT could detect disease in approximately 17% of patients with negative FDG-PET/CT. Binse and colleagues[30] showed that SSTR-based PET should be considered in radio-iodine and FDG-PET-negative DTC patients with elevated and rising Tg levels. This SSTR positivity in thyroid malignancies, especially in diagnostically and therapeutically challenging TENIS syndrome, opens potential avenues for diagnosis and treatment (with [177]Lu to [90]Y), known as peptide receptor radionuclide therapy (PRRT). One recent study by Basu and colleagues[31] has placed PRRT concurrently or ahead of tyrosine kinase inhibitors in the management of TENIS, in eligible patients (showing high-grade SSTR expression, Krenning 3 or 4). In an early study, Jois and colleagues[32] had endeavored to analyze the percentage of TENIS patients who are suitable for PRRT and came to a conclusion that although

63% of patients showed SSTR-positive lesion expression demonstrating uptake ranging from grade I to IV, only 16% showed high enough uptake to qualify for the PRRT.

### Prostate specific membrane antigen
Prostate-specific membrane antigen (PSMA) is a type II transmembrane glycoprotein receptor and a zinc-dependent peptidase having glutamate carboxypeptidase/folate hydrolase enzymatic activity.[33] Derlin and colleagues,[34] Chang and colleagues,[35] Bychkov and colleagues,[36] and Gordon and colleagues[37] demonstrated that PSMA is significantly expressed on the endothelium of the neovasculature of tumor cells in the solid tumors (and not in the blood vessels of normal tissue), except in prostate carcinoma, where it is expressed in cytoplasm and membrane of the epithelium. Bertagna and colleagues[38] in their review article stated that classical papillary thyroid carcinoma, follicular thyroid carcinoma, and radioactive iodine refractory thyroid carcinomas demonstrated the highest percentage of PSMA staining and was greater in distant metastases than lymph nodal metastases. Moore and colleagues[39] demonstrated that compared with normal thyroid tissue PSMA is significantly overexpressed in the neovasculature of DTC, especially in radio-iodine refractory type. Although [68]Ga-PSMA and [177]Lu-PSMA could form a potential theranostic pair in patients with TENIS where there is a paucity of diagnostic and therapeutic options and few such endeavors are done, a well-structured study with statistically significant sample size and critical analysis is needed to effectively draw any conclusions.[40]

### Iodine 124
The main use of [124]I PET/CT in DTC has been for dosimetric studies for determining an accurate and personalized therapeutic dose of radio-iodine.[41] There are 2 ways to determine the dose of [131]I activity to be administered by dosimetry planning: (a) the most efficient absorbed dose in the tumor to reach tumor lysis (100 Gy to distant metastases), and (b) by giving the greatest [131]I activity limited by the threshold toxicity in normal tissues (2 Gy to bone marrow). Its role in TENIS where there is no significant radio-iodine uptake in tumor cells is not well defined and theoretically inappropriate. In DTC, [124]I PET/CT shows better sensitivity than gamma camera-based radio-iodine scan because of better resolution of the PET system, and there are highly variable results on comparing [124]I PET and [131]I after therapy whole-body scan. Furthermore, thyroid hormone withdrawal significantly enhanced the sensitivity

of $^{124}$I PET/CT than rhTSH stimulation. Khorjekar and colleagues[42] demonstrated that a negative $^{124}$I PET failed to rule out the need for empiric radionuclide therapy, as 10/12 patients with negative $^{124}$I PET showed suspicious foci on $^{131}$I after therapy whole-body scan.

### Recommendations

- FDG-PET/CT is the imaging method of choice for TENIS if high-resolution USG is negative. High stimulated Tg increases the sensitivity and specificity of the scan and is greater than 90% in reported literature when stimulated Tg is greater than 20 ng/mL and anti-Tg antibodies are greater than 40 IU/mL.
- Somatostatin receptor analogue (SSA)-based PET/CT may be considered in patients with negative FDG-PET/CT, especially in the setting of TENIS syndrome and while planning patients for PRRT. PSMA-PET/CT showed PSMA expression in radio-iodine refractory metastatic thyroid carcinoma, especially in osseous lesions, and could be considered in radio-iodine refractory disease with high Tg and negative conventional imaging.
- In a vast majority of patients, however, the SSTR and PSMA expression is either absent or low and not suitable for targeting radionuclide therapy.
- $^{124}$I is used for dosimetric studies and has better image resolution and sensitivity than $^{131}$I- and $^{123}$I-based gamma camera scans.

### Fluorodeoxyglucose and Non-Fluorodeoxyglucose-PET Tracers in Aggressive Variants of Differentiated and Poorly Differentiated Thyroid Carcinoma

Aggressive variants of papillary thyroid carcinoma include tall cell, columnar cell, solid, and diffuse sclerosing types and tend to show a more aggressive behavior than classical papillary thyroid carcinoma. Some have included these aggressive variants of papillary thyroid carcinoma with poorly differentiated thyroid carcinoma (PDTC), but this could not be justified. The term poorly differentiated thyroid carcinoma was introduced by Sakamoto and colleagues[43] in 1983 based on the presence of nonglandular components with a solid, trabecular, and/or scirrhous growth pattern and includes insular and other large cell types.[44] PDTC results from dedifferentiation of well-differentiated thyroid carcinoma and is mostly regarded as an intermediate stage in the oncogenesis of anaplastic (undifferentiated) thyroid carcinoma from well-differentiated thyroid carcinoma.[45,46] In the process of dedifferentiation, there is progressive loss of

function: mainly sodium-iodide symporter expression; in relatively smaller cases, there is loss of Tg formation, and BRAF is the most important gene implicated.[47]

Aggressive variants of DTC retain the ability for concentrating radio-iodine; hence, whole-body radio-iodine scan should be considered in all cases for metastatic workup and guides treatment strategy for a patient. At present, there have been few published accounts on the importance and benefits of FDG in aggressive DTC, but in the authors' clinical experience and according to few published case reports and small case series evaluating the patients with tall cell,[48] diffuse sclerosing,[49] solid/trabecular,[50] and insular[51] variants, FDG-PET is useful in staging and restaging of these tumors.

PDTC falls midway between well differentiated and anaplastic thyroid carcinoma (ATC). Albeit they show limited NIS expression and can produce some Tg, radio-iodine scan and Tg are not considered useful for disease assessment, prognostication, and management. FDG-PET scan has been a reliable tool in such patients because of intermediate GLUT1 (glucose transporter 1) expression more than NIS expression and demonstrates a "flip-flop" phenomenon between radio-iodine and FDG, and PDTC often shows considerable FDG-PET positivity than radio-iodine uptake and TSH increases FDG uptake in PDTC cells.[52]

No studies or guidelines suggest or deal with the utility of non-FDG-PET in aggressive variants of DTC and PDTC.

### Recommendations

- FDG-PET/CT is an important tool in staging and restaging of PDTC, as radio-iodine scintigraphy and Tg are both unreliable in disease assessment, prognostication, and treatment and show considerable FDG positivity.
- Role of FDG-PET/CT is not as well defined in cases of DTC with aggressive histology, but FDG-PET/CT is useful in staging and restaging when radio-iodine scan is either negative or discordant to Tg levels.

### Fluorodeoxyglucose and Non-Fluorodeoxyglucose-PET Tracers in Anaplastic (Undifferentiated) Thyroid Carcinoma

ATC is a follicular cell-derived thyroid malignancy and is characterized by rapidly proliferating cells with an extremely aggressive tumor biology that is associated with the highest mortality for any thyroid tumor, but accounts for only a small fraction of overall thyroid cancer cases, approximately 1.3% to 9.8% (median, 3.6%).[53,54] ATC patients have a historical median survival of about 5 months and a 1-year overall survival of 20%.[55] FDG-PET/CT is particularly useful in ATC for disease staging, restaging, metastatic workup, and treatment response evaluation and is the most reliable modality because undifferentiated cells do not express NIS and do not produce Tg, but they abundantly express GLUT1 responsible for avid FDG uptake.[56,57] Approximately 10% of patients present with intrathyroidal tumor, whereas 40% have extrathyroidal invasion and/or lymph nodal metastases, and the remaining patients present with distant metastases; accurate rapid staging is a prerequisite for the most effective treatment planning.[58,59]

Recent ATA guidelines of 2021 recommend FDG-PET/CT as the best modality for staging to classify the disease as IVA, IVB, or IVC and are particularly valuable in identifying the metastatic sites that are sometimes not appreciated on conventional cross-sectional imaging, like CT or MR imaging, especially osseous and marrow involvement.[54,56] FDG-PET/CT has higher sensitivity for detecting metastatic lesions than CT alone (99.6% vs 62% in identifying 265 individual lesions in 18 patients, $P<.002$).[56] Furthermore, FDG-PET/CT findings can potentially alter the management recommendations in approximately 25% to 50% of patients.[54,56] FDG-PET/CT scan scores better than CT scan in treatment response evaluation in ATC patients. Poisson and colleagues[56] demonstrated discordant findings between FDG-PET/CT and CT scan in 45% of the cases, and in each such case, FDG-PET/CT findings were more informative than change in size, as determined by CT scan.

No studies or guidelines suggest or deal with the utility of non-FDG-PET in anaplastic (undifferentiated) thyroid carcinoma.

### Recommendations

- FDG-PET/CT is the best modality for staging ATC and classifying as stage IVA, IVB, and IVC.
- FDG-PET/CT is more sensitive than conventional imaging for detecting metastatic lesions and can potentially alter the management recommendations in approximately 25% to 50% of patients (Fig. 3).
- FDG-PET/CT is also better in treatment response evaluation of ATC.

### Fluorodeoxyglucose and Non-Fluorodeoxyglucose-PET Tracers in Medullary Thyroid Carcinoma

MTC is a neuroendocrine tumor originating from the neural crest–derived para-follicular "C cells"

of the thyroid gland and accounts for about 1% to 2% of thyroid malignancies.[59,60] Most of the MTC are sporadic, and about one-third are hereditary and are associated with multiple endocrine neoplasia (MEN) 2A or 2B syndromes or familial MTC based on specific autosomal dominant germline mutations in rearrangement during transfection (RET) proto-oncogene.[61] MTC frequently has an aggressive clinical course; only about half (48%) of the patients present with localized disease, whereas 35% have locally advanced and invasive disease to lymph nodal metastases and approximately 13% have distant metastases to lungs, liver, or bones.[62] The prognosis depends on the extent of primary tumor: 10-year survival is 90% when the tumor is confined to the thyroid and drops drastically to 70% and 20% with lymph nodal and distant metastases, respectively. Calcitonin and carcinoembryonic antigen (CEA) are sensitive tumor markers, especially calcitonin and CEA doubling times and correlates well with disease/tumor burden. Gradually increasing tumor markers mandate imaging workup to look for residual/recurrent and metastatic disease (Figs. 4 and 5).

Imaging modalities play a crucial role in therapeutic decision making; however, there are still no comprehensive diagnostic imaging modalities to reliably detect all recurrent and metastatic lesions. Therefore, concurrent use of several imaging methods is often required to provide the required information.[63] Functional imaging with PET/CT scans is particularly useful, is more informative than conventional imaging modalities, and provides whole-body assessment in a single modality. Hybrid PET/CT scan also scores higher than other gamma camera-based nuclear medicine imaging owing to higher resolution of PET systems. Tumor markers, particularly serum calcitonin, correlates well with tumor burden and effectively guides the extent of surgery at baseline and appropriate imaging modality in cases with suspected recurrence and also influences the choice of radiopharmaceuticals for PET/CT imaging.[64]

### Fluorodeoxyglucose-PET/Computed Tomography in Medullary Thyroid Carcinoma

FDG is the most commonly available and frequently used radiopharmaceutical in nuclear medicine with PET systems, detects hypermetabolic lesions, and reflects increased expression of glucose transporter proteins (GLUT), which correlate well with rapidly proliferating cells and is associated with poor prognosis. Hence, it is a marker of poor differentiation/dedifferentiation and aggressive clinical behavior. FDG is superior

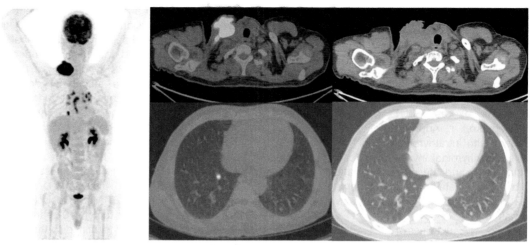

**Fig. 3.** A 56-year-old man presented with neck swelling. The patient underwent total thyroidectomy and central compartment neck dissection. The histopathology was suggestive of metastatic anaplastic carcinoma of the thyroid. He presented with a right supraclavicular mass; on [18]F-FDG, an ill-defined heterogenous exophytic fungating mass was noted in the right cervical level III and IV location measuring ~8.6 × 4.7 × 5.6 cm, with FDG uptake and extending up to the overlying skin. FDG-avid subcentimetric nodules were noted in the bilateral lung lower lobe.

in detecting biochemically progressive disease owing to poorly differentiated/dedifferentiated tumor cell population and has prognostic implications. FDG-PET/CT is more sensitive than anatomic imaging (USG, CT, MR imaging) or SPECT (single photon emission tomography) tracers; however, unlike DTCs, there is relatively less of a role and evidence of increased GLUTs. Hence, the FDG uptake could be highly variable/false negative with significant tumor burden and high tumor markers, and therefore, other tracers, such as fluro-dihydroxyphenylalanine (FDOPA), and different SSTR-based PET/CT have been investigated.

Verbeek and colleagues[64] evaluated outcomes of FDG-PET/CT and FDOPA PET/CT with calcitonin and CEA doubling times in 38 MTC patients and demonstrated FDG-positive disease in patients with shorter calcitonin and CEA doubling times (<24 months) and reported positive and negative predictive values of 77% and 88%, respectively, for biochemically progressive disease.[64] Receiver operating characteristic (ROC) curve analysis showed optimal calcitonin cut off of 874 ng/L for PET positivity with a sensitivity of 69% and specificity of 70%. Ong and colleagues[65] concluded that FDG-PET rarely detects disease in patients with calcitonin less than 500 pg/mL and demonstrated sensitivity of FDG-PET to be 78% and 20% for calcitonin greater than 1000 pg/mL and less than 1000 pg/mL. Overall, the reported patient-based sensitivity and specificity of FDG-

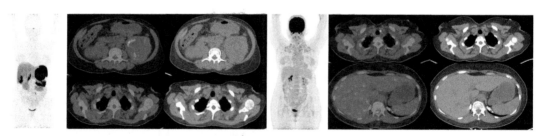

**Fig. 4.** A 33-year-old female patient presented with neck swelling. FNAC revealed medullary carcinoma thyroid. The patient underwent total thyroidectomy in 1995 and was asymptomatic until 2018, when she developed abdominal discomfort, and on evaluation bilateral pheochromocytoma was detected. The patient underwent [68]Ga-DOTATATE PET/CT (*left panel*), which showed bilateral suprarenal soft tissue density mass lesion. The patient underwent bilateral adrenalectomy in 2018 and was under close follow-up. In 2021, the patient presented with raised serum calcitonin level of 2350 pg/mL. On USG, recurrent disease was detected in the neck. [18]F-FDG-PET/CT was performed for restaging, demonstrating neck and upper mediastinal recurrence.

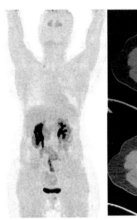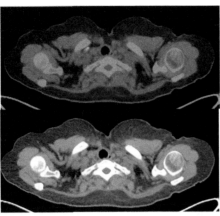

**Fig. 5.** A 55-year-old woman who presented with neck swelling for 3 years underwent total thyroidectomy with bilateral neck dissection. The histopathology proved to be medullary carcinoma of the thyroid. The patient was asymptomatic until 2018, when follow-up calcitonin showed a raising trend with doubling time of 6 months. [18]F-FDOPA PET/CT was performed to detect recurrence, which showed evidence of nodal recurrence in the neck.

PET/CT for recurrent MTC were observed to range between 17% to 93% and 68% to 92%, respectively. Meta-analysis studies showed the patient-based detection rates in recurrent MTC ranged from 59% (95% confidence interval [CI], 54%–63%) to 69% (95% CI, 64%–74%).[66] Treglia and colleagues[67] in their meta-analysis inferred variable detection rates of FDG-PET/CT in MTC according to calcitonin and CEA and their doubling times; overall suspected MTC recurrence was 59%, whereas it increased to 69% when CEA was greater than 5 ng/mL, 75% for patients with serum calcitonin greater than 1000 pg/mL; 76% for calcitonin doubling time of less than 12 months, and 91% when CEA doubling time was less than 24 months. FDG uptake is relatively more when CEA doubling time is less than calcitonin doubling time because CEA is a marker of early dedifferentiation and is retained in poorly differentiated MTC characterized by increased GLUT expression leading to avid FDG uptake, whereas calcitonin being a marker of terminal differentiation is expressed more avidly in well-differentiated MTC.[68] Hence, FDG should not be considered as first-line diagnostic imaging modality in patients with suspected recurrent and metastatic MTC with low serum calcitonin and CEA and their longer doubling times but works well in later stages or rapidly-growing disease.

### Non-Fluorodeoxyglucose-PET Tracers in Medullary Thyroid Carcinoma

#### Fluoro-dihydroxy phenylalanine
Fluoro-dihydroxy phenylalanine ([18]F-FDOPA) PET/CT scan is by far the single best modality for detection of metastatic lesions in MTC and is particularly suitable for detecting small lymph node metastases, as small as 6 mm.[69] Uptake of

[18]F-FDOPA depends on the L-type–amino-acid transporter system, and [18]F-FDOPA is sequestered into cells by cytosolic L-aromatic amino acid decarboxylase.[70] Most of the studies have reported [18]F-FDOPA PET/CT to be highly sensitive to stage MTC at baseline, before primary surgery and restaging MTC in suspected recurrence with better accuracy than FDG-PET/CT at relatively lower calcitonin values. [18]F-FDOPA PET/CT has relatively less prognostic value, but is more accurate in detecting extent of disease and counted more lesions than FDG-PET/CT, especially when serum calcitonin is not very high and is particularly suitable for detection of small metastatic lymph nodes, as small as around 6 mm.[69]

Giovanella and colleagues[71] in their recent practice guidelines for PET/CT imaging in MTC inferred a consistently high specificity with wide patient-based sensitivity ranging from 45% to 93% in patients with suspected recurrence. Treglia and colleagues[67] in their meta-analysis reported per-patient detection rate of [18]F-FDOPA PET/CT to be 66% (95% CI, 58%–74%). The detection rate further improves in patients with higher levels of calcitonin and shorter calcitonin doubling time, reaching as high as 86% with calcitonin doubling time less than 24 months.[72–74] Bovioand colleagues evaluated outcome of FDG and [18]F-FDOPA PET/CT with calcitonin and CEA doubling times in 36 MTC patients and demonstrated positive and negative predictive value of 56% and 75%, respectively, in [18]F-FDOPA PET-positive and -negative patients.[75] In the ROC curve analysis, the calcitonin cutoff was 825 ng/mL to be optimal for PET positivity, with a sensitivity and specificity of 88% and 80%, respectively.[76] Verbeek and colleagues[64] also demonstrated that calcitonin and CEA significantly differed between [18]F-FDOPA PET-positive and -negative patients, but there was no significant difference in doubling times. An analysis based on whole-body metabolic tumor burden (WBMTB), calcitonin, and CEA levels, including 21 patients with both FDG and [18]F-FDOPA PET/CT scans, found that, in PET-positive patients, WBMTB on [18]F-FDOPA significantly correlated with calcitonin levels ($r = 0.82$, $P = .013$) and CEA levels ($r = 0.88$, $P = .004$) but not with doubling times. No significant correlation was found between FDG-PET and calcitonin and CEA and doubling times.[64] In a recent review article by Kushchayev and colleagues,[77] [18]F-FDOPA PET/CT was found superior to FDG-PET/CT in evaluation of metastatic/recurrent MTC with a higher patient and lesion-based sensitivity. The patient-based detection rates improve significantly when calcitonin and CEA cutoff values of 150 pg/mL and 5 ng/mL are used, and Treglia and colleagues demonstrated the sensitivity of 73%.[67] Recent ATA guidelines for MTC recommend [18]F-FDOPA PET/CT at serum calcitonin level greater than 150 pg/mL, and the studies found sensitivity of [18]F-FDOPA PET/CT to be 79% to 100% for recurrent/metastatic MTC. The patient-based detection rates increase significantly with calcitonin levels greater than 150 pg/mL versus less than 150 pg/mL for both [18]F-FDOPA PET/CT (sensitivity 91% vs 29%) and for FDG-PET/CT (sensitivity 73% vs 14%) and with CEA levels greater than 5 ng/mL versus less than 5 ng/mL for both [18]F-FDOPA PET/CT (sensitivity 81% vs 43%) and FDG-PET/CT (sensitivity 73% vs 14%). Albeit [18]F-FDOPA fares better in detection rates than any other imaging modality for MTC, Kauhanen and colleagues[78] and Wong and colleagues[79] stated that combining both [18]F-FDOPA and FDG-PET/CT increases the sensitivity and hence are complementary. Apart from better sensitivity, specificity, and detection accuracy, [18]F-FDOPA PET/CT has the highest sensitivity and specificity (>95%) for detecting pheochromocytoma and paraganglioma and hence is a one-stop shop for MTC with suspected MEN syndromes.[80]

### Somatostatin receptor analogue

Somatostatin is a regulatory peptide, and human tissues express SSTR 1 to 5 and can be targeted by synthetic somatostatin analogue ligands TOC, TATE, and NOC chelated by DOTA (DOTATOC, DOTATATE, and DOTANOC) with each having a unique profile of affinity for SSTRs 1 to 5 and are tagged with [68]Ga for imaging and with [177]Lu/[90]Y for therapeutic purposes. The relative affinities of SSTR analogues are DOTANOC for SSTR 2, 3, and 5, DOTATATE (SSTR 2), and DOTATOC (SSTR 2 and 5). SSA PET/CT in evaluation of

MTC is the natural evolution of octreotide scintigraphy with [111]In, and the reported data range from highly favorable to disappointing and are due in part to heterogeneous SSTR expression, differences in SSA used for PET/CT, patient selection, and use of contrast-enhanced CT (CECT) scan with PET.

Souteiro and colleagues[81] in their study on 13 MTC patients with residual/recurrent/metastatic disease and elevated serum calcitonin and CEA found SSA PET/CT to detect a higher number of lesions than FDG-PET/CT (sensitivity 69.2% vs 53.9% for SSA and FDG). Furthermore, they also inferred that MTC lesions are better detected by SSA PET/CT in whom calcitonin levels are comparatively higher than CEA levels, and FDG-PET/CT fared better in patients with CEA higher than calcitonin. Hence, they hypothesized 2 profiles for metastatic MTC: a high calcitonin burden, well-differentiated, SSA PET-positive MTC with better prognosis and CEA preponderant, poorly differentiated/dedifferentiated, FDG-positive MTC with a worse prognosis. Tuncel and colleagues[82] in their study on 38 MTC patients detecting clinical impact of [68]Ga-DOTATATE PET/CT demonstrated it to be an essential part of MTC workup, as it outperformed conventional imaging in 14/38 (37%) patients and changed the clinical management in 13/38 (34%) patients.[82] They further showed a positive correlation between tumor marker, particularly calcitonin and [68]Ga-DOTATATE PET positivity. Castroneves and colleagues[83] demonstrated that [68]Ga-DOTATATE PET/CT has higher sensitivity (100%) for bone metastases when compared with the bone scintigraphy (44%). On a per-patient based analysis, the detection rate of SSA PET/CT is 63.5% (95% CI, 49%–77%) in suspected recurrent MTC. Positive SSA PET/CT can modify surgical management in a significant number of patients with recurrent MTC.[84] Albeit [18]F-FDOPA PET/CT is the most sensitive and specific imaging modality for detecting MTC lesions, SSA PET/CT has potential to identify patients for PRRT.[69,85]

### [11]C-Methionine

Methionine is an essential amino acid necessary for protein synthesis; however, this tracer has considerable nonprotein metabolites, making correct quantification of protein synthesis difficult.[86] Jang and colleagues[87] reported [11]C-methionine PET/CT scan to be more sensitive than FDG-PET/CT in detecting lymph nodal metastases; however, there was no benefit as compared with USG neck and a combination of USG neck and FDG-PET/CT; moreover, [11]C-methionine PET/CT scan with high physiologic uptake of tracer in the liver limits its use in hepatic metastases. Sensitivity of $^{11}$C-methionine PET/CT scan like that of other molecular imaging modalities increases with an increase in calcitonin, and the cutoff was determined to be 370 pg/mL.

### Immuno-PET using anti-carcinoembryonic antigen antibodies

Immuno-PET using anti-CEA antibodies, using directly labeled antibodies, their fragments, or antibody-derived recombinant constructs tagged with $^{68}$Ga, $^{111}$In, or $^{131}$I against CEA, was reported to be potentially accurate in detecting relapsing MTC; however, further studies are required.

### Recommendations

- $^{18}$F-FDOPA is the single best modality for evaluating disease burden and extent of disease with highest sensitivity in detecting metastatic and recurrent lesions in MTC, reflects well-differentiated phenotype, and should be considered as first-imaging modality when serum calcitonin is greater than 150 pg/mL.
- Furthermore, $^{18}$F-FDOPA has the highest sensitivity and specificity (>95%) for detecting pheochromocytoma and paraganglioma and hence is a one-stop shop for imaging in hereditary MTCs associated with MEN 2 syndromes.
- FDG-PET/CT positivity is a marker of poor differentiation/dedifferentiation reflecting aggressive behavior, has prognostic implications, and should be considered in patients with serum calcitonin greater than 1000 pg/mL; a shorter calcitonin and CEA doubling times (<12–24 months), and serially rising serum calcitonin and CEA levels.
- FDG-PET should not be considered as first-line diagnostic imaging modality in patients with suspected recurrence and metastases.
- SSA PET/CT should be considered in patients with high-serum calcitonin and progressive disease, especially when treatment with PRRT is under consideration.
- Combining $^{18}$F-FDOPA and FDG-PET/CT and also SSA PET/CT and FDG-PET/CT increases the sensitivity, and hence they are complementary.

## FLUORODEOXYGLUCOSE AND NON-FLUORODEOXYGLUCOSE-PET TRACERS IN PARATHYROID NEOPLASMS

Parathyroid neoplasms most commonly constitute adenomas followed by hyperplasia and carcinoma, are responsible for derangements in calcium homeostasis owing to hypersecretion of parathyroid hormone (PTH), also known as hyperparathyroidism (HPT), and are due to hyperfunctioning of one or more parathyroid glands. Hyperfunctioning parathyroid glands are due to solitary adenomas most cases (75%–80%) followed by multiglandular disease characterized by adenoma or hyperplasia (15%–20%), whereas parathyroid carcinoma accounts for less than 1% of cases.[88] Parathyroid neoplasms are broadly classified as primary hyperparathyroidism (pHPT) characterized by elevated or inappropriately normal PTH with hypercalcemia and secondary HPT characterized by elevated serum PTH owing to parathyroid hyperplasia in response to hypocalcemia, hyperphosphatemia, and hypovitaminosis D (mainly owing to chronic renal failure). Rarely, it could be due to paraneoplastic syndrome, and in most cases, is due to overproduction and secretion of parathyroid hormone–related peptide (PTH-rp). In paraneoplastic syndrome, the serum levels of PTH are low with respect to hypercalcemia with no hyperfunctioning parathyroid glands and PTH or both PTH and PTH-rp are produced by the culprit cancer. . Most pHPT are sporadic (95%), but about 5% occur as part of hereditary syndromes of MEN 1, 2, and 4 and HPT-jaw tumor syndrome or as part of nonsyndromic familial pHPT.

### Fluorodeoxyglucose -PET/Computed Tomography in Parathyroid Neoplasm

FDG-PET/CT is not deemed suitable for detection of hyperfunctioning parathyroid glands compared with other conventional imaging modalities, as sensitivity and specificity ranges from 0% to 94% and 62% to 100%, respectively, and varies considerably between available studies.[89] However, FDG-PET/CT is a sensitive tool in imaging parathyroid carcinoma for (a) baseline staging, (b) restaging, and (c) treatment response evaluation. Recent studies have shown choline PET tracers to be more sensitive and specific in imaging parathyroid cancers and detected relatively more lesions than FDG.

### Non-Fluorodeoxyglucose-PET Tracers in Parathyroid Neoplasm

#### Choline based tracers

Recently, 11-carbon and 18-fluorine tagged with choline have shown encouraging results as compared with conventional imaging modalities. Choline is a precursor of phospholipid biosynthesis, which is an essential component of cell membrane. Cells with a high proliferation rate have increased demand for choline, are phosphorylated by enzyme choline kinase, and are retained in the cell.[90] Choline PET has historically been introduced for prostate carcinoma imaging, outperforming FDG-PET, but positive results are seen in various nonmalignant conditions as well, and incidental [11]C-choline uptake was initially reported in parathyroid adenoma by Mapelli and colleagues.[91] [18]F-Fluorocholine is preferred over [11]C-choline owing to its long half-life, which alleviates the need for onsite cyclotron.

Quak and colleagues[92] published a prospective bicentric study on [18]F-fluorocholine PET/CT–guided surgery for pHPT in 25 patients in whom choline PET/CT–guided surgery in 22 patients and bilateral neck exploration could be avoided in 75% patients. In a recent head-to-head comparative study including 103 patients with pHPT, the diagnostic performance of choline PET/CT was found superior to conventional imaging modalities either separately or in combination, with a sensitivity of 92% for choline PET/CT, compared with 39% to 56% for conventional imaging, and 65% for a combination of conventional methods.[93] López-Mora and colleagues[94] in their prospective series of 33 patients found that [18]F-fluorocholine PET/CT in an analog system could detect hyperfunctioning tissue in 22 of 33 patients, whereas a digital PET/CT system detected hyperfunctioning tissue in 30 of 33 patients, and the lesions detected only on digital systems were less than 10 mm in diameter. In view of these unique advantages with [18]F-fluorocholine PET/CT, such as better detection of smaller lesions, low radiation exposure, higher resolution, and shorter acquisition time, it is therefore considered the alternative first-line imaging modality for this indication[95,96] (Fig. 6). Parathyroid carcinoma is also known to accumulate choline; the major limiting factors for choline PET are high cost and limited availability.

### [11]C-Methionine

Methionine is involved in the synthesis of PTH precursor and is trapped in a hyperfunctioning parathyroid gland. Kluijfhout and colleagues[97] in a meta-analysis of 14 studies found a pooled sensitivity of 77% and positive predictive value of 98% for detection of hyperfunctioning parathyroid glands in the correct quadrant. Other studies, however, have reported slightly lower detection rates ranging from 64% to 70% in preoperative scanning of patients with negative results on conventional imaging[98,99] (Fig. 7). The major limitations of this tracer are absolute requirement of onsite cyclotron owing to short half-life of ~20 minutes and lower signal-to-noise ratio owing to higher average positron energy than [18]F.

### Recommendations

- Choline PET/CT should be considered as an alternative first-line imaging modality in

patients with pHPT for preoperative localization. Choline PET/CT using a digital system yields better results, especially in lesions less than 1 cm in size.
- FDG-PET/CT does not show advantage over conventional imaging modalities for detecting hyperfunctioning parathyroid glands. However, FDG-PET/CT could be considered in parathyroid carcinoma.
- Methionine PET/CT may be useful as a second-line imaging modality in pHPT.

## FLUORODEOXYGLUCOSE AND NON-FLUORODEOXYGLUCOSE-PET TRACERS IN ADRENAL NEOPLASMS AND TUMORS OF AUTONOMIC NERVOUS SYSTEM

Clinically symptomatic adrenal diseases are relatively rare in patients when compared with those who are diagnosed with adrenal tumor and are more frequently encountered because of a rapid increase in the use of cross-sectional imaging. The reported incidence extends up to around 5% in CT examinations, and the characterization and follow-up of these "incidentalomas" place increasing demands on health care resources. In healthy individuals, 80% of incidentally found adrenal masses are benign, nonfunctioning adenomas, and even in patients with known malignancy, approximately 40% to 57% of adrenal incidentalomas are benign. These incidentalomas can be accurately classified in most cases as benign and malignant with contrast washout studies on CT scan (adrenal protocol on CECT). The workup of adrenal neoplasms should aim at establishing functional versus nonfunctional phenotype and benign versus malignant features to devise appropriate treatment plans.

USG, CT scan, and MR imaging are the first-line imaging modalities for the evaluation of adrenal neoplasms. CT scan can be used to distinguish between benign and malignant causes with a diagnostic sensitivity of 88%, and small lesions (<4 cm) with homogeneous low HU on unenhanced CT (<10 HU) are usually benign, in which further imaging is not required.[100] Similarly, chemical shift MR imaging identifies high intracellular lipid content with lesion intensity similar to liver on T2-weighted images, confirming benign cause; however, lipid-poor adenomas representing about 30% of all adrenocortical adenomas (ACA) will remain indeterminate by anatomic imaging techniques. Functional imaging modalities provide an edge over anatomic imaging modalities in distinguishing benign and malignant lesions. Metastatic lesions of adrenals should be evaluated with core-needle biopsy or fine-needle aspiration cytology

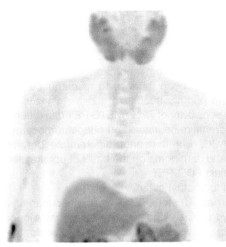
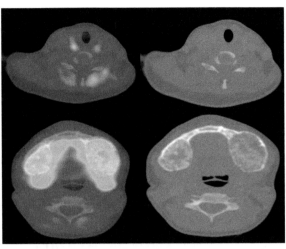

Fig. 6. A 32-year-old woman, with a history of left inferior parathyroid adenoma operated in 2016, presented with bilateral jaw swelling and iPTH = 72.7 pg/mL and serum Ca = 12.2 mg/dL (performed on March 12, 2021). The patient was clinically suspected to have HPT-jaw tumor syndrome, and $^{18}$F-fluorocholine was performed to localize the recurrent parathyroid adenoma. Scan findings were consistent with bilateral superior parathyroid adenoma and brown tumor of the mandible.

(FNAC) for ascertaining the diagnosis and then imaging, once pheochromocytoma has been ruled out biochemically.

## Tumors of Adrenal Cortex

Adrenal cortex comprises 3 distinct histologic and functional regions: zona glomerulosa, zona fasciculata, and zona reticularis, from outside to inside, producing mineralocorticoids, glucocorticoids, and sex steroids. Functioning neoplasms of adrenal gland constitute a smaller proportion of all detected lesions, and approximately 70% to 94% are benign, nonfunctioning adenomas; however, unsuspected adrenal malignancies can be encountered in about 21% of patients, and of these, about 32% to 73% represent metastases.[75,101,102]

## Fluorodeoxyglucose-PET/Computed Tomography in Adrenocortical Neoplasms

Benign ACA demonstrates low-grade to mild FDG uptake in the lesions, and hence, a lower SUV$_{max}$ value points toward benign cause. Metastatic disease, apart from the histopathologic findings, is the most important determinant for malignant tumor. The main utility of functional imaging is to distinguish benign from malignant cause, and FDG-PET/PET/CT is an important tool offering high sensitivity, specificity, and diagnostic accuracy. Adrenocortical carcinoma (ACC) is a rare malignancy with poor prognosis, and overall 5-year survival is 20% to 45% with dismal survival (<12%) in the presence of distant metastases. Primary treatment is adrenalectomy with adjuvant

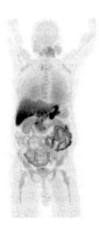
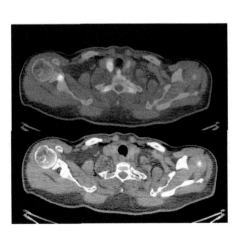

Fig. 7. A 66-year-old man with suspected HPT underwent $^{11}$C-methionine PET/CT, which revealed a hypodense lesion posterior to the upper pole of the right lobe of the thyroid gland with increased radiotracer uptake suggestive of right superior parathyroid adenoma.

antimetabolite mitotane, and recurrence rate is initially high despite complete surgical resection; hence, early detection of recurrence is the key to improved survival.

A recent systemic review and meta-analysis comprising 21 studies published between 1995 and 2009 evaluating a total of 1391 lesions (824 benign and 567 malignant) in 1217 patients showed mean sensitivity of 97% (95% CI, 93%–98%) and specificity of 91% (95% CI, 87%–94%) in differentiating benign from malignant lesions.[103] Becherer and colleagues[104] evaluated FDG-PET in 10 patients with confirmed ACC and reported sensitivity and specificity of 100% and 95%, respectively. They identified additional lesions that were not detected by anatomic imaging alone in approximately 30%, and FDG-PET modified the treatment protocol in about 20% patients.[104] Lebboulleux and colleagues[105] in their study found sensitivity for detection of distinct lesions and the diagnosis of metastases as 90% and 93%, respectively, and demonstrated that tumor $SUV_{max}$ greater than 10 was found to be an adverse prognostic factor. In another study by Tessonnier and colleagues[106] evaluating the role of FDG, including 37 patients of ACC, $SUV_{max}$ correlated with atypical mitosis and Weiss score, but not with overall survival or disease-free survival at a mean follow-up period of 49 months. FDG-PET/PET/CT is advantageous in being (a) able to distinguish effectively between benign and malignant tumors; (b) assessing the malignant potential of adrenal mass that is otherwise deemed indeterminate on anatomic imaging, especially lipid poor adenomas versus malignancy; and (c) having wide availability and relatively longer half-life, providing ease of utilization (**Fig. 8**).

### Non-fluorodeoxyglucose-PET Tracers in Adrenocortical Neoplasms

#### [11]C-Metomidate

Metomidate (METO) is the methyl ester of "etomidate" (ETO, an anesthetic agent), and both are inhibitors of the CYP11B enzymes: 11β-hydroxylase and aldosterone synthase involved in cortisol and aldosterone synthesis, respectively. Based on high affinity to these enzymes and specific adrenocortical binding properties, METO and ETO have been labeled with [11]C and [18]F and are being used as PET tracers for adrenocortical imaging. Hennings and colleagues[107] in their study evaluated correlation with [11]C-METO PET and histopathologic findings on 73 patients with 75 adrenal tumors (26 adenomas, 13 adrenocortical cancers, 8 hyperplasia, 6 pheochromocytoma, 3

metastases, and 19 tumors of nonadrenal origin) with varying sizes ranging from 1 to 20 cm, the sensitivity and specificity were found to be 89% and 96%, respectively, in distinguishing adrenocortical tumors from nonadrenocortical tumors. ACCs have been shown to accumulate [11]C-METO in primary neoplasm and metastases and have a sensitivity of 72%. METO PET can differentiate adrenal metastases and pheochromocytoma from ACC, but it cannot differentiate between ACAs and carcinoma on the basis of uptake alone as against FDG-PET.

#### [18]F-Fluoroethyl ester

Fluoroethyl ester (FETO) is another marker of 11β-hydroxylase, and because of [18]F, has a longer half-life, allows longer imaging protocols than METO, and has experimental importance.

### Recommendations

- FDG-PET/CT is an important tool in distinguishing benign from malignant lesions on a per-lesion basis.
- FDG-PET should be considered for evaluating the malignant potential of adrenal incidentalomas, which appear indeterminate on anatomic imaging as in lipid-poor adenoma versus malignancy (higher $SUV_{max}$ values greater than 10 point toward malignancy).
- FDG-PET could detect the metastatic lesions with high sensitivity but with low specificity and cannot differentiate adrenocortical tumors from PPGL.
- METO and FETO PET can differentiate between adrenocortical and adrenal medullary neoplasms and are of special importance in biochemically silent tumors (parasympathetic PGL).

### Tumors of Adrenal Medulla and Autonomic Nervous System/Neural Crest Neoplasms

Tumors of adrenal medulla are derived from postganglionic sympathetic or parasympathetic neurons; the sympathetic postganglionic neurons are called as "chromaffin" cells (based on characteristic staining on tissue histology) and are derived from neural crest cells and hence have neuroendocrine origin. Neural crest–derived neoplasms have a reported prevalence between 0.2% and 0.6% in patients with hypertension and in nearly 5% of patients with an incidentally discovered adrenal tumor.[108] Phenotypically, these may be sympathetic (catecholamine and dopamine secreting), in adrenal medulla and posterior mediastinum and parasympathetic (nonsecretory), in head and neck and anterior and middle mediastinum and according to location are pheochromocytoma (located in adrenal

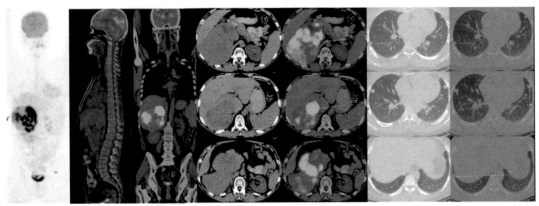

**Fig. 8.** A 19-year-old man, suspected for ACC, presented with facial puffiness of 6 months' duration. Basal S cortisol 36.4 μg/dL LDDS, cortisol 36.6 μg/dL USG abdomen showed a large well-defined lobulated right suprarenal mass. FDG-PETPET/CT scan showed FDG-avid large, ill-defined, lobulated soft tissue density mass with focal areas of calcification and central necrosis in the right suprarenal region with right adrenal gland not separately delineated. Left adrenal appeared unremarkable. Well-circumscribed multiple (at least 8 to 10) pleural-based nodules of varying sizes and minimal FDG uptake were seen involving bilateral lung parenchyma. He underwent right adrenalectomy, and histopathology report was confirmatory for ACC.

gland) and paraganglioma (all extra-adrenal lesions irrespective of being sympathetic or parasympathetic; 85% are intra-abdominal, 15% are intrathoracic, and 1%–3% are paracervical). Both can be termed together and referred to as PPGL. Differential diagnosis may include other tumors of neural crest origin: neuroblastoma, ganglioneuroma, and composite tumors and metastases from these tumors (**Figs. 9 and 10**).

Most of these cells are located in the adrenal medulla or in extra-adrenal locations near the celiac axis. Approximately 5% to 10% of solitary pheochromocytoma are hereditary, whereas the presence of multiple pheochromocytomas or a combination of pheochromocytoma with a synchronous or metachronous extra-adrenal paragangliomas is associated with germline or somatic mutation in greater than 70%. The PPGL susceptibility genes can be classified into 4 major clusters: (a) pseudohypoxia subtype (subdivided into tricarboxylic acid cycle–dependent and Von-Hippel Lindau [VHL]/EPAS-1 dependent), (b) kinase signaling subtype, (c) Wnt signaling subtype, and (d) cortical admixture subtype, and can be driven by either germline mutation (27%), somatic mutation (39%), or fusion gene mutation (7%).[109] Albeit most PPGLs are benign, 10% to 20% are malignant (characterized by presence of distant metastases), of which 10% to 15% of patients present with metastases at diagnosis. Metastatic disease is more commonly found in patients with SDHB and α-thalassemia/mental retardation syndrome X-linked mutations, large tumors (>5 cm), extra-adrenal location, and noradrenergic and dopaminergic phenotype.

## Fluorodeoxyglucose -PET/Computed Tomography in Tumors of Adrenal Medulla and Autonomic Nervous System/Neural Crest Neoplasms

Benign pheochromocytoma can show a high grade of FDG uptake, which is a unique feature for any benign tumor, and which further increases in malignant tumors as the tumor cells are forced to resort to anaerobic glycolysis (Warburg effect). Taieb and colleagues in their early study proposed 2 alternative explanations: an early metabolic switch related to genetic defects (pseudohypoxia model) and an adaptive response to hypoxia, and the fact that these tumors are highly vascularized is indirect evidence of hypoxia.[70] Pseudohypoxia model implies a link between inactivation of SDH and VHL genes and induction of a hypoxic response mediated by inactivation of prolyl hydrolase and consequent stabilization of HIF-2α (hypoxia-inducible factor).[110,111] In general, in malignant cases, FDG uptake is a marker of functional dedifferentiation, but this phenomenon does not hold good for PPGL (as benign pheochromocytoma are FDG avid), and the underlying mechanism could be attributed to "metabolic reprogramming" rather than tumor cell dedifferentiation.

Shulkin and colleagues[76] reported sensitivity of 58% in benign pheochromocytoma and 76% in malignant pheochromocytoma, particularly in meta-iodobenzyl guanidine (MIBG) -negative tumors. Across the spectrum, succinate dehydrogenase (SDH; particularly SDHB) and VHL-related tumors have higher FDG uptake as against neurofibromatosis and MEN-related PPGL. The main advantage of FDG-PET/CT is in patients with

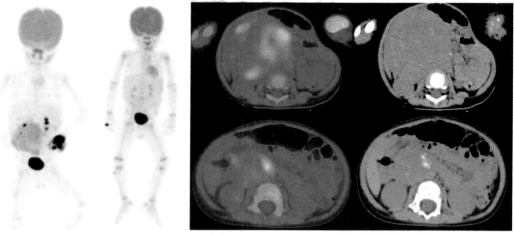

Fig. 9. A 1-year-old male child presented with abdominal distention. On evaluation, he had a right suprarenal mass, which on biopsy proved to be neuroblastoma. $^{18}$F-FDG-PET/CT (dated February 18, 2021) was performed for baseline evaluation and showed metabolically active heterogenous density mass lesion in the suprarenal location with specks of calcification and central necrosis. The patient was started on chemotherapy, and after 4 cycles of chemotherapy, PET/CT was performed for response assessment, which showed a decrease in size and metabolic activity of the primary lesion, suggestive of partial response.

metastatic PPGL related to SDH germline mutation in which FDG has a sensitivity of 100%, which exceeded that of FDOPA (88%), MIBG (80%), and SSA PET (81%), as SDH-related PPGL have larger tumor volumes, greater rates of metastases, multifocal disease, and higher SUVs on FDG.[112]

### Non-Fluorodeoxyglucose-PET Tracers in Tumors of Adrenal Medulla and Autonomic Nervous System/Neural Crest Neoplasms

#### Somatostatin receptor analogue and antagonists

PPGLs are neuroendocrine cell derivatives, hence express SSTR, particularly SSTR 2 and 3, which can be targeted for imaging and therapeutic (theranostic) interventions using somatostatin analogues and antagonists (SSA). As SSTR 2A and 3 are more commonly and avidly expressed in PPGLs than SSTR 5, thus $^{68}$Ga-DOTATATE and $^{68}$Ga-DOTA-NOC are preferred agents[113–115] (Figs. 11 and 12). Tracer binding and retention depend on the density of receptors on cell surface and internalization of ligand-receptor complex. SSTR antagonist NODAGA-JR 11 has recently been developed and is expected to reduce DOTA-peptide washout and hence increase the residency time despite lack of internalization, as the radiopharmaceuticals remain anchored within the cell membrane.

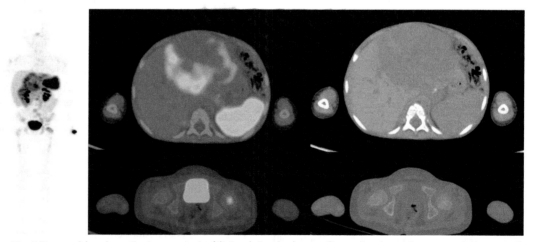

Fig. 10. A 3-year-old male patient presented with an abdominal mass. On evaluation, a large mass lesion was detected in the liver, which on biopsy was proven to be neuroblastoma. The patient was referred for $^{68}$Ga-DOTA-NOC PET/CT, which revealed a tracer-avid large heterogenous mass in the epigastrium and right hypochondrium, involving the segments II, III, IV, V, and VIII of the liver with tracer-avid left para-aortic, pre-aortic, aortocaval, and bilateral common iliac lymph nodes. Multiple skeletal sites with increased uptake were also detected.

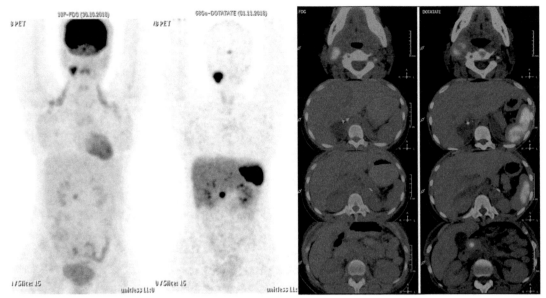

Fig. 11. A 16-year-old woman presented with accelerated hypertension (210/140 mm Hg). CECT scan abdomen showed a large heterogeneously enhancing mass in the bilateral adrenal regions with similar enhancing lesion in right paraaortic region. Laboratory investigations showed the following: PFNMN, 3337 pg/mL; and PFMN, calcitonin, aldosterone, and cortisol all within normal limits. She underwent bilateral adrenalectomy with excision of the right para-aortic lesion. HPR: bilateral pheochromocytoma with right para-aortic paraganglioma. FDG and 68Ga-DOTATATE PET/CT scans were performed to look for other sites of paraganglioma and showed a metabolically active intensely SSTR-expressing lesion in the right carotid space in the region of the angle of mandible encasing the right carotid artery and the right IJV with preserved fat planes with adjacent muscles and prevertebral space suggestive of cervical (extra-adrenal) paraganglioma (carotid body tumor) with metabolically active, intense SSTR expressing a pancreatic head mass. Further histopathologic and chromogranin A correlation was suggested to rule out neuroendocrine involvement. Here, FDG and 68Ga-DOTATATE scans demonstrated other sites of paraganglioma with suspicious neuroendocrine involvement of the pancreatic head mass.

Available literature is scarce on the use of SSA PET in benign pheochromocytoma and primary PPGL, whereas there are excellent results for localizing these lesions when they are malignant and/or extra-adrenal and reported to be more sensitive than MIBG scintigraphy. In a recent systemic review and meta-analysis, pooled detection rate for SSA PET was 93% (95% CI, 91%–95%) and was significantly higher ($P<.001$ for all) than FDOPA (80%; 95% CI, 69%–88%), FDG (74%; 95% CI, 46%–91%), and MIBG scintigraphy (38%; 95% CI, 20%–59%).[116] Several studies compared SSA PET with FDOPA PET and concluded that SSA PET fares better than FDOPA on a per-patient and per-lesion basis, and the statistics were much better in extra-adrenal PGL (98% vs 95% and 99% vs 68%, respectively).[117] In recent noncomparative studies, SSA PET demonstrated sensitivity of 84% for pheochromocytoma and 100% for PGL and as compared with FDG-PET, and SSA PET was more valuable in pediatric patients.[117] SSA PET showed lesser concentration in PPGLs related to EPAS 1 (HIF 2α), PHD 1/2, and FH than SDHx-related PPGLs and

in areas of higher physiologic uptake (eg, liver, adrenals).[118] Furthermore, approximately 50% of metastatic PPGLs related to SDHB mutation do not concentrate MIBG owing to cellular dedifferentiation leading to lack of norepinephrine transporter system but do not show significant loss of SSTR expression, and SDH-deficient tumors show avid SSTR 2A and SSTR 3 expression, making them valid theranostic targets, which has led to treatment changes in up to 60% of patients.

### Fluro-dihydroxyphenylalanine

FDOPA offers high sensitivity and specificity for detecting nonmetastatic pheochromocytoma (both approaching 100%).[119] FDOPA uptake in PPGL is attributed to their property to decarboxylate L-amino acids owing to inherent activity of L-aromatic amino-acid decarboxylase and their uptake and storage in neurosecretory vesicles through L-type amino-acid transporters (LATs), primarily LAT1.

A recent meta-analysis, including 11 studies involving 275 subjects with PPGLs, demonstrated

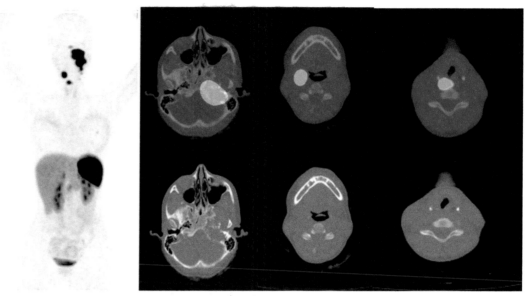

**Fig. 12.** A 21-year-old woman presented with right-sided neck swelling. CECT performed showed a heterogeneously enhancing lesion at the right carotid artery bifurcation causing splaying of the internal and external carotid artery suspicious of carotid body tumor. The patient was referred for [68]Ga-DOTANOC PET/CT to confirm the diagnosis and rule out paraganglioma of any other location. [68]Ga-DOTANOC PET/CT detected SSTR expressing left glomus jugulotympanicum, right carotid body tumor, and right prevertebral paraganglioma.

pooled sensitivity and specificity in lesion-based analysis of FDOPA to be 79% (95% CI, 76%–81%) and 95% (95% CI, 84%–99%), and the most important factors are sympathetic phenotype and being negative for SDHx mutation.[120] In several published studies, the reported patient- and lesion-based specificity of FDOPA is 94% and 100%, respectively, and for sporadic- and MEN 2–associated (almost always sympathetic) pheochromocytoma, the sensitivity for detection approaches 100%.[119,120] For metastatic PPGL, FDOPA performs better in SDHB mutation negative than for SDHB mutation positive (sensitivity: 93% vs 20% respectively).[119] On the other hand, FDOPA shows very high sensitivity for detection of VHL, EPAS (HIF-2α), and FH-related PPGLs, which are often multiple, recurrent, and occasionally exhibit high metastatic potential. The decreased sensitivity in metastatic disease related to SDHB mutation-related PPGL is probably due to dedifferentiation, which might lead to loss of specific norepinephrine transporters in these tumors.

### Fluro-dopamine

Theoretically, fluro-dopamine (FDA) appears to be a promising tool for the detection of PGLs associated with the sympathetic nervous system and is currently used as an experimental tracer with few preliminary studies reported to date. Timmers and colleagues[121] in their prospective study on 52 patients inferred that FDA-PET is the preferred imaging modality for localizing primary PGL and to rule out metastases. For patients with known metastatic PGL, they recommended FDA-PET in patients with an unknown genotype, FDG, or FDA-PET in SDHB mutation and FDOPA or FDA-PET in SDHB mutation-negative patients.[121] In various studies, the sensitivity and specificity of FDA-PET in imaging PPGL ranged from 90% to 100% and 75% to 90%, respectively.[121,122]

### [11]C-Hydroxyephedrine

Hydroxyephedrine (HED) is a norepinephrine analogue that binds to the norepinephrine transporter, is transported to neurosecretory vesicles in presynaptic adrenergic nerve terminals, and is stored there. Vyakaranam and colleagues[123] retrospectively evaluated 102 patients with symptoms suspicious for PPGL and showed sensitivity, specificity, positive predictive value, and negative predictive value of 96%, 99%, 96%, and 99%, respectively, and when correlated with histopathology, the respective parameters were 96%, 93%, 96%, and 93%, respectively. The study further demonstrated that HED-PET effectively ruled out PPGL in 78 patients in whom CT was inconclusive.[123] Few disadvantages associated with HED PET are shorter half-life of [11]C (20 minutes), which mandates the presence of an on-site cyclotron, limited availability, and that it can be used only in patients with sympathetic PGL.

## $^{124}$I-Metaiodobenzyl guanidine

$^{124}$I is a positron-emitting isotope of iodine and holds promise for detection of primary and metastatic sites in malignant PPGLs owing to higher image resolution of PET systems and provides the scope to quantitate the uptake, which is valuable for dosimetric analysis and more objective treatment response evaluation. Few studies have been performed with $^{124}$I-MIBG, and Ott and colleagues[124] used it to predict the absorbed dose of $^{131}$I-MIBG in neural crest tumor sites of 2 patients. Pre-therapeutic imaging of PPGLs to ascertain eligibility for $^{131}$I-MIBG therapy and dosimetry is perhaps the most attractive feature of $^{124}$I-MIBG PET imaging. Disadvantages are limited availability and a longer half-life (4 days) than other PET tracers in use for the indication and hence should be considered only when $^{131}$I-MIBG therapy is being planned.

## Recommendations

- Sporadic nonmetastatic pheochromocytomas: FDOPA PET is the most sensitive tracer, and if available, should be the preferred imaging modality. If not, SSA-PET or MIBG scintigraphy should be considered. FDG-PET can provide genotypic information linked to SDHB mutation. FDA and HED PET are of experimental status, and more data are required for their formal clinical inclusion.
- Head and neck paragangliomas (HNPGLs): SSA-PET should be considered the first imaging modality, as it has high detection efficiency for both SDHx-related and non-SDHx-related tumors, can detect very small lesions that tend to be overlooked by other imaging modalities, and has better availability, followed by FDOPA-PET. FDG has high sensitivity for SDHx-related HNPGLs and can complement SSA and FDOPA PET for detecting additional lesions. As HNPGLs are mostly parasympathetic paragangliomas, tracers targeting adrenergic pathways are of no significant importance.
- Retroperitoneal and other extra-adrenal nonmetastatic paragangliomas: A main objective is to rule out neurogenic tumors, lymphoproliferative disorders, and mesenchymal tumors, and PET tracers with specific targets, SSA > FDOPA should be considered (as the former has high sensitivity and specificity for both SDHx-related and non-SDHx-related tumors, can detect very small lesions, and has better availability). Because most of the extra-adrenal PGLs apart from HNPGLs have sympathetic phenotype, PET tracers targeting adrenergic pathways (FDA and HED) are valid alternatives, mainly of experimental importance.
- Metastatic pheochromocytomas and paragangliomas (PPGLs): SSA PET is the imaging modality of choice owing to the above-mentioned reasons (SDHx-related and non-SDHx-related tumors, can detect very small lesions, and has better availability). FDOPA should be considered as the second-line imaging modality in the absence of SDHB mutation and if the genotype is unknown. FDG-PET is an important imaging tool for SDHB–mutated lesions for detection of metastases. MIBG scintigraphy may cause significant underestimation of the tumor burden and consequent inappropriate management. $^{124}$I-MIBG PET appears promising in this setting and has theranostic implications.
- VHL and RET/MEN 2–associated PPGLs: MEN 2–associated pheochromocytomas are almost always sympathetic (adrenergic phenotype) and are exclusively adrenal; hence, FDOPA is the imaging modality of choice with the exception of larger tumors (>5 cm), which tend to become metastatic. FDG-PET fares better and should be chosen over FDOPA when aggressive metastatic PPGLs are suspected.

## FUTURE DIRECTIONS
### Fibroblast Activation Protein Inhibitor PET

Tumor microenvironment is a complex dynamic framework that plays a crucial role in survival, proliferation, spread, and drug resistance of malignant cells through protumorigenic signaling pathways.[125,126] Fibroblast activation protein (FAP) is overexpressed in stroma of several tumor entities, especially in those that are characterized by a strong desmoplastic reaction, so much so that approximately 90% of the gross tumor mass consists of stromal cells contributed mainly by cancer-associated fibroblasts (CAF) and extracellular fibrosis, and original tumor cells are only in the minority.[127,128] Normal fibroblasts are present ubiquitously in the whole-body and show dipeptidyl peptidase 4 expression (exopeptidase activity) and very low FAP expression, whereas CAFs are specifically characterized by overexpression of FAP (both exo-peptidase and endo-peptidase activity). Hence, FAP provides a promising highly tumor-specific target, and FAP-specific inhibitors (FAPI) have been developed as anticancer drugs.

FAPI are "quinoline"-based agents attached with positron emitters ($^{68}$Ga) to DOTA-containing ligands (universal bifunctional chelators) as tumor targeting radiopharmaceuticals, and the biodistribution suggested that FAPI may be suitable for radioligand therapy and here has over the time developed as one of the most promising theranostic agents.

Published accounts on FAPI-PET being used in endocrine malignancies are extremely deficient, and most of the work is done on metastatic thyroid carcinoma (both differentiated and in TENIS syndrome); however, no publication could be found on FAPI PET being used in adrenal or parathyroid tumors. Wu and colleagues[129] in their study compared FDG and FAPI PET/CT scans in a cohort of 35 patients and demonstrated [68]Ga-DOTA-FAPI-04 detected more lymph nodal and skeletal lesions as compared with FDG (268). The specificity, accuracy, positive predictive value, and negative predictive value of [68]Ga-DOTA-FAPI-04 relative to FDG for detection of metastatic lymph nodes were 84.38% versus 34.38%, 83.10% versus 60.56%, 86.49% versus 59.62%, and 79.41% versus 57.89%, respectively, and were statistically significant ($P = .05$), and for skeletal lesions, the parameters were statistically not significant (268). However, the detection rate of [68]Ga-DOTA-FAPI-04 for skeletal metastases was found to be 96.0% (24/25 lesions) and was significantly higher than FDG 72.0% (18/25 lesions) ($P<.05$) (0.049). The detection rate for lymph nodes was also marginally higher for [68]Ga-DOTA-FAPI-04 (82.05%; 32/39) than for FDG (79.49%; 31/39) and was statistically not significant ($P>.05$) (0.774), and for distant metastases other than bones, [68]Ga-DOTA-FAPI-04 scored 91.07% (51/55) versus FDG 89.09% (49/55) and was statistically not significant ($P>.05$) (0.742). Fu and colleagues[130] in the case report on patients with TENIS syndrome reported intense uptake of [68]Ga-DOTA-FAPI in metastatic lesions demonstrating its usefulness in detecting recurrent/metastatic lesions in patients with TENIS. Furthermore, [68]Ga-DOTA-FAPI uptake qualifies the patients for radioligand therapy and will be a valuable addition to the limited therapeutic intervention against TENIS.

## DISCLOSURE

The authors have nothing to disclose.

## REFERENCES

1. Hundahl SA, Fleming ID, Fremgen AM, et al. A National Cancer Data Base report on 53,856 cases of thyroid carcinoma treated in the U.S., 1985-1995. Cancer 1998;83(12):2638–48.
2. Iñiguez-Ariza NM, Brito JP. Management of low-risk papillary thyroid cancer. Endocrinol Metab 2018; 33:185.
3. Lan W, Gege Z, Ningning L, et al. Negative remnant 99mTc-pertechnetate uptake predicts excellent response to radioactive iodine therapy in low- to intermediate-risk differentiated thyroid cancer patients who have undergone total thyroidectomy. Ann Nucl Med 2019;33:112–8.
4. Soelberg KK, Bonnema SJ, Brix TH, et al. Risk of malignancy in thyroid incidentalomas detected by 18F-fluorodeoxyglucose positron emission tomography: a systematic review. Thyroid 2012;22:918–25.
5. Buyukdereli G, Aktar Y, Kara E, et al. Role of 18F-fluorodeoxyglucose positron emission tomography/computed tomography in the evaluation of cytologically indeterminate thyroid nodules. Iran J Radiol 2016;13(1):e21186.
6. Castellana M, Trimboli P, Piccardo A, et al. Performance of 18F FDG PET/CT in selecting thyroid nodules with indeterminate fine-needle aspiration cytology for surgery: a systematic review and a meta-analysis. J Clin Med 2019;8(9):1333.
7. Yen TC, Lin HD, Lee CH, et al. The role of technetium-99m sestamibi whole-body scan in diagnosing metastatic hurtle cell carcinoma of thyroid gland after total thyroidectomy: a comparison with iodine-131 and thallium-201 whole-body scans. Eur J Nucl Med 1994;21:980–3.
8. Pryma DA, Schoder H, Gonen M, et al. Diagnostic accuracy and prognostic value of 18F-FDG PET in Hurthle cell thyroid cancer patients. J Nucl Med 2006;47:1260–6.
9. Plotkin M, Hautzel H, Krause BJ, et al. Implication of 2-18fluor-2-deoxyglucose positron emission tomography in the follow-up of Hurthle cell thyroid cancer. Thyroid 2002;12:155–61.
10. Gasparre G, Porcelli AM, Bonora E, et al. Disruptive mitochondrial DNA mutations in complex I subunits are markers of oncocytic phenotype in thyroid tumors. Proc Natl Acad Sci U S A 2007;104: 9001–6.
11. Nascimento C, Borget I, Al Ghuzlan A, et al. Postoperative fluorine-18-fluorodeoxyglucose positron emission tomography/computed tomography: an important imaging modality in patients with aggressive histology of differentiated thyroid cancer. Thyroid 2015;25(4):437–44.
12. Feine U, Lietzenmayer R, Hanke JP, et al. Fluorine-18-FDG and iodine-131-iodide uptake in thyroid cancer. J Nucl Med 1996;37:1468–72.
13. Lazar V, Bidart JM, Caillou B, et al. Expression of the Na?/I-symporter gene in human thyroid tumors: a comparison study with other thyroid-specific genes. J Clin Endocrinol Metab 1999;84:3228–34.
14. Ma C, Kuang A, Xie J, et al. Possible explanations for patients with discordant findings of serum

thyroglobulin and 131I whole body scanning. J Nucl Med 2005;46:1473–80.

15. Silberstein EB. The problem of the patient with thyroglobulin elevation but negative iodine scintigraphy: the TENIS syndrome. Semin Nucl Med 2011;41:113–20.

16. Sherman SI. Thyroid carcinoma. Lancet 2003;361:501–11.

17. American Thyroid Association (ATA), Guidelines Taskforce on thyroid nodules and differentiated thyroid cancer, Cooper DS, Doherty GM, et al. Revised American Thyroid Association management guidelines for patients with thyroid nodules and differentiated thyroid cancer. Thyroid 2009;19(11):1167–214.

18. Özdemir E, Yildirim Poyraz N, Polat SB, et al. Diagnostic value of 18F-FDG PET/CT in patients with TENIS syndrome: correlation with thyroglobulin levels. Ann Nucl Med 2014;28(3):241–7.

19. Finkelstein SE, Grigsby PW, Siegel BA, et al. Combined [18F]fluorodeoxyglucose positron emission tomography and computed tomography (FDG-PET/CT) for detection of recurrent, 131I-negative thyroid cancer. Ann Surg Oncol 2008;15(1):286–92.

20. Bannas P, Derlin T, Groth M, et al. Can (18)F-FDG-PET/CT be generally recommended in patients with differentiated thyroid carcinoma and elevated thyroglobulin levels but negative I-131 whole body scan? Ann Nucl Med 2012;26(1):77–85.

21. Na SJ, Yoo IeR, O JH, et al. Diagnostic accuracy of (18)F-fluorodeoxyglucose positron emission tomography/computed tomography in differentiated thyroid cancer patients with elevated thyroglobulin and negative (131)I whole body scan: evaluation by thyroglobulin level. Ann Nucl Med 2012;26(1):26–34.

22. Deichen JT, Schmidt C, Prante O, et al. Influence of TSH on uptake of 18Ffluorodeoxyglucose in human thyroid cells in vitro. Eur J Nucl Med Mol Imaging 2004;31:507–12.

23. Filetti S, Damante G, Foti D. Thyrotropin stimulates glucose transport in cultured rat thyroid cells. Endocrinology 1987;120:2576–81.

24. Trybek T, Kowalska A, Lesiak J, et al. The role of 18F-fluorodeoxyglucose positron emission tomography in patients with suspected recurrence or metastatic differentiated thyroid carcinoma with elevated serum thyroglobulin and negative I-131 whole body scan. Nucl Med Rev Cent East Eur 2014;17(2):87–93.

25. Asa S, Aksoy SY, Vatankulu B, et al. The role of FDG- PET/CT in differentiated thyroid cancer patients with negative iodine-131 whole-body scan and elevated anti-Tg level. Ann Nucl Med 2014;28(10):970–9.

26. Pazaitou-Panayiotou K, Tiensuu Janson E, Koletsa T, et al. Somatostatin receptor expression in non-medullary thyroid carcinomas. Hormones (Athens) 2012;11(3):290–6.

27. Pisarek H, Stepień T, Kubiak R, et al. Expression of somatostatin receptor subtypes in human thyroid tumors: the immunohistochemical and molecular biology (RT-PCR) investigation. Thyroid Res 2009;2(1):1.

28. Antunes P, Ginj M, Zhang H, et al. Are radiogallium labelled DOTA-conjugated somatostatin analogues superior to those labelled with other radiometals? Eur J Nucl Med Mol Imaging 2007;34:982–93.

29. Mourato AM, Almeida MA, Brito AET, et al. FDG PET/CT versus somatostatin receptor PET/CT in TENIS syndrome: a systematic review and meta-analysis. Clin Translational Imaging 2020;20:390–400.

30. Binse I, Poeppel TD, Ruhlmann M, et al. 68Ga-DOTATOC PET/CT in patients with iodine- and 18F-FDG-negative differentiated thyroid carcinoma and elevated serum thyroglobulin. J Nucl Med 2016;57(10):1512–7.

31. Basu S, Dandekar M, Joshi A, et al. Defining a rational step-care algorithm for managing thyroid carcinoma patients with elevated thyroglobulin and negative on radioiodine scintigraphy (TENIS): considerations and challenges towards developing an appropriate roadmap. Eur J Nucl Med Mol Imaging 2015;42(8):1167–71.

32. Jois B, Asopa R, Basu S. Somatostatin receptor imaging in non-(131)I-avid metastatic differentiated thyroid carcinoma for determining the feasibility of peptide receptor radionuclide therapy with (177)Lu-DOTATATE: low fraction of patients suitable for peptide receptor radionuclide therapy and evidence of chromogranin A level-positive neuroendocrine differentiation. Clin Nucl Med 2014;39(6):505–10.

33. Pinto JT, Suffoletto BP, Berzin TM, et al. Prostate-specific membrane antigen: a novel folate hydrolase in human prostatic carcinoma cells. Clin Cancer Res 1996;2:1445–51.

34. DerlinT, Kreipe HH, Schumacher U, et al. PSMA expression in tumor neovasculature endothelial cells of follicular thyroid adenoma as identified by molecular imaging using 68Ga-PSMA ligand PET/CT. Clin Nucl Med 2017;42:e173–4.

35. Chang SS, Reuter VE, Heston WD, et al. Five different anti-prostate-specific membrane antigen (PSMA) antibodies confirm PSMA expression in tumor associated neovasculature. Cancer Res 1999;59:3192–8.

36. Bychkov A, Vutrapongwatana U, Tepmongkol S, et al. PSMA expression by microvasculature of thyroid tumors - potential implications for PSMA theranostics. Sci Rep 2017;7:5202.

37. Gordon IO, Tretiakova MS, Noffsinger AE, et al. Prostate-specific membrane antigen expression in regeneration and repair. Mod Pathol 2008;21(12):1421–7.

38. Bertagna F, Albano D, Giovanella L, et al. 68Ga-PSMA PET thyroid incidentalomas. Hormones (Athens) 2019;18(2):145–9.

39. Moore M, Panjwani S, Mathew R, et al. Well-differentiated thyroid cancer neovasculature expresses prostate-specific membrane antigen-a possible novel therapeutic target. Endocr Pathol 2017;28(4):339–44.

40. de Vries LH, Lodewijk L, Braat AJAT, et al. 68Ga-PSMA PET/CT in radioactive iodine-refractory differentiated thyroid cancer and first treatment results with 177Lu-PSMA-617. EJNMMI Res 2020;10(1):18.

41. Freudenberg LS, Jentzen W, Stahl A, et al. Clinical applications of 124I-PET/CT in patients with differentiated thyroid cancer. Eur J Nucl Med Mol Imaging 2011;38:S48–56.

42. Khorjekar GR, Van Nostrand D, Garcia C, et al. Do negative 124I pretherapy positron emission tomography scans in patients with elevated serum thyroglobulin levels predict negative 131I posttherapy scans? Thyroid 2014;24:1394–9.

43. Sakamoto A, KasaiN Sugano H. Poorly differentiated carcinoma of the thyroid. A clinicopathologic entity for a high-risk group of papillary and follicular carcinomas. Cancer 1983;52:1849–55.

44. Sanders EM Jr, LiVolsi VA, Brierley J, et al. An evidence-based review of poorly differentiated thyroid cancer. World J Surg 2007;31:934–45.

45. Volante M, Papotti M. Poorly differentiated thyroid carcinoma: 5 years after the 2004 WHO classification of endocrine tumours. Endocr Pathol 2010;21:1–6.

46. Durante C, Puxeddu E, Ferretti E, et al. BRAF mutations in papillary thyroid carcinomas inhibit genes involved in iodine metabolism. J Clin Endocrinol Metab 2007;92:2840–3.

47. Ghossein R, Livolsi VA. Papillary thyroid carcinoma tall cell variant. Thyroid 2008;18(11):1179–81.

48. Kuo CS, Tang KT, Lin JD, et al. Diffuse sclerosing variant of papillary thyroid carcinoma with multiple metastases and elevated serum carcinoembryonic antigen level. Thyroid 2012;22(11):1187–90.

49. Giovanella L, Fasolini F, Suriano S, et al. Hyperfunctioning solid/trabecular follicular carcinoma of the thyroid gland. J Oncology 2010;4:635984.

50. Diehl M, Graichen S, Menzel C, et al. F-18 FDG PET in insular thyroid cancer. Clin Nucl Med 2003;28(9):728–31.

51. Treglia G, Muoio B, Giovanella L, et al. The role of positron emission tomography and positron emission tomography/computed tomography in thyroid tumours: an overview. Eur Arch Otorhinolaryngol 2013;270(6):1783–7.

52. Kim CH, Yoo IR, Chung YA, et al. Influence of thyroid stimulating hormone on 18F-fluorodeoxyglucose and 99mTc-methoxyisobutylisonitrile uptake in human poorly differentiated thyroid cancer cells in vitro. Ann Nucl Med 2009;23(2):131–6.

53. Smallridge RC, Copland JA. Anaplastic thyroid carcinoma: pathogenesis and emerging therapies. Clin Oncol 2010;22:486–97.

54. Bogsrud TV, Karantanis D, Nathan MA, et al. 18F-FDG PET in the management of patients with anaplastic thyroid carcinoma. Thyroid 2008;18:713–9.

55. Khan N, Oriuchi N, Higuchi T, et al. Review of fluorine-18-2-fluoro-2-deoxy-D-glucose positron emission tomography (FDG-PET) in the follow-up of medullary and anaplastic thyroid carcinomas. Cancer Control 2005;12:254–60.

56. Poisson T, Deandreis D, Leboulleux S, et al. 18F-fluorodeoxy-glucose positron emission tomography and computed tomography in anaplastic thyroid cancer. Eur J Nucl Med Mol Imaging 2010;37:2277–85.

57. Samih N, Hovsepian S, Notel F, et al. The impact of N- and O-glycosylation on the functions of Glut-1 transporter in human thyroid anaplastic cells. Biochim Biophys Acta 2003;1621:92–101.

58. Bible KC, Kebebew E, Brierley J, et al. American Thyroid Association Guidelines for management of patients with anaplastic thyroid cancer. Thyroid 2021;31(3):337–86.

59. Trimboli P, Giovanella L, Crescenzi A, et al. Medullary thyroid cancer diagnosis: an appraisal. Head Neck 2014;36:1216–23.

60. Guyetant S, Rousselet MC, Durigon M, et al. Sex-related C cell hyperplasia in the normal human thyroid: a quantitative autopsy study. J Clin Endocrinol Metab 1997;82:42–7.

61. Roy M, Chen H, Sippel RS. Current understanding and management of medullary thyroid cancer. Oncologist 2013;18:1093–100.

62. Roman S, Lin R, Sosa JA. Prognosis of medullary thyroid carcinoma: demographic, clinical, and pathologic predictors of survival in 1252 cases. Cancer 2006;107:2134–42.

63. Kushchayev SV, Kushchayeva YS, Tella SH, et al. Medullary Thyroid carcinoma: an update on imaging. J Thyroid Res 2019 2019;7:1893047.

64. Verbeek HHG, Plukker JTM, Koopmans KP, et al. Clinical relevance of 18F-FDG PET and18FDOPA PET in recurrent medullary thyroid carcinoma. J Nucl Med 2012;53:1863–71.

65. Ong SC, Schöder H, Patel SG, et al. Diagnostic accuracy of 18F-FDG PET in restaging patients with

medullary thyroid carcinoma and elevated calcitonin levels. J Nucl Med 2007;48(4):501–7.

66. Rubello D, Rampin L, Nanni C, et al. The role of 18F-FDG-PET/CT in detecting metastatic deposits of recurrent medullary thyroid carcinoma: a prospective study. Eur J Surg Oncol 2008;34(5):581–6.

67. Treglia G, Villani MF, Giordano A, et al. Detection rate of recurrent medullary thyroid carcinoma using fluorine-18 fluorodeoxyglucose positron emission tomography: a meta-analysis. Endocrine 2012;42(3):535–45.

68. Mendelsohn G, Wells SA Jr, Baylin SB. Relationship of tissue carcinoembryonic antigen and calcitonin to tumor virulence in medullary thyroid carcinoma. An immunohistochemical study in early, localized, and virulent disseminated stages of disease. Cancer 1984;54:657–62.

69. Romero-Lluch AR, Cuenca-Cuenca JI, Guerrero-Vázquez R, et al. Diagnostic utility of PET/CT with 18F-DOPA and 18F-FDG in persistent or recurrent medullary thyroid carcinoma: the importance of calcitonin and carcinoembryonic antigen cutoff. Eur J Nucl Med Mol Imaging 2017;44(12):2004–13.

70. Taieb D, Timmers HJ, Hindie E, et al. EANM 2012 guidelines for radionuclide imaging of phaeochromocytoma and paraganglioma. Eur J Nucl Med Mol Imaging 2012;39:1977–95.

71. Giovanella L, Treglia G, Iakovou I, et al. EANM practice guideline for PET/CT imaging in medullary thyroid carcinoma. Eur J Nucl Med Mol Imaging 2020;47(1):61–77.

72. Archier A, Heimburger C, Guerin C, et al. 18)18F-FDOPA PET CT in the diagnosis and localization of persistent medullary thyroid carcinoma. Eur J Nucl Med Mol Imaging 2016;43(6):1027–33.

73. Gómez-Camarero P, Ortiz-de Tena A, Borrego-Dorado I, et al. Evaluation of efficacy and clinical impact of 18F-FDG PET in the diagnosis of recurrent medullary thyroid cancer with increased calcitonin and negative imaging test. Rev Esp Med Nucl Imagen Mol 2012;31(5):261–6.

74. Rasul S, Hartenbach S, Rebhan K, et al. [18F]DOPA PET/ceCT in diagnosis and staging of primary medullary thyroid carcinoma prior to surgery. Eurj Nucl Med Mol Imaging 2018;45(12):2159–69.

75. Bovio S, Cataldi A, Reimondo G, et al. Prevalence of adrenal incidentaloma in a contemporary computerized tomography series. J Endocrinol Invest 2006;29:298–302.

76. Shulkin BL, Thompson NW, Shapiro B, et al. Pheochromocytomas: imaging with 2-[fluorine-18]fluoro-2-deoxy-D-glucose PET. Radiology 1999;212:35–41.

77. Kushchayev SV, Kushchayeva YS, Tella SH, et al. Medullary thyroid carcinoma: an update on imaging. J Thyroid Res 2019;2019:1893047.

78. Kauhanen S, Schalin-Jantti C, Seppanen M, et al. Complementary roles of 1818F-FDOPA PET/CT and 18F- FDG PET/CT in medullary thyroid cancer. J Nucl Med 2011;52:1855–63.

79. Wong KK, Laird AM, Moubayed A, et al. How has the management of medullary thyroid carcinoma changed with the advent of 18F-FDG and non-18F-FDG PET radiopharmaceuticals. Nucl Med Commun 2012;33(7):679–88.

80. Lussey-Lepoutre C, Hindié E, Montravers F, et al. The current role of 18F-FDOPA PET for neuroendocrine tumor imaging. Médecine Nucl 2016;40:20–30.

81. Souteiro P, Gouveia P, Ferreira G, et al. 68Ga-DOTANOC and 18F-FDG PET/CT in metastatic medullary thyroid carcinoma: novel correlations with tumoral biomarkers. Endocrine 2019;64(2):322–9.

82. Tuncel M, Kılıçkap S, Süslü N. Clinical impact of 68Ga-DOTATATE PET-CT imaging in patients with medullary thyroid cancer. Ann Nucl Med 2020;34(9):663–74.

83. Castroneves LA, Coura Filho G, de Freitas RMC, et al. Comparison of 68Ga PET/CT to other imaging studies in medullary thyroid cancer: superiority in detecting bone metastases. J Clin Endocrinol Metab 2018;103:3250–9.

84. Soussan M, Nataf V, Kerrou K, et al. Added value of early 18F-FDOPA PET/CT acquisition time in medullary thyroid cancer. Nucl Med Commun 2012;33(7):775–9.

85. Skoura E. Depicting medullary thyroid cancer recurrence: the past and the future of nuclear medicine imaging. Int J Endocrinol Metab 2013;11(4):e8156.

86. Jager PL, Vaalburg W, Pruim J, et al. Radiolabeled amino acids: basic aspects and clinical applications in oncology. J Nucl Med 2001;42(3):432–45.

87. Jang HW, Choi JY, Lee JI, et al. Localization of medullary thyroid carcinoma after surgery using (11)C-methionine PET/CT: comparison with (18)F-FDG PET/CT. Endocr J 2010;57(12):1045–54.

88. Silverberg SJ, Lewiecki EM, Mosekilde L, et al. Presentation of asymptomatic primary hyperparathyroidism: proceedings of the third international workshop. J Clin Endocrinol Metab 2009;94(2):351–65.

89. Evangelista L, Sorgato N, Torresan F, et al. FDG-PET/CT and parathyroid carcinoma: review of literature and illustrative case series. World J Clin Oncol 2011;2(10):348–54.

90. Jadvar H. Prostate cancer: PET with 18F-FDG, 18F- or 11C-acetate, and 18F- or 11C-choline. J Nucl Med 2011;52:81–9.

91. Mapelli P, Busnardo E, Magnani P, et al. Incidental finding of parathyroid adenoma with 11C-choline PET/CT. Clin Nucl Med 2012;37:593–5.

92. Quak E, Blanchard D, Houdu B, et al. F18-choline PET/CT guided surgery in primary hyperparathyroidism when ultrasound and MIBI SPECT/CT are negative or inconclusive: the APACH1 study. Eur J Nucl Med Mol Imaging 2017;45:658–66.

93. Cuderman A, Senica K, Rep S, et al. 18F-fluorocholine PET/CT in primary hyperparathyroidism: superior diagnostic performance to conventional scintigraphic imaging for localization of hyperfunctioning parathyroid glands. J Nucl Med 2020;61(4):577–83.

94. López-Mora DA, Sizova M, Estorch M, et al. Superior performance of 18F-fluorocholine digital PET/CT in the detection of parathyroid adenomas. Eur J Nucl Med Mol Imaging 2020;47(3):572–8.

95. Broos WAM, Wondergem M, Knol RJJ, et al. Parathyroid imaging with 18F fluorocholine PET/CT as a first- line imaging modality in primary hyperparathyroidism: a retrospective cohort study. EJNMMI Res 2019;9(1):72.

96. Giovanella L, Bacigalupo L, Treglia G, et al. Will 18F-fluorocholine PET/CT replace other methods of preoperative parathyroid imaging? Endocrine 2021;71(2):285–97.

97. Kluijfhout WP, Pasternak JD, Drake FT, et al. Use of PET tracers for parathyroid localization: a systematic review and meta-analysis. Langenbeck's Arch Surg 2016;401(7):925–35.

98. Noltes ME, Coester AM, van der Horst-Schrivers ANA, et al. Localization of parathyroid adenomas using 11C-methionine pet after prior inconclusive imaging. Langenbeck's Arch Surg 2017;402(7):1109–17.

99. Weber T, Gottstein M, Schwenzer S, et al. Is C-11 methionine PET/CT able to localise sestamibi-negative parathyroid adenomas? World J Surg 2017;41(4):980–5.

100. Mackie GC, Shulkin BL, Ribeiro RC, et al. Use of [18F]fluorodeoxyglucose positron emission tomography in evaluating locally recurrent and metastatic adrenocortical carcinoma. J Clin Endocrinol Metab 2006;91:2665–71.

101. Aron DC. The adrenal incidentaloma: disease of modern technology and public health problem. Rev Endocr Metab Disord 2001;2:335–42.

102. Kloos RT, Gross MD, Francis IR, et al. Incidentally discovered adrenal masses. Endocr Rev 1995;16:460–84.

103. Boland GW, Dwamena BA, Jagtiani Sangwaiya M, et al. Characterization of adrenal masses by using FDG PET: a systematic review and meta-analysis of diagnostic test performance. Radiology 2011;259:117–26.

104. Becherer A, Vierhapper H, Pötzi C, et al. FDG-PET in adrenocortical carcinoma. Cancer Biother Radiopharm 2001;16:289–95.

105. Leboulleux S, Dromain C, Bonniaud G, et al. Diagnostic and prognostic value of 18 fluorodeoxyglucose positron emission tomography in adrenocortical carcinoma: a prospective comparison with computed tomography. J Clin Endocrinol Metab 2006;91:920–5.

106. Tessonnier L, Ansquer C, Bournaud C, et al. (18)F-FDG uptake at initial staging of the adrenocortical cancers: a diagnostic tool but not of prognostic value. World J Surg 2013;37:107–12.

107. Hennings J, Lindhe O, Bergstrom M, et al. [11C] metomidate positron emission tomography of adrenocortical tumors in correlation with histopathological findings. J Clin Endocrinol Metab 2006;91:1410–4.

108. Lenders JW, Duh QY, Eisenhofer G, et al. Pheochromocytoma and paraganglioma: an endocrine society clinical practice guideline. J Clin Endocrinol Metab 2014;99:1915–42.

109. Fishbein L, Leshchiner I, Walter V, et al. Comprehensive molecular characterization of pheochromocytoma and paraganglioma. Cancer Cell 2017;31:181–93.

110. Pollard PJ, Briere JJ, Alam NA, et al. Accumulation of Krebs cycle intermediates and over expression of HIF1alpha in tumours which result from germline FH and SDH mutations. Hum Mol Genet 2005;14:2231–9.

111. Selak MA, Armour SM, MacKenzie ED, et al. Succinate links TCA cycle dysfunction to oncogenesis by inhibiting HIF-alpha prolyl hydroxylase. Cancer Cell 2005;7:77–85.

112. Timmers HJ, Kozupa A, Chen CC, et al. Superiority of fluorodeoxyglucose positron emission tomography to other functional imaging techniques in the evaluation of metastatic SDHB-associated pheochromocytoma and paraganglioma. J Clin Oncol 2007;25:2262–9.

113. Venkatesan AM, Trivedi H, Adams KT, et al. Comparison of clinical and imaging features in succinate dehydrogenase- positive versus sporadic paragangliomas. Surgery 2011;150:1186–93.

114. Wild D, Macke HR, Waser B, et al. 68Ga-DOTA-NOC: a first compound for PET imaging with high affinity for somatostatin receptor subtypes 2 and 5. Eur J Nucl Med Mol Imaging 2005;32:724.

115. Wild D, Schmitt JS, Ginj M, et al. DOTA-NOC, a high affinity ligand of somatostatin receptor subtypes 2, 3 and 5 for labelling with various radiometals. Eur J Nucl Med Mol Imaging 2003;30:1338–47.

116. Chang CA, Pattison DA, Tothill RW, et al. 68)Ga-DOTATATE and (18)F-FDG PET/CT in Paraganglioma and Pheochromocytoma: utility, patterns and heterogeneity. Cancer Imaging 2016;16:22.

117. Taieb D, Jha A, Guerin C, et al. 18F-FDOPA PET/CT imaging of MAX-Related Pheochromocytoma. J Clin Endocrinol Metab 2018;103:1574–82.

118. Gild ML, Naik N, Hoang J, et al. Role of DOTATATE-PET/CT in preoperative assessment of phaeochromocytoma and paragangliomas. Clin Endocrinol 2018;89(2):139–47.

119. Hoegerle S, Nitzsche E, Altehoefer C, et al. Pheochromocytomas: detection with 18F DOPA whole body PET—initial results. Radiology 2002;222:507–12.

120. Treglia G, Cocciolillo F, de Waure C, et al. Diagnostic performance of 18F-dihydroxyphenylalanine positron emission tomography in patients with paraganglioma: a meta-analysis. Eur J Nucl Med Mol Imaging 2012;39:1144–53.

121. Timmers HJ, Chen CC, Carrasquillo JA, et al. Comparison of 18F-fluoro-L-DOPA, 18F-fluoro-deoxyglucose, and 18F-fluorodopamine PET and 123I-MIBG scintigraphy in the localization of pheochromocytoma and paraganglioma. J Clin Endocrinol Metab 2009;94:4757–67.

122. Pacak K, Eisenhofer G, Carrasquillo JA, et al. 6-[18F]Fluorodopamine positron emission tomographic (PET) scanning for diagnostic localization of pheochromocytoma. Hypertension 2001;38:6–8.

123. Vyakaranam AR, Crona J, Norlén O, et al. 11C-hydroxy-ephedrine-PET/CT in the diagnosis of pheochromocytoma and paraganglioma. Cancers 2019;11(6):847.

124. Ott RJ, Tait D, Flower MA, et al. Treatment planning for 131I-mIBG radiotherapy of neural crest tumours using 124I-mIBG positron emission tomography. Br J Radiol 1992;65:787–91.

125. Balkwill FR, Capasso M, Hagemann T. The tumor microenvironment at a glance. J Cell Sci 2012;125:5591–6.

126. Zhang Y, Weinberg RA. Epithelial-to-mesenchymal transition in cancer: complexity and opportunities EMT: a naturally occurring transdifferentiation program. Front Med 2018;12:1–13.

127. Hamson EJ, Keane FM, Tholen S, et al. Understanding fibroblast activation protein (FAP): substrates, activities, expression and targeting for cancer therapy. Proteomics Clin Appl 2014;8:454–63.

128. Garin-Chesa P, Old LJ, Rettig WJ. Cell surface glycoprotein of reactive stromal fibroblasts as a potential antibody target in human epithelial cancers. Proc Natl Acad Sci USA 1990;87:7235–9.

129. Wu J, Ou L, Zhang C. Comparison of 68Ga-FAPI and 18F-FDG PET/CT in metastases of papillary thyroid carcinoma, Endocrine 2021;73:767–8.

130. Fu H, Fu J, Huang J, et al. 68Ga-FAPI PET/CT in thyroid cancer with thyroglobulin elevation and negative iodine scintigraphy. Clin Nucl Med 2021;46(5):427–30.

# 18F-Fluorodeoxyglucose-PET-Computerized Tomography and non-Fluorodeoxyglucose PET-Computerized Tomography in Hepatobiliary and Pancreatic Malignancies

Gopinath Gnanasegaran, MSc, MD, FRCP[a],*, Kanhaiyalal Agrawal, MD[b],
Simon Wan, FRCR[c]

## KEYWORDS

• Hepatocellular cancer • Gall bladder cancer • Pancreatic cancer • Cholangiocarcinoma

## KEY POINTS

- PET-CT plays important role in the management of patients with hepatobiliary and pancreatic malignancies.
- There is good evidence to support the use of FDG PET-CT in the management of patients with hepatobiliary and pancreatic cancers in various clinical settings.
- A multitude of non-FDG and novel tracers are in the pipeline with seemingly promising results.

## INTRODUCTION

Hepatobiliary and pancreatic malignancies constitute a range of pathologic processes. Hepatobiliary malignancies include liver tumors, gallbladder cancers (GCs), and cholangiocarcinoma's.[1,2] Pancreatic malignancies include exocrine tumors such as adenocarcinomas and endocrine pancreatic tumors (neuroendocrine tumors [NETs]). Radiological imaging such as triple-phase contrast-enhanced computerized tomography (CT) and magnetic resonance imaging (MRI) plays a vital role in diagnosis and management. In general, MRI techniques have relatively improved the ability to differentiate benign and malignant lesions.[1–5] Radionuclide molecular imaging using Positron Emission Tomography (PET) tracers in hepatobiliary and pancreatic cancers is evolving. PET-CT using 18F-fluorodeoxyglucose (FDG) as radiopharmaceutical plays a vital role in managing tumors in various clinical scenarios. Historically and clinically, FDG tracer is the most available and commonly used molecular tracer in PET-CT imaging and deserves full credit in taking radionuclide imaging to a higher level. There is ample evidence supporting the established use of FDG PET in managing patients with pancreatic cancer, cholangiocarcinoma, and GC. More recently, several non-FDG tracers have been studied and were found to be potentially useful in imaging hepatobiliary and pancreatic cancers, such as 68Ga-DOTA, 11C-acetate, 11C-choline, 18F-dihydroxyphenylalanine (18F-DOPA), and 18F- or 68-Ga prostate-specific membrane antigen (18F/68Ga-PSMA). This chapter will summarize the role, advantages, and limitations of FDG and non-FDG tracers in hepatobiliary and pancreatic cancers and discuss its role in

[a] Royal Free NHS Foundation Trust, London, United Kingdom; [b] All India Institute of Medical Sciences, Bhubaneswar, India; [c] University College London Hospitals NHS Foundation Trust, London, United Kingdom
* Corresponding author.
E-mail address: gopinath.gnanasegaran@nhs.net

PET Clin 17 (2022) 369–388
https://doi.org/10.1016/j.cpet.2022.03.007
1556-8598/22/

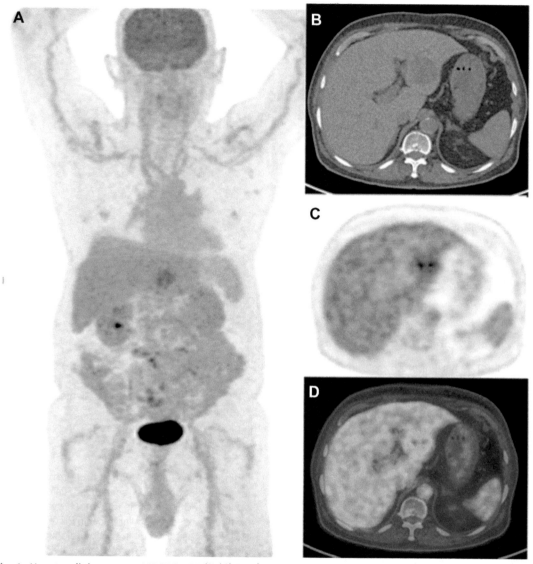

**Fig. 1.** Hepatocellular cancer: 18F-FDG PET-CT (*A*) on the MIP image, there is low to moderate increased tracer uptake in the left lobe of the liver. On the trans axial images, there is a focal area of low to moderate heterogeneous tracer uptake in segment II/III (*C, D*) posteriorly, which corresponds to the lesion seen on the unenhanced CT (*B*). The liver lesion demonstrated arterialization with washout on the portal venous and delayed phases on the contrast enhanced CT (*not shown*). There is no evidence of hypermetabolic extrahepatic disease. Histology confirmed HCC.

staging, assessment of treatment response, and surveillance.

## Hepatocellular Cancer

### Fluorodeoxyglucose-PET-computerized tomography in hepatocellular cancer

18F-FDG uptake within hepatocellular cancers (HCCs) is variable due to varying expressions of glucose-6-phosphatase activity and glucose transporters.[1,2,5–9] The reported overall sensitivity of 50%–65% is insufficient to support the use of 18F-FDG PET-CT in the diagnostic algorithm for detection of HCCs[9–11] (**Fig. 1**). Moreover, 18F-FDG PET-CT is better than 18F-FDG PET in differentiating pathologic and physiologic processes and can be used for problem solving in lesion characterization. In general, malignant liver lesions take uptake tracer more than benign lesions. Benign hepatic tumors such as hemangiomas, focal nodular hyperplasia (FNH), and hepatocellular adenomas are reported to take up FDG similarly to normal liver tissue[1,2,6] (see **Fig. 1**).

Furthermore, within the spectrum of HCC, FDG PET can act as a marker of tumor differentiation. Tumors with a higher density of glucose receptors expression (manifesting as having higher FDG uptake) tend to be more aggressive, and tumors with less FDG uptake have better clinical outcomes than FDG avid tumors. In addition, tumors with a higher FDG uptake tend to show a shorter doubling time and often present with a higher stage of disease.[12–16] In FDG negative liver tumors, the CT component might help as 70% of the HCCs are often seen as hypodense lesions on unenhanced CT and 20% as hyperdense lesions.[17]

18F-FDG PET is useful in detecting extrahepatic disease in patients with primary HCC. 18F-FDG PET plays an important complementary role in detecting unsuspected regional and distant metastases at primary staging.[10,18] A meta-analysis reviewing the role of 18F-FDG PET and PET-CT in assessing extra-hepatic metastases reported a sensitivity of 76.6%, specificity of 98%.[19]

In a post-treatment scenario, using change in lesion size and enhancement features as a surrogate marker for tumor response may be difficult due to post-treatment inflammatory changes and the heterogeneous nature of the tumor environment. Therefore, functional imaging, such as diffusion-weighted magnetic resonance (DWMRI) or 18F-FDG PET-CT, is often recommended. 18F-FDG PET-CT shows a higher sensitivity in detecting residual disease than contrast-enhanced CT (CECT).[20,21] Secondly, several studies have shown better survival and event-free rates in patients with a significant reduction in the FDG uptake at the tumor sites.[22,23] The ideal time to assess response is 3 months post-therapy to avoid false positive or equivocal findings. In general, 18F-FDG PET might change management in approximately 30% of high-risk patients.[24]

## Non-fluorodeoxyglucose-PET-Computerized Tomography in Hepatocellular Cancer

Given the limited sensitivity of 18F-FDG PET in detecting HCC, 11C-acetate and choline PET tracers have been explored as an alternative or a complementary tracer.[6] Well-differentiated HCCs preferentially accumulate 11C-acetate. In contrast, poorly differentiated tumors tend to accumulate FDG.[6,11,25] Based on this analogy, it is suggested that when the tumor accumulates both tracers, or only 11C-acetate, HCC is high on the differential. Secondly, lesions accumulating only FDG could represent a non-HCC malignancy (eg, metastases or lymphoma), and lastly, if the lesions are negative on both tracers, this could imply a benign process.[6,11,25] These tracers may

therefore help improve the detection and characterization of HCC. In well-differentiated HCC, 11C-acetate detects tumor better than FDG (87% vs 47%).[11] Overall reported sensitivities of 18F-FDG, 11C-acetate, and dual-tracer PET-CT in evaluating lesions in patients with primary HCC were 61%, 75%, and 83%, respectively.[13] Nonetheless, despite the addition of 11C-acetate to FDG PET-CT increases the overall sensitivity for detecting primary HCC, this addition did not lead to an increase detection of extrahepatic metastases.[1,2,6] One possible valid explanation is that 18F-FDG PET is sensitive in detecting poorly differentiated HCC tumors, which are more aggressive and associated with metastases.

68Ga-PSMA or 18F-PSMA PET tracers, currently used in imaging of prostate cancer, is reported to accumulate in several solid tumors, including in HCC.[26] Kesler and colleagues have reported in their small prospective pilot study that Ga-PSMA PET-CT is superior to 18F-FDG PET-CT in imaging patients with HCC.[26] HCC lesions being more hypervascular, generally take up 68Ga-PSMA in tumoral microvessels.[26] The fibroblast activation protein (FAP) is commonly expressed in activated stromal fibroblasts in several epithelial tumors. The radiolabeled Fibroblast-activation-protein inhibitors (FAPI) PET-CT (eg, 68Ga-FAPI) has been used for tumor imaging, and initial reports suggest 68Ga-FAPI-04 PET-CT is more sensitive than 18F-FDG PET-CT in detecting HCC lesions.[27–29] At this stage, clinical data for use of these non-FDG PET tracers to image HCC is limited, but this is evolving and seems to show potential. The false positive, false negative, and current evidence of FDG and non-FDG tracers are summarized in **Tables 1 and 2**.[1,2,5,30–33]

## Hepatic Metastases

The liver is the most common site of hematogenous metastatic spread and is more common than primary liver cancer. Several cancers metastasize to the liver such as primary colorectal, breast, lung cancers, and the most common being colorectal cancer.[34] In general, liver metastases are FDG avid. 18F-FDG PET and PET-CT are found to be useful in evaluating liver metastases and several studies have found 18F-FDG PET to be sensitive (90%–95%) in the diagnosis of liver metastases arising from cancers such as colorectal, gastric, esophageal[1,2,35,36] (**Fig. 2**). 18F-FDG PET is reported to have higher sensitivity (95%) in comparison with conventional radiological modalities such as ultrasound (55%), CT (65%), 1.5-T MRI (76%).[27,36] 18F-FDG is reported to have better sensitivity (96%) and specificity

**Table 1**
Summary of false positive and false negative on 18F-FDG studies in hepatobiliary and pancreatic cancers

| Cancer Type | 18F-FDG False Positive | 18F-FDG False Negative |
|---|---|---|
| Hepatocellular cancer | Infective or inflammatory causes (eg, abscesses)<br>Postprocedural inflammatory or reactive changes<br>Misregistration of lung lesions secondary to respiratory motion<br>Hepatoblastoma<br>Hepatic adenoma<br>Hemangioendotheliomas<br>Focal nodular hyperplasia<br>Angiomyolipoma<br>Focal hepatic steatosis | Well-differentiated tumors<br>Small-sized lesions<br>Infiltrative tumors<br>Hyperglycemia |
| Pancreatic cancer | Postprocedural inflammatory or reactive changes<br>Pancreatitis<br>Serous cystadenomas | Well-differentiated tumors<br>Mucin-producing tumors |
| Cholangiocarcinoma | Infection<br>Inflammation | Mucin-producing tumors<br>Small-sized lesion<br>Infiltrative tumors<br>Hyperglycemia |
| Gall bladder cancer | Cholecystitis<br>Adenomyomatosis<br>Postprocedural inflammatory or reactive changes<br>Misregistration of liver lesion or bowel uptake | Mucin-producing tumors<br>Small-sized lesion |

(75%) in comparison with CECT in untreated metastases (sensitivity 88% and specificity 25%).[37] In the colorectal group, 18F-FDG PET-CT showed a 94% sensitivity and 75% specificity, while CECT had 91% sensitivity and 25% specificity. Overall, 18F-FDG-PET-CT altered patient management over CECT in 25% of patients.[37] 18F-FDG PET has also been shown to be useful in assessing the chemotherapy treatment response or after localized treatment such as radiofrequency ablation (RFA) of hepatic metastases. 18F-FDG PET-CT is found to be more accurate than CECT in surveillance after RFA (65% vs 44%).[38] The sensitivity of 18F-FDG PET is found to be lower in neoadjuvant chemotherapy settings than CT and possible explanations include (a) reduced metabolic activity within the metastases (thus reduced standardized uptake value (SUV) compared with background uptake) and (b) reduction in the size of the lesions that might be below the resolution of PET.[39]

## Pancreatic Cancer

### 18F-fluorodeoxyglucose PET-computerized tomography in pancreatic cancer

Pancreatic cancer is often diagnosed at an advanced stage, and the 5-year survival is approximately 6%, and only 20% are eligible for resection at the time of diagnosis.[40,41] In general, pancreatic tumors are exocrine, and 85% are invasive ductal adenocarcinoma[42]; endocrine tumors such as pancreatic neuroendocrine tumors (PNETs) constitute 3%–4%, and less than 2% of pancreatic tumors originate from endocrine cells.[41–45] The remaining pancreatic tumor types include exocrine acinar cell neoplasms, cystic pancreatic neoplasms, and neoplasms of epithelial origin and mixed differentiation.[41]

In general, radiological imaging modalities for assessment include CT, MRI, ultrasound, endoscopic ultrasound, endoscopic retrograde cholangiopancreatography (ERCP), and magnetic resonance cholangiopancreatography (MRCP). CT or MRI is recommended for the evaluation of patients in whom pancreatic cancer is clinically suspected.[41,44] The potential indications of 18F-FDG PET-CT in pancreatic cancer include diagnosis, staging, or re-staging of pancreatic adenocarcinomas and evaluating treatment response.[41,45]

In staging pancreatic cancer, CECT is commonly used for the initial assessment of locoregional and nodal disease. MRI is also often used, especially if when patients are unable to undergo a CT scan (eg, patients with allergy to iodinated contrast agents). Currently, the National Institute for Health

**Table 2**
**Summary of current evidence of18F-FDG and non-FDG PET-CT in hepatocellular cancers**

| 18F-FDG PET-CT | Non-FDG Tracers |
| --- | --- |
| 18F-FDG uptake by HCC varies according to histologic differentiation of the tumor. | $^{11}$C-acetate tracer used in conjunction with FDG increases the detection of HCC. |
| Not recommended as a standard imaging modality for the early diagnosis of HCC. | 11C-choline is relatively better than FDG in well to moderately differentiated lesions. FNH is one of the reported false-positive findings |
| Mixed role in the detection of HCC and larger tumor is better seen than smaller tumors | 18F or Ga-PSMA PET-CT is superior to FDG PET-CT in imaging patients with HCC *(limited evidence)* |
| 18F-PET-CT combination has a role in detecting vascular invasion, regional, and extrahepatic metastatic lesions. | 68Ga-FAPI PET-CT is more sensitive than FDG PET-CT in detecting HCC lesions *(limited evidence)* |
| Higher FDG uptake correlates with higher-grade cancers and often predicts prognosis. | |
| 18F-FDG-PET can predict the risk of early recurrence or poor survival after surgical resection or liver transplantation. | |
| Incremental value in patients with elevated tumor marker and negative cross-sectional imaging | |
| Benign tumors of the liver take up 18F-FDG at a similar rate to surrounding tissue. | |
| The sensitivity of detecting liver metastases is found to be equal or superior to CT and MRI. | |
| 18F-FDG PET and 18F-FDG PET-CT can be used for follow up after treatment of liver metastases to both assess for success and recurrence, | |
| Sensitivity of 18F-FDG PET for detecting liver metastases is generally lower in neoadjuvant chemotherapy settings | |
| FDG is more sensitive than 11C-acetate in the detection of extrahepatic metastases | |

and Care Excellence Guidelines in the United Kingdom recommends 18F-FDG PET-CT in adults with localized pancreatic cancer on CT to have staging using FDG positron emission tomography/CT (18F-FDG PET-CT) before they have surgery, radiotherapy, or systemic therapy.[46] Change in management of approximately 36% is seen if PET-CT is used in the staging algorithm.[47] In the preoperative assessment of resection, the reported sensitivity and specificity of 18F-FDG PET-CT are 100% and 56%, respectively, and in CE 18F-FDG PET-CT, sensitivity, and specificity are 96% and 82%, respectively[41,48] (Fig. 3).

Differentiating benign and malignant lymph nodes on CT is challenging as reactive nodes are often seen in the pancreas region, especially after the placement of a biliary stent or in the presence of stricture-induced cholangitis.[45] 18F-FDG PET-CT for nodal staging in the pancreas is evolving and is relatively better than CT with a sensitivity ranging from 30% to 49% and specificity of 63%–93%.[45] Overall, the current consensus is 18F-FDG PET-CT may improve the specificity of nodal staging compared with CT alone.[41,45]

In the detection of liver metastases, a study comparing the performance of hepatobiliary CE MR imaging and 18F-FDG PET showed MR imaging to be more accurate in depicting small liver metastases (97%), compared with 18F-FDG PET-CT (85%).[44,45,49] However, in assessing extrahepatic distant metastases, 18F-FDG PET-CT sensitivity was 88%, superior to CECT and MR imaging.[44,45,49] The evaluation of peritoneal metastases with 18F-FDG-PET-CT is evolving. Overall, 18F-FDG PET-CT is valuable in assessing distant metastases and helps avoid unnecessary surgery.[41,45]

Most recurrent disease presents itself within 2 years postresection of pancreatic adenocarcinoma (72%–92%).[45,50] 18F-FDG PET-CT is useful in detecting and confirming recurrence when conventional modalities are equivocal. Abnormally increased uptake in the resection bed represents recurrent disease in most cases if the scan is performed 3 months postsurgery, and the sensitivity is 96% and far superior to CT and MR imaging (39%).[45,51–53] In addition, recurrence is often seen earlier on PET-CT (sensitivity 98% and specificity 98%) compared with CT alone.[53]

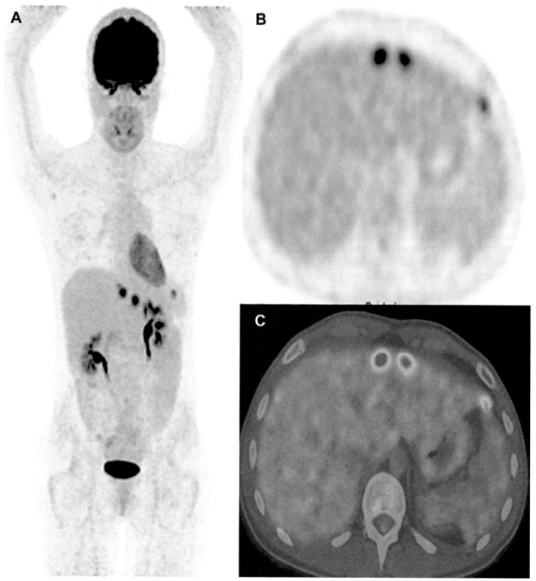

**Fig. 2.** Colorectal cancer with liver metastases. (*A*) MIP and (*B*) trans axial PET images. There are two foci of intense increased tracer uptake in the liver and an additional focus in the left hypochondrium. (*C*) On the fused PET-CT image, the increased foci correspond to the left lobe of the liver, consistent with metastases.

FDG PET-CT is also reported to be helpful in the assessment of treatment response in pancreatic cancer. In patients with locally advanced pancreatic cancer, tumors with a higher baseline SUV-max is more likely to recur in the early postoperative period; FDG PET-CT is also an independent predictor for overall survival.[45,54,55] Finally, FDG PET-CT is also reported to be helpful in delineating the gross tumor volume for radiotherapeutic planning and said to increase the gross tumor volume by 30%.[56,57]

Besides aiding management of cases with an established diagnosis of pancreatic cancer, FDG

PET can often help in the characterization and differentiation of benign inflammatory from malignant etiology of pancreatic lesions in challenging cases. In particular, combined imaging modality often helps in characterization without tissue confirmation.[41] FDG PET-CT is used to differentiate benign from malignant pancreatic lesions such as chronic pancreatitis from pancreatic cancer and pancreatic cancer from autoimmune pancreatitis (AIP). In general, pancreatic adenocarcinoma manifests as a focal area of increased uptake within the pancreas. This is not exclusive and pancreatic ductal adenocarcinoma may

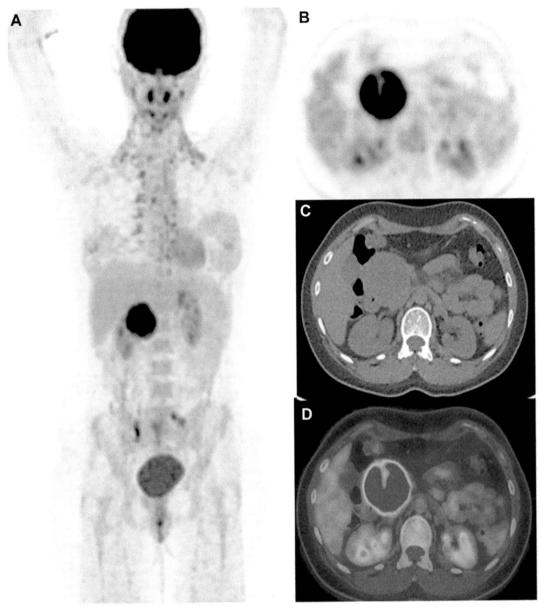

Fig. 3. Pancreatic cancer: 18F-FDG PET-CT. (A) MIP and (B) trans axial PET images-There is a large focal area of increased FDG uptake in the abdomen. (C, D) Increased tracer uptake in the abdomen corresponds to a large pancreatic head mass. There is no evidence of abnormal hypermetabolic distant metastatic disease. Histology confirmed pancreatic adenocarcinoma.

demonstrate a low level or FDG negative.[45] In general, the maximum SUV is higher in malignant lesions, irrespective of the size of the tumor. The sensitivity of 18F-FDG PET is approximately 100%. It is only 40% for CECT for lesions smaller than 2 cm.[45,58] 18F-FDG PET-CT has been used in differentiating mass forming pancreatitis (MFP) from pancreatic adenocarcinoma. The pancreatic adenocarcinoma tends to demonstrate higher FDG uptake compared with MFP. Although sensitivity is higher, the specificity is low because both

inflammation and neoplasms show low FDG uptake. Overall, focal increased FDG uptake is suspicious for malignancy and requires further investigation in most cases.[45] The lack of FDG uptake in euglycemic patients suggests MFP.[45] In patients with suspected pancreatic cancer, the reported sensitivity is 89%, and specificity is 74%.[49,59] AIP is a subtype of chronic pancreatitis and accounts for approximately 2% −11% of all cases of chronic pancreatitis. Type 1 AIP is reported to be part of the immunoglobulin G4–

related disease spectrum[60]—in addition to pancreatic disease, other systems or organs, such as bile ducts, salivary and lacrimal glands, lymph nodes, and retroperitoneal tissue, are concurrently involved in 30%.[60–62] FDG uptake and intensity in pancreatitis are often related to the cause or severity, for example, low-grade acute or subacute pancreatitis or AIP often show diffuse uptake, and no significant uptake is seen in chronic pancreatitis.[45,63,64] Pancreatic ductal

adenocarcinoma and AIP can both be FDG avid, but the patterns of uptake such as longitudinal shape, heterogeneous or diffuse accumulation, and multifocal localization favor AIP.[45] Further supplementary findings in extrapancreatic organs such as salivary glands and bile ducts point toward a systemic cause than cancer.[45,56,65]

Another diagnostic challenge is with cystic neoplasms of the pancreas, which constitute less than 10% of all pancreatic neoplasms. This includes

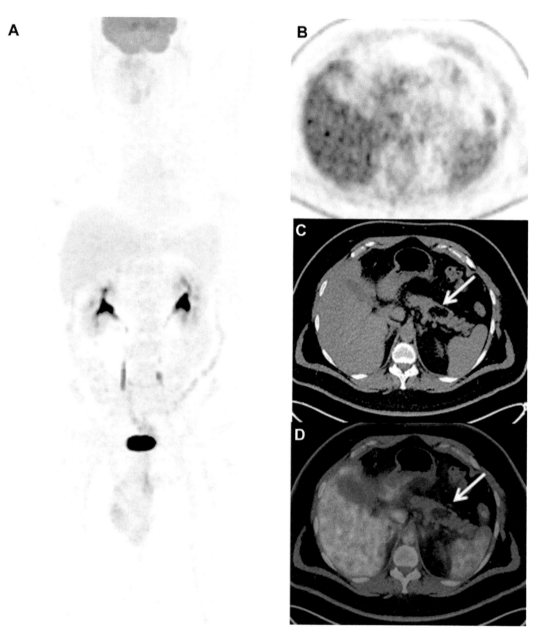

Fig. 4. Pancreatic lipoma: 18F-FDG PET-CT. No abnormal focal increased tracer uptake seen in the abdomen on both (A) MIP and (B) trans axial PET images. The tail of pancreas lesion (arrow) with macroscopic fat (C) does not show increased metabolic activity (D). No metabolically active foci elsewhere. Scan finding suggestive of a pancreatic lipoma.

serous cystadenomas, malignant, potentially malignant, and borderline tumors (NETs with cystic features, mucinous cystic neoplasms, and intraductal papillary mucinous neoplasms (IPMNs)).[7,45,66] Differentiating benign from the malignant disease within this spectrum is challenging.[3] Initial evaluations are often performed with CECT and MR imaging. Several radiological features such as mural nodules/irregularity, calcifications, and heterogenous soft-tissue relative to the rest of the pancreas are useful but not always diagnostic due to overlap of features.[41,45,66] In general, 18F-FDG PET-CT is reported to be comparable or superior to PET or CT alone in determining the presence of malignancy in cystic pancreatic lesions[67] (**Fig. 4**). 18F-FDG-positive cystic neoplasms are often malignant or invasive, and FDG-negative lesions may be benign, borderline malignant, or noninvasive malignant.[45,48] IPMNs are epithelial pancreatic cystic tumors of mucin-producing cells that arise from the pancreatic ducts. SUV max often helps differentiate benign from malignant IPMNs. The malignant lesions show significantly higher SUVmax than benign lesions. The reported sensitivity (94%) and specificity (100%) of PET-CT for depicting

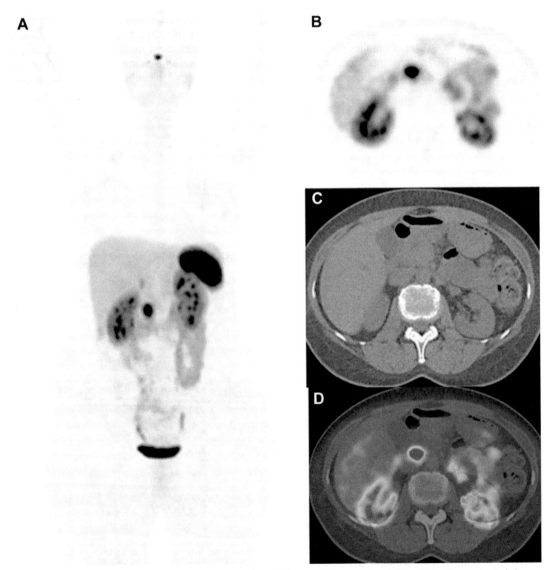

**Fig. 5.** PNET: 68Gallium-DOTATATE scan. (*A*) MIP: There is intense increased uptake within the central abdomen. (*B–D*) The focus of increased uptake in the abdomen corresponds to the mass in the head of the pancreas. The scan appearance is compatible with a somatostatin receptor-positive pancreas mass. There is no evidence of tracer avid metastatic disease.

malignant cystic pancreatic lesions are superior to FDG PET and CT.[45,68] With current evolving evidence and intrinsic limitations of CT and PET-CT, combining the morphologic features and functional information might improve the diagnosis of malignant or invasive mucinous neoplasms of the pancreas. Several non-FDG tracers are also used in distinguishing tumor from inflammatory tissue, for example, 18F 3′-fluoro-3′-deoxy-L-thymidine (FLT) is more tumor specific than FDG in animal models and performs better than FDG in distinguishing tumor from inflammatory tissue.[69,70]

### Non-fluorodeoxyglucose PET-Computerized Tomography in Various Pancreatic Cancer Types

NETs represent 3% of pancreatic neoplasms. 60%–80% of PNETs are nonfunctional.[71–73] PNETs can be categorized based on the predominant hormone they produce. Most of the well-differentiated PNETs express somatostatin receptors (SSTRs) and can be visualized by binding to radioactive somatostatin analogs (SSAs). The SSTR-based functional imaging with 68Ga-labeled peptides, 68Ga-DOTATATE, 68Ga-DOTA-TOC, and 68Ga-DOTANOC is the current clinical gold standard in diagnosing NETs. The 68Ga-DOTATATE has the strongest SSTR2-binding affinity, compared with 68Ga-DOTATOC (SSTR2, SSTR5) and 68Ga-DOTANOC (SSTR2, SSTR3, and SSTR5) (45, 74). However, the three analogs have shown no clinical practice differences by some authors.[72] The indications of SSTR-based functional imaging with 68Ga-labeled peptides include to (a) localize primary tumors and detect sites of metastatic disease (staging), (b) follow up patients by detecting residual, recurrent, or progressive disease (re-staging), (c) monitor the effects of therapy, (d) select patients for peptide

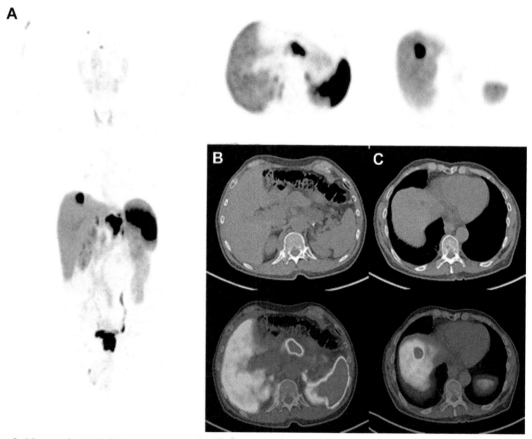

**Fig. 6.** Metastatic PNET: 68Ga-DOTATATE. (*A*) MIP: There is intense focal increased tracer uptake in the liver and in the central abdomen. There is intense DOTATATE uptake in the body of pancreas. (*B*) The uptake extends into the root of the small bowel mesentery and into the adjacent left gastric node (not shown). Solitary intense tracer avid focus in the liver. (*C*) Focal uptake at the junction between the skull and the right frontal cortex represents a meningioma. Scan findings consistent with primary PNET extending into the root of the small bowel mesentery and with liver metastasis.

receptor radionuclide therapy, and (e) provide a prognosis or predictive parameter for the response of subsequent therapy[74] (**Figs. 5** and **6**).

The pancreas shows variable uptake of 68Ga-DOTA-conjugate peptides, and all five subtypes of SSTR are present in the pancreas. In general, SSTR2 receptor is preferably found in the islets. Accumulation of tracer in the pancreatic head/uncinate process may mimic focal tumor disease in the pancreas,[74] suggesting caution is needed for scan interpretation in this region. In general, 18F-FDG uptake is a useful prognostic marker and

---

**Table 3**
**Summary of current evidence of 18F-FDG and non-FDG PET tracers in pancreatic cancer**

| 18F-FDG PET-CT | Non-FDG Tracers |
|---|---|
| Valuable in the management of pancreatic ductal adenocarcinoma. | SSTR-based functional imaging with 68Ga-labeled peptides is the gold standard in the diagnosis of the PNETs |
| The average sensitivity and specificity in detecting pancreatic ductal adenocarcinoma are 94% and 90%, respectively. | 68Ga-labeled peptide measurements of SUV in tumor and normal tissues are not entirely reliable |
| Malignant lesions are often 18F-FDG avid, whereas most benign lesions show minimally increased FDG accumulation or normal uptake(similar to background uptake) | Dual-tracer (68Gallium-labeled peptides and 18F-FDG) PET-CT imaging has a complementary role in the diagnostic workup of PNETs |
| Focal abnormal increased uptake is considered suspicious for malignant disease and requires further investigation. | 18F-FDG PET-CT is a surrogate measure of tumor aggressiveness, and 68Ga-labeled peptides have prognostic value and predict the histopathological tumor grade. |
| False-positive and false-negative results occur with 18F-FDG PET | 11C-5-HTP is an alternative tracer when SSR imaging is negative. The sensitivity is higher for PNETs, as opposed to carcinoids, because there is no intracellular saturation from endogenous serotonin |
| Serum glucose levels can affect 18F-FDG PET findings. | 18F-DOPA can be of value as an alternative or problem-solving tool when SSR imaging is negative or assessment of treatment response. |
| Sensitivity is 83%–86% for tumor depiction in euglycemic patients and is 42%–69% in those with elevated glucose levels. | 18 FLT is more tumor specific than FDG in animal models and performed better than FDG in distinguishing tumor from inflammatory tissue |
| Maximum SUV is higher in malignant lesions, irrespective of the size of the tumor. | GLP-1R imaging: 68Ga-labeled exendin-4 is a sensitive tool for preoperatively localizing insulinoma. |
| Pancreatic adenocarcinoma tends to demonstrate higher 18F-FDG uptake than MFP. | Pancreatic cancers take up radiolabeled PSMA (limited evidence) |
| Fused 18F-PET-CT may improve the specificity of nodal staging compared with CT alone. | Radiolabeled FAPI uptake is directly associated with the degree of fibrosis in PDAC. (limited evidence) |
| MR imaging is reported to be more accurate in depicting small liver metastases than 18F-FDG PET. | Radiolabeled FAPI imaging might help differentiate inflammation from pancreatic tumor lesions (limited evidence) |
| 18F-FDG PET-CT is superior to CECT and MR imaging in the depiction of distant metastases. | |
| 18F-FDG PET-CT improves the selection of patients for surgery and helps in avoiding unnecessary surgical procedures. | |
| 18F-FDG PET-CT is useful in detecting recurrence and the sensitivity and specificity are higher than conventional radiological modalities. | |
| Postoperative inflammatory changes secondary to radiation therapy or stent placement show increased tracer uptake in the pancreas and are the common false positives (pitfalls). To minimize errors in interpretation, PET-CT should be performed at least 6 weeks after surgery. | |
| Diffuse 18F-FDG uptake may be seen in low-grade acute or subacute pancreatitis or AIP patients. In contrast, increased radiotracer uptake generally is not seen in patients with conventional chronic pancreatitis. | |

can demonstrate NET aggression; well-differentiated, slow-growing NETs demonstrate little or no FDG uptake. The reported sensitivity of 68 Ga DOTA-TATE uptake in low-grade and well-differentiated tumors is 82%, whereas the sensitivity of FDG in high-grade and poorly differentiated NETs is 66%.[75] Dual-tracer PET-CT imaging has a complementary role, and it enables the detection of a potentially aggressive disease during the diagnostic workup of well-differentiated PNETs.

There are several newer tracers such as 64Cu-labeled SSA, novel SSA antagonists, GLP-1 receptor peptides (68Ga-NODAGA-Excedin 4) in imaging NETs, and their advantages and limitations are described in **Table 3**.[76–81] L-DOPA and carbon-11-labeled 5-hydroxytryptophan (11C-5-HTP) can be used as an alternative or problem-solving tool when radiolabeled SSR imaging is negative or in assessing response to treatment.[76,77] The sensitivity of 11C-5-HTP is higher for PNETs than midgut carcinoids because there is no intracellular saturation from endogenous serotonin.[77] In PNETs (per lesion analysis), the sensitivity of 11C-5-HTP; 18F-DOPA is 96% and 80%,[77] but the production of 11C-5-HTP is complex with the need for onsite cyclotron. Its limited availability makes its use in routine practice challenging. 18F-DOPA PET-CT is often used in the localization of focal pancreatic lesions in patients

**Table 4**
**Summary of advantages and limitations of FDG and non-FDG PET tracers in pancreatic neuroendocrine tumors**

| Tracer | Advantages | Limitations |
|---|---|---|
| 18F-FDG: Glucose analog and localizes in the tumor cells and is proportionally to their glucose metabolic activity Marker of glucose consumption | Prognostic evaluation Imaging of high-grade G2 and G3 NET tumors | Imaging well-differentiated NETs |
| 68Ga-labeled peptides: Bind with varying affinity to SSTRs expressed on NETs | Localization, staging, restaging Selecting patients for radionuclide peptide therapy Detecting unexpected sites of disease (eg, bones, peritoneum, the heart, soft tissues, etc.) Possibility of labeling the same peptide used for PRRT (theragnostic) Modifies therapeutic management | Requires generator Limited availability |
| 18F-FLT: Marker of cell proliferation and intracellular localization | Tailoring therapy for neuroendocrine tumor patients through early identification of responders and nonresponders | Limited availability Requires validation |
| 11C-5-HTTP: Targets the serotonin production pathway. Serotonin precursor with irreversible trapping in NETs | High sensitivity for PNETs Alternative or a problem-solving tool when radiolabeled SSTR imaging is negative | Requires on-site cyclotron Limited availability Requires validation No therapeutic application. |
| 18F-DOPA: Based on the biochemical pathway in dopamine synthesis. | Alternative or a problem-solving tool when radiolabeled SSTR imaging is negative Localization of pancreatic lesions in patients with hyperinsulinemic hypoglycemia | Requires on-site cyclotron Limited availability Requires validation No therapeutic application cost |
| 68Ga- exendin-4 (GLP-1R imaging): Targets GLP1R of pancreatic β-cells. | Sensitive tool for preoperatively localizing insulinoma (sensitivity = 98%) | Limited availability Requires generator |

with congenital hyperinsulinemic hypoglycemia. Adult patients with suspected insulinoma are challenging as imaging with radiolabeled SSA is insufficiently sensitivity. 68Ga-NOTA-exendin-4 PET-CT is a more novel agent with promise for sensitive localization of insulinoma.[82] The reported sensitivity of 68Ga-NOTA-exendin-4 PET-CT in localizing insulinoma is 98%.[82]

Pancreatic cancer is a source of potential PSMA-expressing lesion because these tumors have high expression of PSMA in their neovasculature, and there are several case reports of incidental detection of pancreatic cancer on 18F-PSMA PET-CT.[83–85] 68Ga-FAPI-04 is a tumor imaging agent that targets FAP, and uptake of FAPI is directly associated with the degree of fibrosis.[86–89] Pancreatic ductal carcinoma (PDAC) typically has a prominent stroma, including cancer-associated fibroblasts that express FAP. In a small cohort of patients, 68Ga-FAPI PET-CT led to a change in staging in half of the patients with PDAC and most patients with the recurrent disease, compared with standard of care imaging with CECT.[90] In addition, where 18F-F-FDG imaging provides inconclusive information in differentiating inflammation from tumor lesions, FAPI

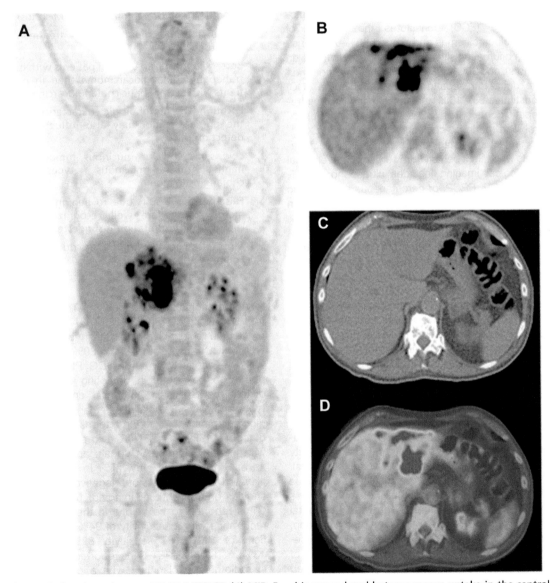

Fig. 7. Cholangiocarcinoma: 18F-FDG PET-CT. (A) MIP: Focal increased and heterogeneous uptake in the central abdomen. (B–D) The increased heterogeneous tracer uptake in the abdomen corresponds to the left lobe of the liver extending into the hepatic hilum. There is no evidence of hypermetabolic distant metastatic disease. Histology confirmed cholangiocarcinoma.

imaging might offer an important clue and yield a more accurate diagnosis.[86–90] Clinical data for PSMA and FAPI tracers are emerging with currently only limited evidence; further test performance data and ultimately whether their roles may expand and change the imaging landscape of patients with pancreatic malignancy remains to be seen. Current evidence of FDG and non-FDG tracers is summarized in **Tables 1, 3,** and **4.**

## Cholangiocarcinoma

Cholangiocarcinoma (CCA) accounts for <2% of all malignancies and is the second most common primary hepatic cancer.[91,92] Extrahepatic cholangiocarcinoma (ECC) constitutes the majority of cholangiocarcinomas and around 60%–70% arise at the bifurcation site of the hepatic ducts (Klatskin tumors), and 20%–30% occur in the distal common bile duct. Intrahepatic cholangiocarcinoma (ICC) constitutes 5%–10% and arises in the liver's intrahepatic ducts.[92] The ICC is subdivided into peripheral and perihilar cholangiocarcinomas (PCC).[93] Accurate tumor staging is essential to select patients who might benefit from surgery. Conventional radiological imaging includes ultrasound, CECT, MRI, MRCP, ERCP, or percutaneous transhepatic cholangiography.[91] 18F-FDG PET-CT is vital in detecting occult metastasis or characterizing indeterminate lesions seen on CT or MRI. However, histopathological subtypes and the anatomic location of the tumor need to be considered when performing 18F-FDG PET-CT to obtain the best possible results. In the primary staging of cholangiocarcinoma, a large meta-analysis of 23 studies showed overall that the pooled results indicate that sensitivity is 81% and specificity is 82% in evaluating primary tumors in patients with cholangiocarcinoma.[94] Sensitivity was 95%, 84%, and 76%, and specificity was 83%, 95%, and 74% for ICC, PCC, and ECC, respectively[94] **(Fig. 7).**

In patients with suspected ECC, the sensitivity of 18F-FDG-PET was 85% for nodular and 18% for infiltrating morphology[95] as the infiltrating tumors have relatively slight structural abnormality and lower tumor cell density per voxel. In general, 18F-FDG PET-CT has low sensitivity for mucinous types of cholangiocarcinoma.[96] Reasons for false negative include infiltrative growth, periductal sclerosing, and tumors with a high mucin fraction, and small tumors.[93,94,97] Reasons for false-positive results include inflammatory changes of the bile ducts, caused either by tumor-induced bile retention or by chemotherapy or following invasive procedures such as implantation of intraluminal bile duct stents.[95,97,98] 18F-FDG PET-CT has a significantly higher specificity and accuracy

---

**Box 1**
**Summary of current evidence of 18F-fluorodeoxyglucose PET-computerized tomography (PET-CT) in cholangiocarcinoma**

- Significant influence on clinical decision making in primary biliary malignancy both as part of initial workup and for identifying recurrent disease.
- Low sensitivity for regional lymph node metastases from cholangiocarcinoma and gallbladder cancer but specificity is high.
- Helpful in identifying recurrent disease.
- Promising diagnostic tool in the primary staging of cholangiocarcinoma (N and M status).
- Useful for the monitoring of treatment response.
- Better diagnostic accuracy in patients with intrahepatic cholangiocarcinoma than in patients with extrahepatic cholangiocarcinoma.
- Location, the morphologic characteristics of the primary tumor may also influence its detection rate.
- Low sensitivity for mucinous tumors and might miss mucinous types of cholangiocarcinoma.
- False-positive results due to benign inflammatory causes are well recognized, and caution in interpretation is suggested.
- Most false-negative findings are due to small volume peritoneal disease.

---

for nodal staging than CT alone.[97,99] The sensitivity and specificity of 18F-FDG PET-CT in detecting metastatic regional lymph nodes in the peripheral type of ICC range from 74% to 80% and 90% to 92%, respectively.[92,99] 18F-FDG PET-CT is reported to be useful in detecting unsuspected distant metastasis in both hilar and peripheral types and plays a crucial role in managing cholangiocarcinoma.[92,100–102] In terms of patient outcome, 18F-FDG PET-CT avid primary tumors with higher SUVmax, SUVpeak, and SUV mean have poorer overall survival.[92] In patients with elevated tumor markers but negative or equivocal findings on conventional imaging, 18F-FDG PET-CT is reported to be helpful in the detection of recurrence with a sensitivity of 94% and a specificity of 100% (CT sensitivity 82%, specificity 43%).[95] 18F-FDG PET-CT is reported to be helpful in radiotherapy planning, with a possible dose reduction for adjacent organs at risk by 17%.[103] The false positive, false negative, and current evidence of FDG and non-FDG tracers are summarized in Table 1 and **Box 1.**

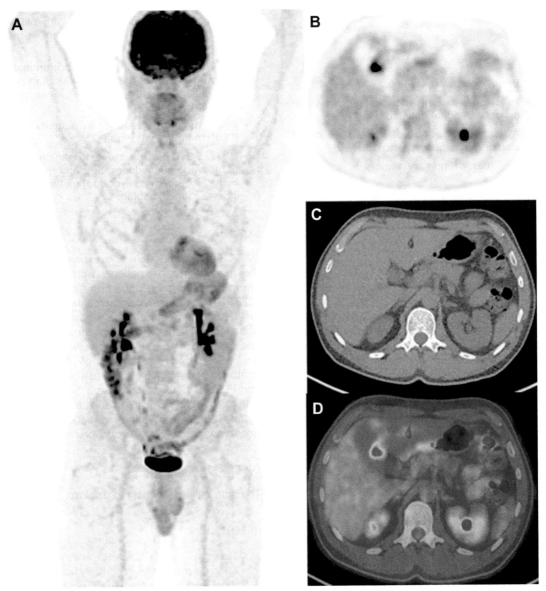

**Fig. 8.** Gall bladder cancer: 18F-FDG PET-CT. (*B-D*) There is an intense hypermetabolic focus within the gallbladder. (*A*) focal uptake in the right hypochondrium is not clearly seen on MIP image due to overlapping tracer activity from the bowel and right kidney. There is no evidence of hypermetabolic distant metastatic disease. Histology confirmed adenocarcinoma.

## Gall Bladder Cancer

GC is an aggressive malignancy and is often diagnosed at an advanced stage. In general, only 15%–47% of patients are eligible for radical resection at the time of diagnosis.[104] Incidental detection of GC with elective resection might have a better prognosis.[105] In patients undergoing radical surgical treatment, around 15% (T1b tumor), 40% (T2), and 80% (T3) tumors often develop recurrent disease.[106] Conventional radiological modalities as CT and MRI are used to evaluate locoregional or distant metastases and assess the involvement of locoregional vascular structures.[106,107] However, common limitations of these radiological modalities include differentiating residual/recurrent tumor from postoperative changes.[98] The role of 18F-FDG PET-CT scan in gall bladder cancer is evolving, and it plays an essential role in staging[107–109] (**Fig. 8**). In general, in staging GC, the reported sensitivity is 87%, and specificity is 78%.[107] 18F-FDG PET-CT scan is also helpful in detecting locoregional and distant metastases. Over the accuracy of FDG PET-CT in detecting nodal and distant metastases is 86% and 96%,

---

**Box 2**
**Summary of current evidence of 18F-fluorodeoxyglucose PET-computerized tomography (PET-CT) in gall bladder cancer**

- Useful in accurate staging.
- Indicated in patients equivocal for metastases on cross sectional imaging.
- Assessment of abnormal nodes seen on CT scan or magnetic resonance imaging.
- SUV max of primary tumors is related to survival.
- Management change is seen in approximately 23%.
- Useful in assessment of recurrent disease.

- SSTR-based functional imaging with 68Ga-labeled peptides is the gold standard in the diagnosis of the PNETs.
- FDG PET-CT is useful in clinical decision making both as part of the initial workup in primary biliary malignancy and for identifying recurrent disease.
- Better diagnostic accuracy in patients with ICC than in patients with ECC.
- FDG PET-CT useful in accurate in staging in patients with gall bladder cancer and indicated in the assessment equivocal for metastases on cross-sectional imaging.

---

respectively.[109] Goel and colleagues have reported detecting additional findings in 31%, which led to change in management in 23% of their patients due to the presence of distant metastases.[110] In addition, the impact of change in staging was higher in patients having positive node disease on CECT than negative node patients. 18F-FDG PET-CT scan is also helpful in detecting recurrence and is reported to be more specific than conventional radiological techniques. Lastly, several false-positive FDG PET findings such as cholecystitis and adenomyomatosis should be considered while interpreting increased FDG uptake in the gall bladder.[111] The false positive, false negative, and current evidence of FDG and non-FDG tracers are summarized in **Table 1** and **Box 2**.

## CLINICS CARE POINTS

- There is ample evidence to support the use of FDG PET-CT in the management of patients with hepatobiliary and pancreatic cancers in various clinical settings.
- Several non-FDG PET tracers are available in the assessment hepatobiliary and pancreatic cancers and the evidence is evolving.
- FDG uptake by HCC varies according to histologic differentiation of the tumor and is not recommended as a standard imaging modality for the early diagnosis of HCC.
- FDG PET-CT has a valuable in the management of pancreatic ductal adenocarcinoma.
- FDG PET-CT is superior to CECT and MR imaging in the depiction of distant metastases in pancreatic cancer.

## SUMMARY

PET-CT plays important and expanding roles in the management of patients with hepatobiliary and pancreatic malignancies. In many instances, FDG PET-CT provides complementary information for lesion characterization, staging (especially nodal and distant staging), response evaluation, and detection of recurrent disease, where there are recognized limitations of conventional anatomic imaging in mainstay use. A multitude of non-FDG and novel tracers are in the pipeline with seemingly promising results as summarized in this article and further validation would be necessary before clinical adoption.

## DISCLOSURE

The authors have nothing to disclose.

## REFERENCES

1. Sacks A, Peller PJ, Surasi DS, et al. Value of PET/CT in the management of primary hepatobiliary tumors, part 2. AJR Am J Roentgenol 2011;197(2):W260–5.
2. Sacks A, Peller JP, Surasi DS, et al. Value of PET/CT in the management of liver metastases, part 1. AJR Am J Roentgenol 2011;197:W256–9.
3. Seale MK, Catalano OA, Saini S, et al. Hepatobiliary-specific MR contrast agents: role in imaging the liver and biliary tree. RadioGraphics 2009;29:1725–48.
4. Parikh U, Marcus C, Sarangi R, et al. FDG PET/CT in pancreatic and hepatobiliary carcinomas: value to patient management and patient outcomes. PET Clin 2015;10(3):327–43.
5. Rezaee A, Subramaniam R, Raderer M, et al. Hepatobiliary cancer. In: Behesti M, Rezaee A, Langsteteger W, editors. PET-CT In cancer; an interdisciplinary approach to individualised imaging. Elsevier Inc; 2018. p. 127–48.

6. Tamaki N, Inokuma T, et al. In Vivo assessment of glucose metabolism in hepatocellular carcinoma with FDG-PET. J Nucl Med 1995;36:1811–7.

7. Salem N, MacLennan GT, Kuang Y, et al. Quantitative evaluation of 2-deoxy-2[F-18]fluoro-D-glucose-positron emission tomography imaging on the woodchuck model of hepatocellular carcinoma with histological correlation. Mol Imaging Biol 2007;9:135–43.

8. Lee JD, Yang WI, Park YN, et al. Different glucose uptake and glycolytic mechanisms between hepatocellular carcinoma and intrahepatic mass- forming cholangiocarcinoma with increased (18) F-FDG uptake. J Nucl Med 2005;46:1753–9.

9. Roh MS, Jeong JS, Kim YH, et al. Diagnostic utility of GLUT1 in the differential diagnosis of liver carcinomas. Hepatogastroenterology 2004;51:1315–8.

10. Khan MA, Combs CS, Brunt EM, et al. Positron emission tomography scanning in the evaluation of hepatocellular carcinoma. J Hepatol 2000;32:792–7.

11. Ho CL, Yu SC, Yeung DW. [11]C-acetate PET imaging in hepatocellular carcinoma and other liver masses. J Nucl Med 2003;44:213–21.

12. Kwee TC, Basu S, Saboury B, et al. A new dimension of FDG-PET interpretation: assessment of tumor biology. Eur J Nucl Med Mol Imaging 2011; 38:1158–70.

13. Park JW, Kim JH, Kim SK, et al. A prospective evaluation of [18]F-FDG and [11]C-acetate PET/CT for detection of primary and metastatic hepatocel- lular carcinoma. J Nucl Med 2008;49:1912–21.

14. Kong YH, Han CJ, Lee SD, et al. Positron emission tomography with fluorine-18-fluorodeoxyglucose is useful for predicting the prognosis of patients with hepatocellular carcinoma (in Korean). Korean J Hepatol 2004;10:279–87.

15. Shiomi S, Nishiguchi S, Ishizu H, et al. Usefulness of positron emission tomography with fluorine-18-fluorodeoxyglucose for predicting outcome in patients with hepatocellular carcinoma. Am J Gastroenterol 2001;96:1877–80.

16. Cho E, Jun CH, Kim BS, et al. 18F-FDG PET CT as a prognostic factor in hepatocellular carcinoma. Turk J Gastroenterol 2015;26(4):344–50.

17. Iannaccone R, Piacentini F, Murakami T, et al. Hepatocellular carcinoma in patients with non-alcoholic fatty liver disease: helical CT and MR imaging findings with clinical-pathologic com- parison. Radiology 2007;243:422–30.

18. Yoon KT, Kim JK, Kim do Y, et al. Role of [18]F- fluorodeoxyglucose positron emission tomography in detecting extrahepatic metastasis in pre- treatment staging of hepatocellular carcinoma. Oncology 2007;72(suppl 1):104–10.

19. Lin CY, Chen JH, Liang JA, et al. 18F-FDG PET or PET/CT for detecting extrahepatic metastases or recurrent hepatocellular carcinoma: a systematic review and meta-analysis. Eur J Radiol 2012; 81(9):2417–22.

20. Kim HO, Kim JS, Shin YM, et al. Evaluation of metabolic characteristics and viability of lipiodolized hepatocellular carcinomas using 18F-FDG PET/CT. J Nucl Med 2010;51:1849–56.

21. Song HJ, Cheng JY, Hu SL, et al. Value of 18F-FDG PET/CT in detecting viable tumour and predicting prognosis of hepatocellular carcinoma after TACE. Clin Radiol 2014;70(2):128–37.

22. Song MJ, Bae SH, Lee SW, et al. 18F-fluorodeoxy-glucose PET/CT predicts tumour progression after transarterial chemoembolization in hepatocellular carcinoma. Eur J Nucl Med Mol Imaging 2013; 40(6):865–73.

23. Ma W, Jia J, Wang S, et al. The prognostic value of 18F-FDG PET/CT for hepatocellular carcinoma treated with transarterial chemoembolization (TACE). Theranostics 2014;4(7):736–44.

24. Wudel LJ Jr, Delbeke D, Morris D, et al. The role of [18F]fluorodeoxyglucose positron emission tomography imaging in the evaluation of hepatocellular carcinoma. Am Surg 2003;69(2):117–24.

25. Delbeke D, Pinson CW. [11]C-acetate: a new tracer for the evaluation of hepatocellular carcinoma. J Nucl Med 2003;44:222–3.

26. Kesler M, Levine C, Hershkovitz D, et al. 68Ga-PSMA is a novel PET-CT tracer for imaging of hepatocellular carcinoma: a prospective pilot study. J Nucl Med 2019;60(2):185–91.

27. Wang H, Zhu W, Ren S, et al. 68Ga-FAPI-04 versus 18F-FDG PET/CT in the detection of hepatocellular carcinoma. Front Oncol 2021;11:693640.

28. Shi X, Xing H, Yang X, et al. Comparison of PET imaging of activated fibroblasts and 18F-FDG for diagnosis of primary hepatic tumours: a prospective pilot study. Eur J Nucl Med Mol Imaging 2021;48(5):1593–603.

29. Guo W, Pang Y, Yao L, et al. Imaging fibroblast activation protein in liver cancer: a single-center post hoc retrospective analysis to compare [68Ga]Ga-FAPI-04 PET/CT versus MRI and [18F]-FDG PET/CT. Eur J Nucl Med Mol Imaging 2021;48(5): 1604–17.

30. Abdelhalim H, Houseni M, Elsakhawy M, et al. Role of 18F-FDG PET-CT in initial staging of hepatocellular carcinoma and its impact on changing clinical decision. Egypt Liver J 2020;10:3.

31. European Association for the Study of the Liver. EASL clinical practice guidelines: management of hepatocellular carcinoma. J Hepatol 2018;69: 182–236.

32. Ida Y, Tamai H, Shingaki N, et al. Prognostic value of 18F-fluorodeoxyglucose positron emission tomography in patients with small hepatocellular carcinoma treated by radiofrequency ablation. Cancer Imaging 2020;20:74.

33. Kim MJ, Kim YS, Cho YH, et al. Use of 18F-FDG PET to predict tumor progression and survival in patients with intermediate hepatocellular carcinoma treated by transarterial chemoembolization. Korean J Intern Med 2015;30:308–15.

34. Zhang Yan-Nan, Lu Xin, Lu Zhen-Guo, et al. Evaluation of hybrid PET/MRI for gross tumor volume (GTV) delineation in colorectal cancer liver metastases radiotherapy. Cancer Manag Res 2021;13: 5383–9.

35. Ekhlas Abdelmonem Ibrahem Nasr Shaban. Can fluorine-18-fluorodeoxyglucose positron emission tomography/computed tomography detect hepatocellular carcinoma and its extrahepatic metastases? Egypt J Radiol Nucl Med 2018;49(1):196–201.

36. Safaie E, Matthews R. Metastatic breast cancer to the liver. In: PET/MR imaging. Cham: Springer; 2018. https://doi.org/10.1007/978-3-319-65106-4_42. Available at.

37. Chua SC, Groves AM, Kayani I, et al. The impact of 18F-FDG PET/CT in patients with liver metastases. Eur J Nucl Med Mol Imaging 2007;34(12): 1906–14.

38. Veit P, Antoch G, Stergar H, et al. Detection of residual tumor after radiofre- quency ablation of liver metastasis with dual-modali- ty PET/CT: initial results. Eur Radiol 2006;16:80–7.

39. Lubezky N, Metser U, Geva R, et al. The role and limitations of 18-fluoro-2-deoxy-D-glucose positron emission tomography (FDG-PET) scan and computerized tomography (CT) in restaging patients with hepatic colorectal metastases following neoadjuvant chemotherapy: comparison with oper- ative and pathological findings. J Gastrointest Surg 2007;11:472–8.

40. Gress TM, Michl P, Pauls S. Evidence-based diagnosis and staging of pancreatic cancer. Best Pract Res Clin Gastroenterol 2006;20:227–51.

41. Dibble EH, Karantanis D, Mercier G, et al. PET/CT of cancer patients: part 1, pancreatic neoplasms. AJR Am J Roentgenol 2012;199(5):952–67.

42. Klimstra DS, Pitman MB, Hruban RH. An algorithmic approach to the diagnosis of pancreatic neo- plasms. Arch Pathol Lab Med 2009;133: 454–64.

43. Tempero MA, Malafa MP, Chiorean EG, et al Pancreatic Adenocarcinoma, Version 1.2019. J Natl Compr Canc Netw. 2019 1;17(3):202-210.

44. Kauhanen SP, Komar G, Seppänen MP, et al. A prospective diagnostic accuracy study of 18F-fluo- rodeoxyglucose positron emission tomography/com- puted tomography, multidetector row computed tomography, and magnetic resonance imaging in primary diagnosis and staging of pancreatic cancer. Ann Surg 2009;250(6):957–63.

45. Sahani DVBonaffini PA, Catalano OA, et al. State-of-the-Art PET/CT of the pancreas: current role

and emerging indications. RadioGraphics 2012; 32:1133–58.

46. National Institute of Clinical Excellence. Available at: http://nice.org.uk/guidance/qs177/resources/pancreatic-cancer-pdf Quality standard. 2018.

47. Gambhir SS, Czernin J, Schwimmer J, et al. A tabulated sum- mary of the FDG PET literature. J Nucl Med 2001;42(5 suppl):1S–93S.

48. Strobel K, Heinrich S, Bhure U, et al. Contrast-enhanced F-18-FDG PET/CT: 1-stop-shop imaging for assessing the resectability of pancreatic cancer. J Nucl Med 2008;49:1408–13.

49. Sahani DV, Kalva SP, Fischman AJ, et al. Detection of liver metastases from adenocarcinoma of the colon and pancreas: comparison of mangafodipir trisodium-enhanced liver MRI and whole-body FDG PET. AJR Am J Roentgenol 2005;185(1):239–46.

50. Kleeff J, Reiser C, Hinz U, et al. Surgery for recurrent pancreatic ductal adenocarcinoma. Ann Surg 2007;245(4):566–72.

51. Casneuf V, Delrue L, Kelles A, et al. Is combined 18F-fluorodeoxyglucose-positron emission tomography/computed tomography superior to positron emission tomography or computed tomography alone for diagnosis, staging and restaging of pancre- atic lesions? Acta Gastroenterol Belg 2007; 70(4):331–8.

52. Ruf J, Lopez Hänninen E, Oettle H, et al. Detection of recurrent pancreatic cancer: comparison of FDG- PET with CT/MRI. Pancreatology 2005;5(2– 3):266–72.

53. Sperti C, Bissoli S, Pasquali C, et al. 18-fluorodeoxyglucose positron emission tomography enhances computed tomography diagnosis of malignant in- traductal papillary mucinous neoplasms of the pancreas. Ann Surg 2007;246(6):932–7.

54. Schellenberg D, Quon A, Yuriko Minn A, et al. 18 Fluorodeoxyglucose PET is prognostic of progression-free and overall survival in locally advanced pancreas cancer treated with stereotactic radiotherapy. Int J Radiat Oncol Biol Phys 2010; 77(5):1420–5.

55. Okamoto K, Koyama I, Miyazawa M, et al. Preoperative 18[F]-fluorodeoxyglucose positron emission tomography/computed tomography predicts early recurrence after pancreatic cancer resection. Int J Clin Oncol 2011;16(1):39–44.

56. Ford EC, Herman J, Yorke E, et al. 18)F- FDG PET/CT for image-guided and intensity- modulated radiotherapy. J Nucl Med 2009;50:1655–65.

57. Topkan E, Yavuz AA, Aydin M, et al. Comparison of CT and PET-CT based planning of radiation therapy in locally advanced pancreatic carcinoma. J Exp Clin Cancer Res 2008;27:41.

58. Lemke AJ, Niehues SM, Hosten N, et al. Retrospective digital image fusion of multidetector CT and 18F-FDG PET: clinical value in pancreatic

lesions—a prospective study with 104 patients. J Nucl Med 2004;45(8):1279–86.

59. Schick V, Franzius C, Beyna T, et al. Diagnostic impact of 18F-FDG PET-CT evaluating solid pancreatic lesions versus endosonography, endoscopic ret- rograde cholangio-pancreatography with intraductal ultrasonography and abdominal ultrasound. Eur J Nucl Med Mol Imaging 2008;35(10):1775–85.

60. Vlachou PA, Khalili K, Jang HJ, et al. IgG4-related sclerosing disease: autoimmune pancreatitis and extrapancreatic manifestations. RadioGraphics 2011;31(5):1379–402.

61. Zen Y, Nakanuma Y. IgG4-related disease: a cross-sectional study of 114 cases. Am J Surg Pathol 2010;34(12):1812–9.

62. Finkelberg DL, Sahani D, Deshpande V, et al. Autoimmune pancreatitis. N Engl J Med 2006;355(25): 2670–6.

63. Lee TY, Kim MH, Park H, et al. Utility of 18F- FDG PET/CT for differentiation of autoimmune pancreatitis with atypical pancreatic imaging find- ings from pancreatic cancer. AJR Am J Roentgenol 2009;193(2):343–8.

64. Jeong Yoon S, Lee B, Park CH. Imaging diagnosis of post-ERCP focal pancreatitis mimicking pancreatic carcinoma by follow-up F-18 FDG PET/CT. Clin Nucl Med 2011;36(1):70–2.

65. Kamisawa T, Takum K, Anjiki H, et al. FDG-PET/CT findings of autoimmune pancreatitis. Hepatogastroenterology 2010;57(99–100):447–50.

66. Brugge WR, Lauwers GY, Sahani D, et al. Cystic neoplasms of the pancreas. N Engl J Med 2004; 351(12):1218–26.

67. Tann M, Sandrasegaran K, Jennings SG, et al. Positron- emission tomography and computed tomography of cystic pancreatic masses. Clin Radiol 2007;62:745–51.

68. von Schulthess GK, Steinert HC, Hany TF. Integrated PET/CT: current applications and future directions. Radiology 2006;238(2):405–22.

69. van Waarde A, Cobben DC, Suurmeijer AJ, et al. Selectivity of 18F-FLT and 18F-FDG for dif- ferentiating tumor from inflammation in a rodent model. J Nucl Med 2004;45(4):695–700.

70. van Waarde A, Jager PL, Ishiwata K, et al. Comparison of sigma-ligands and metabolic PET tracers for differentiating tumor from inflammation. J Nucl Med 2006;47(1):150–4.

71. Hruban RH, Klimstra DS, Pitman MB. AFIP atlas of tumor pathology: tumors of the pancreas—series 4. Washington, DC: AFIP; 2007. p. 23–376.

72. Majala S, Seppänen H, Kemppainen J, et al. Prediction of the aggressiveness of non-functional pancreatic neuroendocrine tumors based on the dual-tracer PET/CT. EJNMMI Res 2019;9(1):116.

73. Yao JC, Hassan M, Phan A, et al. One hundred years after "carcinoid": epidemiology of and prognostic factors for neuroendocrine tumors in 35,825 Cases in the United States. JCO 2008; 26:3063–72.

74. Bozkurt MF, Virgolini I, Balogova S, et al. Guideline for PET/CT imaging of neuroendocrine neoplasms with 68Ga-DOTA-conjugated somatostatin receptor targeting peptides and 18F–DOPA. Eur J Nucl Med Mol Imaging 2017;44:1588–601.

75. Kayani I, Bomanji JB, Groves A, et al. Functional imaging of neuroendocrine tumors with combined PET/CT using 68Ga-DOTATATE (DOTA- DPhe1,Tyr3-octreotate) and 18F-FDG. Cancer 2008;112(11): 2447–55.

76. Ambrosini V, Fanti S. 68Ga-DOTA-peptides in the diagnosis of NET. PET Clin 2014;9:37–42.

77. Koopmans KP, Neels OC, Kema IP, et al. Improved staging of patients with carcinoid and islet cell tumors with 18F-dihydroxy-phenyl- alanine and 11C-5-hydroxy-tryptophan positron emission tomography. J Clin Oncol 2008;26:1489–95.

78. Bombardieri E, Maccauro M, De Deckere E, et al. Nuclear medicine imaging of neuroen- docrine tumours. Ann Oncol 2001;12(Suppl 2):S51–61.

79. Ichikawa T, Peterson MS, Federle MP, et al. Islet cell tumor of the pancreas: biphasic CT versus MR imaging in tumor detection. Radiology 2000; 216(1):163–71.

80. Nakamoto Y, Higashi T, Sakahara H, et al. Evaluation of pancreatic islet cell tumors by fluorine-18 fluorodeoxyglucose positron emission tomography: comparison with other modalities. Clin Nucl Med 2000;25(2):115–9.

81. Bodei L, Sundin A, Kidd M, et al. The status of neuroendocrine tumor imaging: from darkness to light? Neuroendocrinology 2015;101:1–17.

82. Luo Y, Pan Q, Yao S, et al. Glucagon-like peptide-1 receptor PET/CT with 68Ga-NOTA-exendin-4 for detecting localized insulinoma: a prospective cohort study. J Nucl Med 2016;57(5):715–20.

83. Haffner MC, Kronberger IE, Ross JS, et al. Prostate-specific membrane antigen expression in the neovasculature of gastric and colorectal cancers. Hum PatholElsevier Inc 2009;40: 1754–61.

84. de Galiza Barbosa F, Queiroz MA, Nunes RF, et al. Nonprostatic diseases on PSMA PET imaging: a spectrum of benign and malignant findings. Cancer Imaging 2020;20:23.

85. Poels TT, Vuijk FA, de Geus-Oei LF, et al. Molecular targeted positron emission tomography imaging and radionuclide therapy of pancreatic ductal adenocarcinoma. Cancers (Basel) 2021;13(24):6164.

86. Loktev A, Lindner T, Mier W, et al. A tumor-imaging method targeting cancer-associated fibroblasts. J Nucl Med 2018;59:1423–9.

87. Lindner T, Loktev A, Altmann A, et al. Development of quinoline-based theranostic ligands for the

targeting of fibroblast activation protein. J Nucl Med 2018;59(9):1415–22.

88. Luo Y, Pan Q, Yang H, et al. Fibroblast activation protein targeted PET/CT with 68Ga-FAPI for imaging IgG4-related disease: comparison to 18F-FDG PET/CT. J Nucl Med 2020;62(2):266–71.

89. Kratochwil C, Flechsig P, Lindner T, et al. 68Ga-FAPI PET/CT: tracer uptake in 28 different kinds of cancer. J Nucl Med 2019;60(6):801–5.

90. Röhrich M, Naumann P, Giesel FL, et al. Impact of 68Ga-FAPI PET/CT imaging on the therapeutic management of primary and recurrent pancreatic ductal adenocarcinomas. J Nucl Med 2021;62(6):779–86.

91. Breitenstein S, Apestegui C, Clavien PA. Positron emission tomography (PET) for cholangiocarcinoma. HPB (Oxford) 2008;10(2):120–1.

92. Lee Y, Yoo IR, Boo SH, et al. The role of F-18 FDG PET/CT in intrahepatic cholangiocarcinoma. Nucl Med Mol Imaging 2017;51(1):69–78.

93. Olthof SC, Othman A, Clasen S, et al. Imaging of cholangiocarcinoma. Visc Med 2016;32(6):402–10.

94. Annunziata S, Caldarella C, Pizzuto DA, et al. Diagnostic accuracy of fluorine-18-fluorodeoxyglucose positron emission tomography in the evaluation of the primary tumor in patients with cholangiocarcinoma: a meta-analysis. Biomed Res Int 2014; 2014:247693.

95. Seo S, Hatano E, Higashi T, et al. Fluorine-18 fluorodeoxyglucose positron emission tomography predicts lymph node metastasis, P-glycoprotein expression, and recurrence after resection in mass-forming intrahepatic cholangiocarcinoma. Surgery 2008;143:769–77.

96. Jadvar H, Henderson RW, Conti PS. [F-18]fluorodeoxyglucose positron emission tomography and positron emission tomography: computed tomography in recurrent and metastatic cholangiocarcinoma. J Comput Assist Tomogr 2007;31:223–8.

97. Kim JY, Kim MH, Lee TY, et al. Clinical role of 18F-FDG PET-CT in suspected and potentially operable cholangiocarcinoma: a prospective study compared with conventional imaging. Am J Gastroenterol 2008;103:1145–51.

98. Anderson CD, Rice MH, Pinson CW, et al. Fluorodeoxyglucose PET imaging in the evaluation of gallbladder carcinoma and cholangiocarcinoma. J Gastrointest Surg 2004;8:90–7.

99. Park TG, Yu YD, Park BJ, et al. Implication of lymph node metastasis detected on 18F-FDG PET/CT for surgical planning in patients with peripheral intrahepatic cholangiocarcinoma. Clin Nucl Med 2014; 39:1–7.

100. Kim YJ, Yun M, Lee WJ, et al. Usefulness of 18F-FDG PET in intrahepatic cholangiocarcinoma. Eur J Nucl Med Mol Imaging 2003;30:1467–72.

101. Jo I, Won KS, Kim SH, et al. Catheter tract implantation metastasis diagnosed by F-18 FDG PET/CT after percutaneous transhepatic biliary drainage for hilar cholangiocarcinoma. Nucl Med Mol Imaging 2014;48:326–7.

102. Fritscher-Ravens A, Bohuslavizki KH, Broering DC, et al. FDG PET in the diagnosis of hilar cholangiocarcinoma. Nucl Med Commun 2001;22:1277–85.

103. Onal C, Topuk S, Yapar AF, et al. Comparison of computed tomography- and positron emission tomography-based radiotherapy planning in cholangiocarcinoma. Onkologie 2013;36:484–90.

104. Mekeel K, Hemming A. Surgical management of gallbladder carcinoma: a review. J Gastrointest Surg 2007;11:1188–93.

105. Pawlik T, Gleisner A, Vigano L, et al. Incidence of finding residual disease for incidental gallbladder carcinoma: implications for re-resection. J Gastrointest Surg 2007;11:1478–86.

106. Butte JM, Redondo F, Waugh E, et al. The role of PET-CT in patients with incidental gallbladder cancer. HPB (Oxford) 2009;11(7):585–91.

107. Annunziata S, Pizzuto DA, Caldarella C, et al. Diagnostic accuracy of fluorine-18-fluorodeoxyglucose positron emission tomography in gallbladder cancer: a meta-analysis. World J Gastroenterol 2015; 21(40):11481–8.

108. RCP and the Royal College of Radiologists (RCR). Evidence-based indications for the use of PET-CT in the UK. 2016

109. Ramos-Font C, Gómez-Rio M, Rodríguez-Fernández A, et al. Ability of FDG-PET/CT in the detection of gallbladder cancer. J Surg Oncol 2014;109(3):218–24.

110. Goel S, Aggarwal A, Iqbal A, et al. 18-FDG PET-CT should be included in preoperative staging of gall bladder cancer. Eur J Surg Oncol 2020;9(01):1711–6.

111. Maldjian PD, Ghesani N, Ahmed S, et al. Adenomyomatosis of the gallbladder: another cause for a "hot" gallbladder on 18F-FDG PET. AJR Am J Roentgenol 2007;189(1):W36–8.

# Molecular Imaging Assessment of Androgen Deprivation Therapy in Prostate Cancer

Hossein Jadvar, MD, PhD, MPH, MBA[a,b,*], Patrick M. Colletti, MD[a]

## KEYWORDS

• Prostate • Hormone • Androgen • Imaging • Choline • Fluciclovine • PSMA • FDG

## KEY POINTS

- Hormonal manipulation is central in management of prostate cancer.
- It is important to understand the effect of androgen deprivation therapy on PET imaging with various radiotracers.
- Prospective studies are needed to characterize the dynamic behavior of ADT on imaging and how it can be leveraged optimally.

Prostate cancer is a prevalent disease. In the Unites States in 2021, the estimated new cases of and estimated deaths from prostate cancer are 248,530 (13.1% of all new cancers) and 34,130 (5.6% of cancer deaths), respectively. The lifetime risk of developing prostate cancer is 12.5% (1 in 8).[1] Prostate cancer is a remarkably heterogenous disease. However, the many strides in understanding the complex biology of prostate cancer and the development of novel diagnostic tools and therapeutic regimens have contributed to decline in age-adjusted rates for new prostate cancer cases by an annual average of 3.1% and age-adjusted death rates by an annual average of 1.8% when compared with the data during 2009 to 2018 decade.

## ANDROGEN AND PROSTATE CANCER

Prostate gland biology is intimately intertwined with the androgen signaling axis that includes effectors (eg, testosterone, dihydrotestosterone), and response elements including the androgen receptor (AR). The interaction between the androgens and the AR leads to nuclear translocation of the receptor ensuing the binding to androgen response elements and initiating transcription of genes responsible for regulation of cellular proliferation, differentiation, and apoptosis.[2] Given the central role of the androgens in prostate pathophysiology, the androgen regulatory axis has been a key target for therapy in prostate cancer.[3,4] Huggins and Hodges were first to note that patients with symptomatic metastatic prostate cancer benefit from androgen deprivation therapy (ADT).[5] Charles B. Huggins received the Nobel Prize in Physiology or Medicine in 1966 for his initial discovery of the hormonal control of prostate cancer in 1941.

In the postprostate-specific antigen (PSA) screening era, most prostate cancers at initial diagnosis are localized and androgen dependent (castrate sensitive). Depending on the stage and grade of the disease and, if applicable, the type of primary definitive therapy, ADT may be used to reduce serum androgens and induce AR inhibition at some point along the treatment course of

For inclusion in: PET Clinics: FDG vs. non-FDG Tracers in Less Explored Domains: An Appraisal (Basu S, Kumar R, Alavi A – eds.)

[a] Division of Nuclear Medicine, Department of Radiology, USC Keck School of Medicine, University of Southern California, Los Angeles, CA, USA; [b] Kenneth Norris Jr. Comprehensive Cancer Center, University of Southern California, Los Angeles, CA, USA

* Corresponding author. 2250 Alcazar Street, CSC 102, Los Angeles, CA.

E-mail address: jadvar@med.usc.edu

the man with prostate cancer, including both the castrate-sensitive and the castrate-resistant phases of the disease. ADT may be accomplished surgically (orchiectomy) or medically through several medications. Medical castration includes luteinizing hormone-releasing hormone (or gonadotropin releasing hormone) agonists or antagonists that affect the testicles, drugs that block adrenal gland sourcing of androgens (eg, abiraterone acetate blocking CYP17 enzyme, ketoconazole), and AR antagonists (eg, first-generation antiandrogens including flutamide, bicalutamide, and nilutamide and second-generation antiandrogens including enzalutamide, apalutamide, and darolutamide). There remain some debates with regard to ADT in prostate cancer including early versus late, intermittent versus continuous, and combined blockade treatments.

## ANDOGEN DEPRIVATION THERAPY AND [18]F-FLUORODEOXYGLUCOSE

PET with 18F-fluorodeoxyglucose (FDG) is standard-of-care imaging in many cancers for staging, restaging, treatment response evaluation, and prognostication. In prostate cancer, FDG PET is most relevant in patients with metastatic disease.[6] The number and hypermetabolism of metastatic lesions are predictive of time to hormonal treatment failure in castrate-sensitive and of overall survival in castrate-resistant disease.[7–10] FDG PET/computed tomography (CT) may have utility in (1) patients with biochemical recurrence and negative prostate-specific membrane antigen (PSMA) PET/CT[11] and (2) stratification of patients before receiving PSMA-targeted radioligand therapy.[12,13] Extent of discordant FDG-positive and PSMA-negative metastatic lesions may also be predictive of limited response to PSMA radioligand therapy and poor prognosis.[14,15]

In preclinical models of prostate cancer, Wang and colleagues showed that FDG accumulation was higher in castrate-resistant than in castrate-sensitive tumors and that GLUT1 was an AR target.[16] The metabolic reprogramming with AR re/activation and antagonism drives progression to castration resistance with high tumoral FDG uptake, which is further enhanced with the loss of AR signaling and neuroendocrine dedifferentiation.[17,18] The effect of ADT on tumoral FDG uptake has been investigated. Emond and colleagues showed that FDG uptake was lower in xenograft tumors implanted in nude mice after surgical castration compared with those tumors implanted in noncastrated animals.[19] Other investigators have shown similar results demonstrating the

modulatory effect of androgen on FDG uptake in prostate tumors.[20,21] Jadvar and colleagues showed that FDG PET may be useful in the imaging evaluation of response to ADT using murine-implanted androgen-sensitive CWR22 and androgen-independent PC-3 xenografts.[22] The preclinical findings of ADT suppressive effect on tumor glucose utilization have also been observed clinically in patients with decline in FDG uptake in both the primary and the metastatic tumor sites 1 to 5 months after initiation of ADT[23] (Fig. 1).

## ANDROGEN DEPRIVATION THERAPY AND RADIOLABELED CHOLINE

There are numerous studies including systematic reviews and meta-analyses that have demonstrated the utility of radiolabeled (with 11C or 18F) choline in the imaging evaluation of patients with prostate cancer, particularly in the clinical setting of biochemical recurrence.[24–27] In fact, in some parts of the world, radiolabeled choline is currently routinely used, although this is not the case in the United States in view of the availability and accessibility logistics and reimbursement issues and despite the regulatory approval of 11C-choline for evaluation of biochemical recurrence.

The effect of ADT on choline uptake in prostate tumor has been investigated in several studies (Fig. 2).[28] One study showed that ADT decreases the visual contouring of the boost intraprostatic tumor volume at the time of dose painting for radiotherapy, and therefore for this purpose, choline PET/CT should be performed before ADT.[29] Evangelista and colleagues reported similar findings in the neoadjuvant ADT setting and observed a significant decline in maximum standardized uptake value and metabolic tumor volume in the prostate tumor with ADT (5.34 vs 7.72, and 3.66 vs 6.86 cm3, respectively, both $P < 0.05$).[30] Similar to these 2 reports that were performed in the castrate-sensitive setting, the Italian investigators confirmed that ADT induces a decline in tumor uptake in the castrate-sensitive patients.[31] After a literature review, Dost and colleagues also concluded that in order to prevent false-negative findings, ADT should be withheld before choline PET/CT in hormone-naïve patients.[32] In contrast, a retrospective investigation of biochemically recurrent castrate-resistant patients concluded that ADT does not negatively influence the detection rate of choline PET/CT, and therefore, in the castrate-resistant setting it is unnecessary to withdraw ADT before PET/CT.[33] Beheshti and colleagues reported similar findings in a prospective study in that ADT did not impair choline uptake in castrate-resistant tumors.[34]

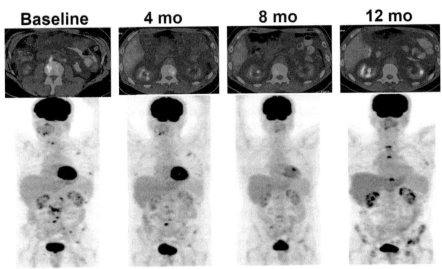

**Fig. 1.** This 70-year-old man with mCSPC (PSA 43.6 ng/mL) was treated with ADT. Sequential 18F-FDG PET/CT examinations demonstrated multifocal stable and improving lesion concordant with decline in serum PSA level from baseline to 8-month time frame. At 12 months, there were new lesions with increasing serum PSA level, and the patient transitioned from CS to CR state and was subsequently treated with docetaxel chemotherapy.

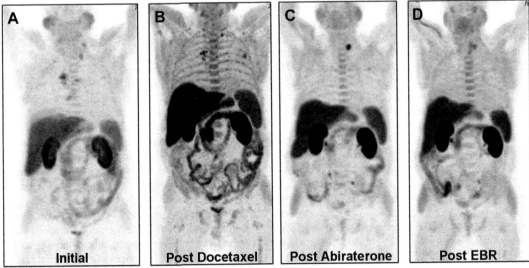

**Fig. 2.** This 62-year-old man had Gleason score of 4 + 4 and pT3b N1(8/24)Mx cancer. Initial PSA was 18 ng/mL. He was treated with RP. BCR occurred 8 months after RP, and ADT was administered. After 26 months, he developed CRPC (PSA, 14 ng/mL; PSA doubling time, 3.2 months). (*A*) 11C-choline PET/CT (maximum-intensity-projection [MIP] images) showed positive lymph nodes in paratracheal region and left supraclavicular lymph node, and docetaxel was administered. (*B*) Subsequent 11C-choline PET/CT (MIP images) showed progression of disease (in mediastinal lymph nodes and third left rib) despite PSA response (PSA, 10 ng/mL). He was given abiraterone; PSA response occurred after 6 mo (PSA, 4 ng/mL). (*C*) 11C-choline PET/CT (MIP images) showed response of mediastinal lymph nodes and rib but increased uptake in supraclavicular lymph node. (*D*) He was given metastasis-directed external-beam radiotherapy; PSA response (PSA, 1 ng/mL) and partial response on 11C-choline PET/CT (MIP images) occurred. (*From* Ceci F, Castellucci P, Mapelli P, et al. Evaluation of prostate cancer with 11C-choline PET/CT for treatment planning, response assessment, and prognosis. J Nucl Med. 2016; 57(suppl):49S–54S; with permission.)

## ANDROGEN DEPRIVATION THERAPY AND [18]F-FLUCICLOVINE

18F-fluciclovine is a synthetic amino acid analogue PET radiotracer that has been approved for the imaging evaluation of men with suspected BCR of prostate cancer after definitive primary therapy. Numerous studies have demonstrated the competitive advantage of 18F-fluciclovine PET/CT over conventional imaging (bone scan, contrast-enhanced abdomen, and pelvis CT) with significant implications on subsequent management strategy.[35–37] The LOCATE trial was a prospective multicenter US trial designed to assess the impact of 18F-fluciclovine PET/CT in men with BCR after primary therapy with curative intent.[38] This trial involved 213 patients with a median PSA level of 1.00 ng/mL and negative or equivocal findings on conventional imaging. Overall, 59% of patients had a change in management informed by PET/CT (25% from salvage or systemic therapy to watchful waiting, 24% from systemic therapy to salvage therapy, and 9% from salvage therapy to systemic therapy). The UK site FALCON trial reported similar findings in 104 patients with BCR of prostate cancer with overall 64% postscan management change (65% salvage or systemic therapy to watchful waiting, 24% salvage therapy to systemic therapy, and 17% alternative changes to treatment modality). Moreover, 18F-fluciclovine–guided salvage therapy was associated with higher PSA response rate than those salvage therapies that did not incorporate the PET/CT findings.[39] There are currently several ongoing or planned clinical trials involving 18F-fluciclovine PET/CT in various prostate cancer clinical settings (eg, salvage radiotherapy, oligorecurrent disease, staging high-risk primary cancer).

There are only a few reports dedicated to study the influence of ADT on the tumoral 18F-fluciclovine uptake (Fig. 3). The investigation on expression levels of amino acid transporters in response to ADT has shown that LAT1 levels are relatively high in 22Rv1 castration-resistant tumors following chronic ADT, whereas ASCT2 levels are preferentially expressed in hormone-sensitive CWR22Res tumors following acute ADT.[40] The latter finding seems contrary to the results of another preclinical study that showed enhancement of ASCT2 expression level with dihydrotestosterone in AR-positive hormone-sensitive LNCaP cells.[41] The clinical implication of these preclinical findings warrants additional studies. A prospective single-center study in the clinical setting of staging newly diagnosed high-risk prostate cancer has also reported decreased 18F-fluciclovine uptake in the primary lesion and the suspicious metastatic nodes following ADT.[42]

## ANDROGEN DEPRIVATION THERAPY AND RADIOLABELED PROSTATE-SPECIFIC MEMBRANE ANTIGEN AGENTS

Radiolabeled small molecular inhibitors of the external moiety of the PSMA have improved the imaging evaluation of all phases of prostate cancer in substantive way over conventional imaging and other approved molecular imaging agents including radiolabeled choline and 18F-fluciclovine.[43–45] The increasing clinical interest in PSMA theranostics has led to a relatively large number of clinical trials in various clinical settings (eg, proPSMA, PRIMARY, LIGHTHOUSE, OSPREY, CONDOR, SPOTLIGHT, etc.).[46] Recently, the US Food and Drug Administration approved 68Ga-PSMA-11 (available at the University of California, San Francisco, and the University of California, Los Angles) and 18F-DCFPyL (national availability) for imaging evaluation of men with suspected metastasis who are candidates for initial definitive therapy and for suspected recurrence based on elevated serum PSA level. It is anticipated that PSMA PET imaging will be incorporated into clinical guidelines that will have significant ramifications on clinical practice.[46,47] Likewise, with the recent favorable results of the VISION trial, the theranostic pair, 177Lu-PSMA-617, will likely be on its way to regulatory approval for targeted radioligand therapy for metastatic castrate-resistant prostate cancer.[48]

The effect of ADT on PSMA expression is relatively complex and may depend on therapy duration and tumor type (castrate sensitive vs castrate resistant). A preclinical investigation of a panel of implanted AR-positive prostate cancer cell lines showed that PSMA expression is suppressed by androgens, whereas androgen deprivation increases PSMA expression as evidenced by PET imaging with 64Cu-J591.[49] In a recent study, enzalutamide (an AR antagonist) induced an increase in PSMA expression in the androgen-independent 22Rv1 xenograft tumor.[50] Similar findings have been reported with C4-2 human castrate-resistant prostate cancer xenografts displaying up to 2.3-fold increase in PSMA expression when subjected to enzalutamide treatment.[51] Hope and colleagues reported a 1.5- to 2.0-fold increase in PSMA uptake in castrate-sensitive LNCaP-AR xenografts with ARN-509 AR inhibition.[52] They also observed 7-fold higher PSMA uptake in tumor sites in one patient with castrate-sensitive prostate cancer after receiving 4 weeks of ADT compared with baseline before ADT. In contrast to these observations, an in-vitro study of hormonally sensitive LNCaP cells when subjected to continuous ADT demonstrated significant downregulation in both AR and PSMA

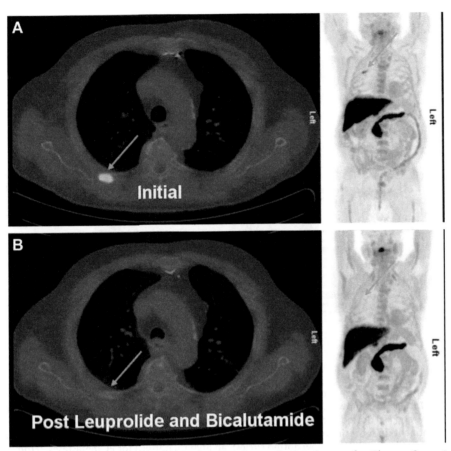

**Fig. 3.** This 78-year-old man presented with BCR 2 years after radiation therapy for Gleason 9 prostate cancer, with initial PSA of 9 ng/mL. After radiation therapy PSA nadir was 1.43 ng/mL. At the time of first scan (*A*), his PSA was elevated to 4.34 ng/mL. This initial scan demonstrated a CT negative right fifth rib with positive 18F-fluciclovine uptake in and scattered bilateral pulmonary nodules (not shown). After his first 18F-fluciclovine PET/CT scan, he was placed on hormonal therapy (Leuprolide acetate [Lupron] and Abiroterone Acetate [Zytiga]). PSA level during follow-up scan was 0.05 ng/mL. Follow-up scan (*B*) showed complete resolution of all lesions with a residual sclerotic lesion at the rib with no focal tracer uptake. (*Courtesy of* E Bulbul, MD, and B Savir-Baruch, MD, Maywood, IL.)

levels.[53] Roy and colleagues showed that in a patient-derived xenograft mouse model using 18F-DCFPyL, there were heterogeneity of responses to ADT.[54]

Mathy and colleagues demonstrated that in androgen-sensitive LNCaP cells, abiraterone acetate upregulates PSMA expression but blocks PSA secretion.[55] Another study found that regardless of hormone sensitivity of the tumor, ongoing ADT was not significant in high detection rate of lesions in patients with metastatic disease, even in very low PSA levels less than 1 ng/mL.[56] This notion was supported by another study in the clinical setting of BCR after primary curative therapy that indeed the detection rate of tumor recurrence was higher in the group with ADT (within 6 months before imaging) and recommended that withdrawal of ADT before PSMA PET imaging would

be unnecessary.[57] In contrast, in nonmetastatic hormone-naïve neoadjuvant clinical setting, Onal and colleagues showed that ADT leads to significant decrease in serum PSA and PSMA uptake in both the primary tumor and in nonconfirmed but suspect metastatic lymph nodes.[58] Similarly, a retrospective study of 21 therapy-naive patients with oligometastatic disease showed that long-term (range 61–289 days) ADT resulted in decline in lesion count compared with baseline before ADT.[59] However, new lesions on PSMA PET following ADT (bipolar or with abiraterone/enzalutamide) in the clinical setting of mCRPC seemed to be suspect for progression of disease[60–62] (**Fig. 4**). Another study suggested that simply early increases in lesion PSMA uptake, both in the castrate-sensitive and castrate-resistant settings, may indicate a flare effect.[63]

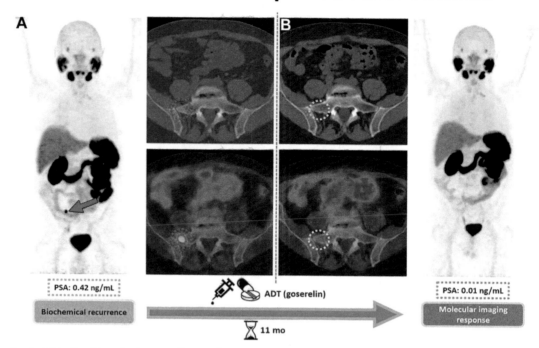

**Fig. 4.** BCR after RP and salvage radiation therapy (performed 15 and 13 years before PET/CT, respectively). (*A*) 68Ga-PSMA PET/CT images show PSMA-avid right sacral bone metastasis with a corresponding sclerotic lesion on CT (red *arrow* and red dotted circles). (*B*) Response assessment 68Ga-PSMA PET/CT images obtained 11 months later, after treatment with continuous ADT, show complete molecular and biochemical responses. However, the bone lesion became less sclerotic (yellow dotted circles), an atypical pattern for PC metastases. (*From* Barbosa FG, Queiroz MA, Ferraro DA, et al. Prostate specific Membrane Antigen PET: Therapy Response Assessment in Metastatic Prostate Cancer. Radiographics 2020; 40(5):1412 – 1430; with permission.)

In summary, the current evidence suggests heterogeneity of PSMA expression response to androgen blockade, although overall it seems that short-term ADT (2–6 weeks) may enhance PSMA expression (flare) regardless of tumor type (castrate sensitive vs castrate resistant), whereas long-term ADT (12 weeks to 7 months) reduces the level of PSMA expression, probably as a consequence of both PSMA downregulation and cell death.[64–66] The temporal effect of ADT on PSMA expression may then need to be considered at the time of PSMA PET imaging for both appropriate interpretation and also potentially as leverage before PSMA radioligand therapy.

centered over various methods of androgen signaling blockade. In this clinical setting, then it is important to understand how androgens and ADT affect the tumor uptake of new-generation imaging agents. ADT typically decreases the uptake of metabolic tracers such as FDG, radiolabeled choline, and fluciclovine, whereas the effect on the expression of transmembrane proteins such as PSMA is more complex and may depend on the tumor biology and the time of imaging after the start of ADT. Additional prospective studies are needed to understand this dynamic behavior and how it may be leveraged optimally for imaging and for radioligand therapy.

## SUMMARY

Androgens, whether sourced from the testes, adrenal glands, or from within the prostate tumor sites, play important role in the pathogenesis of prostate cancer. Since the momentous discovery of Huggins that hormonal manipulation can affect the prostate tumor biological behavior, a central theme in the clinical management of prostate cancer has

## CLINICS CARE POINTS

- Hormonal therapy is a common management strategy in prostate cancer.
- Androgen axis therapies may impact the imgaing evaluation of prostate cancer.

## DISCLOSURE

HJ is on the advisory board of Radiomedix, Inc., a consultant to Blue Earth Diagnostics, on speaker's bureau for Lantheus, and is an investigator with ImaginAb, all unrelated to this submission.

## ACKNOWLEDGMENTS

H. Jadvar was supported in part by grants R01-CA111613, R21-CA142426, R21-EB017568, and P30-CA014089 from the U.S. National Institutes of Health.

## REFERENCES

1. Cancer stat facts: prostate cancer. Available at. https://seer.cancer.gov/statfacts/html/prost.html. Accessed August 21, 2021.
2. Heinlein CA, Chang C. Androgen receptor in prostate cancer. Endocr Rev 2004;25:276–308.
3. Senapati D, Kumari S, Heemers HV. Androgen receptor c0-regulation in prostate cancer. Asian J Urol 2020;7:219–32.
4. Aurilio G, Cimadamore A, Mazzuccheelli R, et al. Androgen receptor signaling pathway in prostate cancer: from genetics to clinical applications. Cells 2020;9:2653.
5. Huggins C, Hodges CU. Studies on prostate cancer. I. The effect of castration, of estrogen and of androgen injection on serum phosphatases in metastatic carcinoma of the prostate. Cancer Res 1941;1:293.
6. Jadvar H. Imaging of prostate cancer with 18F-fluorodeoxyglucose PET/CT: utility and limitations. Eur J Nucl Med Mol Imaging 2013;40(Suppl 1):S5–10.
7. Jadvar H, Velez EM, Desai B, et al. Prediction of time to hormonal treatment failure in metastatic castration-sensitive prostate cancer with 18F-FDG PET/CT. J Nucl Med 2019;60:1524–30.
8. Jadvar H, Desai B, Ji L, et al. Baseline 18F_FDG PET/CT parameters as imaging biomarkers of overall survival in castrate-resistant metastatic prostate cancer. J Nucl Med 2013;54:1195–201.
9. Velez EM, Desai B, Ji L, et al. Comparative prognostic implication of treatment response assessments in mCRPC: PERCIST 1.0, RECIST 1.1, and PSA response criteria. Theranostics 2020;10:3254–62.
10. Fox JJ, Gavane SC, Balnc-Autran E, et al. Positron emission tomography/computed tomography-based assessments of androgen receptor expression and glycolytic activity as a prognostic biomarker for metastatic castration-resistant prostate cancer. JAMA Oncol 2018;4:217–24.
11. Chen R, Wang Y, Zhu Y, et al. The added value of 18F-FDG PET/CT compared to 68Ga-PSMA PET/CT in patients with castration-resistant prostate cancer. J Nucl Med 2021. [Epub ahead of print].
12. Thang SP, Violet J, Sandhu S, et al. Poor outcomes for patients with metastatic castration-resistant prostate cancer with low prostate-specific membrane antigen (PSMA) expression deemed ineligible for 177Lu-labelled PSMA radioligand therapy. Eur Urol Oncol 2019;2:670–6.
13. Chen R, Wang Y, Shi Y, et al. Diagnostic value 18F-FDG PET/CT in patients with biochemical recurrent prostate cancer and negative 68Ga-PSMA PET/CT. Eur J Nucl Med Mol Imaging 2021;48:2970–7.
14. Shen K, Liu B, Zhou Z, et al. The evolving role of 18F-FDG PET/CT in diagnosis and prognosis prediction in progressive prostate cancer. Front Oncol 2021;29(11):683793.
15. Baucknheht M, Bertagna F, Donegani MI, et al. The prognostic power of 18F_FDG PET/CT extends to estimating systemic treatment response duration in metastatic castration-resistant prostate cancer patients. Prostate Cancer Prostatic Dis 2021;24(4):1198–207. [Epub ahead of print].
16. Wang J, Xu W, Wang B, et al. GLUT1 is an AR target contributing to tumor growth and glycolysis in castration-resistant and enzalutamide-resistant prostate cancer. Cancer Lett 2020;485:45–55.
17. Uo T, Sprenger C, Plymate SR. Androgen receptor signaling and metabolic and cellular plasticity during progression to castration resistant prostate cancer. Front Oncol 2020;10:580617.
18. Bakht MK, Lovinski JM, Tubman J, et al. Differential expression of glucose transporters and hexokinases in prostate cancer with a neuroendocrine gene signature: a mechanistic perspective for 18F-FDG imaging of PSMA-suppressed tumors. J Nucl Med 2020;61:904–10.
19. Emonds KM, Swinnen J, Lerut E, et al. Evaluation of androgen-induced effects on the uptake of 18F-FDG, 11C-choline, and 11C-acetate in an androgen-sensitive and androgen-independent prostate cancer xenograft model. EJNMMI Res 2013;3:31.
20. Kukuk D, Reischl G, Raguin O, et al. Assessment of PET tracer uptake in hormone-independent and hormone-dependent xenograft prostate cancer models. J Nucl Med 2011;52:1654–63.
21. Emonds KM, Swinnen JV, van Weerden W, et al. Do androgens control the uptake of 18F-FDG, 11C-acetate in human prostate cancer cell lines? Eur J Nucl Med Mol Imaging 2011;38:1842–53.
22. Jadvar H, Xiankui L, Shahinian A, et al. Glucose metabolism of human prostate cancer mouse xenografts. Mol Imaging 2005;4:91–7.
23. Oyama N, Akino H, Suzuki Y, et al. FDG PET for evaluating the change of glucose metabolism in prostate cancer after androgen ablation. Nucl Med Commun 2001;22:963–99.

24. Fanti S, Minozzi S, catellucci P, et al. PET/CT with 11C-choline for evaluation of prostate cancer patients with biochemical recurrence: meta-analysis and critical review of available data. Eur J Nucl Med Mol Imaging 2016;43:55–69.

25. Von Eyben FE, Kairemo K. Meta-analysis of 11C-choline and 18F-choline PET/CT for management of patients with prostate cancer. Nucl Med Commun 2014;35:221–30.

26. Evangelista L, Guttilla A, Zattoni F, et al. Utility of choline positron emission tomography/computed tomography for lymph node involvement identification in intermediate-to high-risk prostate cancer: a systematic literature review and meta-analysis. Eur Urol 2013;63:1040–8.

27. Zattoni F, Ravelli I, Rensi M, et al. 10-year clinical experience with 18F0choline PET/CT: an Italian multicenter retrospective assessment of 3343 patients. Clin Nucl Med 2020;45:594–603.

28. Ceci F, Castellucci P, Mapelli P, et al. Evaluation of prostate cancer with 11C-choline PET/CT for treatment planning, response assessment, and prognosis. J Nucl Med 2016;57(suppl):49S–54S.

29. Chan J, Carver A, Brunt JNH, et al. Effect of androgen deprivation therapy on intraprostatic tumor volume identified on 18F-choline PET/CT for prostate dose painting radiotherapy. Br J Radiol 2017;90:20160818.

30. Evangelista L, Zattoni F, Guttilla A, et al. The effects of androgen deprivation therapy on the 18F-choline uptake in prostate cancer patients undergoing neoadjuvant treatment. Q J Nucl Med Mol Imaging 2019;63:278–83.

31. Fuccio C, Schiavina R, Castellucci P, et al. Androgen deprivation therapy influences the uptake of 11C-choline in patients with recurrent prostate cancer: the preliminary results of a sequential PET/Ct study. Eur J Nucl Med Mol Imaging 2011;38:1985–9.

32. Dost RJ, Glaudemans AWJM, Breeuwsma AJ, et al. Influence of androgen deprivation therapy on choline PET/CT in recurrent prostate cancer. Eur J Nucl Med Mol Imaging 2013;40(Suppl 1):S41–7.

33. Chondrogiannis S, Marzola MC, Ferretti A, et al. Is the detection of 18F-choline PET/CT influenced by androgen-deprivation therapy. Eur J Nucl Med Mol Imaging 2014;41:1293–300.

34. Beheshti M, Haim S, Zakavi R, et al. Impact of 18F-choline PET/Ct in prostate cancer patients with biochemical recurrence: influence of androgen deprivation therapy and correlation with PSA kinetics. J Nucl Med 2013;54:833–40.

35. Biscontini G, Romagnolo C, Cottignoli C, et al. 18F-fluciclovine positron emission tomography in prostate cancer: a systematic review and diagnostic meta-analysis. Diagnostics (Basel) 2012;11(2):304.

36. Rais-Bahrami S, Efstathiou JA, Turnbull CM, et al. 18F-fluciclovine PET/CT performance in biochemical recurrence of prostate cancer: a systematic review. Prostate Cancer Prostatic Dis 2021;11:304. [Epub ahead of print].

37. Savir-Baruch B, Zanoni L, Schuster DM. Imaging of prostate cancer sing fluciclovine. Urol Clin North Am 2018;45:489–502.

38. Andriole GL, Kostakoglu L, Chau A, et al. The impact of positron emission tomography with 18F-fluciclovine on the treatment of biochemical recurrence of prostate cancer: results from the LOCATE trial. J Urol 2019;201:322–31.

39. Scarsbrook AF, Bottomley D, Teoh EJ, et al. Effect of 18F-fluciclovine positron emission tomography on the management of patients with recurrence of prostate cancer: results from the FALCON trial. Int J Radiat Oncol Biol Phys 2020;10:316–24.

40. Malviya G, Patel R, Salji M, et al. 18F-fluciclovine PET metabolic imaging reveals prostate cancer tumor heterogeneity associated with disease resistance to androgen deprivation. EJNMMI Res 2020;10:143.

41. Okudaira H, Oka S, Ono M, et al. Accumulation of trans-1-amino-3-18F-flurocyclobutanecarboxylic acid in prostate cancer due to androgen-induced expression of amino acid transporters. Mol Imaging Biol 2014;16:756–64.

42. Galagno SJ, McDonald AM, Rais-Bahrami S, et al. Utility of 18F-fluciclovine PET/MRI for staging newly diagnosed high-risk prostate cancer and evaluating response to initial androgen deprivation therapy: a prospective single-arm pilot study. AJR Am J Roentgenol 2021;217(3):720–9. [Epub ahead of print].

43. Lawhn-Heath C, Salavti A, Behr SC, et al. Prostate-specific membrane antigen PET in prostate cancer. Radiology 2021;299:248–60.

44. Hernes E, Revheim ME, Hole KH, et al. Prostate-specific membrane antigen PET for assessment of primary and recurrent prostate cancer with histopathology as reference standard: a systematic review and meta-analysis. PET Clin 2021;16:147–65.

45. Wang R, Shen G, Huang M, et al. The diagnostic role of 18F-choline, 18F-fluciclovine and 18F-PSMA PET/CT in the detection of prostate cancer with biochemical recurrence: a meta-analysis. Front Oncol 2021;11:684629.

46. Jadvar H. Competitive advantage of PSMA theranostics in prostate cancer. Radiology 2021;299:261–3.

47. Trabulsi EJ, Rumble RB, Jadvar H, et al. Optimum imaging strategies for advanced prostate cancer: ASCO guideline. J Clin Oncol 2020;38:1963–96.

48. Sartor O, de Bono J, Chi KN, et al. Leutetium-177-PSMA-617 for metastatic castration-resistant prostate cancer. N Engl J Med 2021;385(12):1091–103. [Epub ahead of print].

49. Evans MJ, Smith-Jones PM, Wongvipat J, et al. Noninvasive measurement of androgen receptor

signaling with a positron-emitting radiopharmaceutical that targets prostate-specific membrane antigen. Proc Natl Acad Sci USA 2011;108:9578–82.

50. Stanicszweska M, Costa PF, Eiber M, et al. Enzalutamide enhances PSMA expression of PSMA-low prostate cancer. Int J Mol Sci 2021;22:7431.

51. Luckerath K, Wei L, Fendler WP, et al. Preclinical evaluation of PSMA expression in response to androgen receptor blockade for theranostics in prostate cancer. EJNMMI Res 2018;8:96.

52. Hope TA, Truillet C, Ehman EC, et al. 68Ga-PSMA-11 PET imaging of response to androgen inhibition: first human experience. J Nucl Med 2017;58:81–4.

53. Liu T, Wu LY, Futon MD, et al. Prolonged androgen deprivation leads to downregulation of androgen receptor and prostate-specific membrane antigen in prostate cancer cells. Int J Oncol 2012;41:2087–92.

54. Roy J, White ME, Basuli F, et al. Monitoring PSMA responses to ADT in prostate cancer patient-derived xenograft mouse models using 18F-DCFPyL PET imaging. Mol Imaging Biol 2021;23(5):745–55. [Epub ahead of print].

55. Mathy CS, Mayr T, Kurpig S, et al. Antihormone treatment differentially regulates PSA secretion, PSMA expression and 68Ga-PSMA uptake in LNCaP cells. J Cancer Res Clin Oncol 2021;147:1733–43.

56. Fassbind S, Ferraro D, Stelmes J-J, et al. Ga-PSMA-11 PET imaging in patients with ongoing androgen deprivation therapy for advanced prostate cancer. Ann Nucl Med 2021;5(10):1109–16. [Epub ahead of print].

57. Bumberg J, Beckl M, Dierks A, et al. Detection rate of 68Ga-PSMA ligand PET/CT in patients with recurrent prostate cancer and androgen deprivation therapy. Biomedicines 2020;8:511.

58. Onal C, Guler OC, Torun N, et al. The effect of androgen deprivation therapy on 68Ga-PSMA tracer uptake in non-metastatic prostate cancer patients. Eur J Nucl Med Mol Imaging 2020;47:632–41.

59. Hoberuck S, Lock S, Winzer R, et al. 68Ga-PSMA-11 PET before and after initial long-term androgen deprivation in patients with newly diagnosed prostate cancer: a retrospective single-center study. EJNMMI Res 2020;10:135.

60. Zukotynski KA, Emmenegger U, Hotte S, et al. Prospective, single-arm trial evaluating changes in uptake patterns on prostate-specific membrane antigen (PSMA)-targeted 18F-DCFPyL PET/CT in patients with castration-resistant prostate cancer starting abiraterone or enzalutamide. J Nucl Med 2021;62(10):1430–7. [Epub ahead of print].

61. Markowski MC, Velho PI, Eisenberger MA, et al. Detection of early progression with 18F-DCFPyL PET/CT in men with metastatic castration-resistant prostate cancer receiving bipolar androgen therapy. J Nucl Med 2021;62(9):1270–3. [Epub ahead of print].

62. Barbosa FG, Queiroz MA, Ferraro DA, et al. Prostate specific membrane antigen PET: therapy response assessment in metastatic prostate cancer. Radiographics 2020;40(5):1412–30.

63. Aggarwal R, Wei X, Kim W, et al. Heterogeneous flare in prostate-specific membrane antigen positron emission tomography tracer uptake with initiation of androgen pathway blockade in metastatic prostate cancer. Eur Urol Oncol 2018;1:78–82.

64. Afshar-Oromieh A, Debus N, Uhrig M. Impact of long-term androgen deprivation therapy on PSMA ligand PET/CT in patients with castration-sensitive prostate cancer. Eur J Nucl Med Mol Imaging 2018;45:2045–54.

65. Emmett L, Yin C, Crumbaker M. Rapid modulation of PSMA expression by androgen deprivation: serial 68Ga-PSMA-11 PET in men with hormone-sensitive and castrate-resistant prostate cancer commencing androgen blockade. J Nucl Med 2019;60:950–4.

66. Vaz S, Hadaschik B, Gabriel M, et al. Influence of androgen deprivation therapy on PSMA expression and PSMA-ligand PET imaging of prostate cancer patients. Eur J Nucl Med Mol Imaging 2020;47:9–15.

# Molecular Imaging Assessment of Hormonally Sensitive Breast Cancer

## An Appraisal of 2-[18F]-Fluoro-2-Deoxy-Glucose and Newer Non-2-[18F]-Fluoro-2-Deoxy-Glucose PET Tracers

Divya Yadav, MD[a], Rakesh Kumar, MBBS, DRM, DNB, MNAMS, PhD[b],*,
Ankita Phulia, MBBS[c], Sandip Basu, MBBS, DRM, DNB, MNAMS[d,e],
Abass Alavi, MD[f]

KEYWORDS

• FDG • FES • Estrogen receptor imaging • Progesterone receptor imaging • Breast cancer

## KEY POINTS

- 2-[18F]-Fluoro-2-deoxy-glucose-PET/computed tomography scans provide valuable information about tumor metabolism and remain a cornerstone modality for staging, response assessment, and prognostication in all breast malignancies.
- 16α-[18F]-fluoro-17β-estradiol and [18F]-fluoro-furanyl-norprogesterone are specific PET tracers targeting hormonal receptors like estrogen and progesterone receptor expression in breast cancer.
- 16α-[18F]-fluoro-17β-estradiol and [18F]-fluoro-furanyl-norprogesterone can provide in vivo information about heterogeneity of receptor status and predictive information regarding endocrine resistance.
- Further application of molecular PET imaging with 16α-[18F]-fluoro-17β-estradiol and 2-[18F]-Fluoro-2-deoxy-glucose can optimize their clinical potential in characterizing the tumor and thereby guiding patient management.

## INTRODUCTION

Molecular imaging with PET has undoubtedly revolutionized the evaluation of in vivo biological processes. 2-[18F]-Fluoro-2-deoxy-glucose (FDG) PET imaging tracks glucose metabolism in both physiologic and pathologic states, for example, cancer cells. The role of FDG-PET in staging and response assessment is well documented in breast cancer.[1,2] Determination of the hormonal receptor status including estrogen receptor (ER), progesterone receptor (PR) positivity and Human epidermal growth factor receptor-2 (HER2) HER2-neu (ERB-B2 gene) expression provides valuable diagnostic, therapeutic, and prognostic information for breast cancer. Patients wit hormonally sensitive breast cancer with hormone receptor-positivity (ER/PR+) will benefit from endocrine

[a] MD Anderson Cancer Center, University of Texas, Houston, TX, USA; [b] Division of Diagnostic Nuclear Medicine, Department of Nuclear Medicine, All India Institute of Medical Sciences, Ansari Nagar, New Delhi 110029, India; [c] Maulana Azad Medical College, New Delhi, 110002, India; [d] Radiation Medicine Centre (B.A.R.C), Tata Memorial Centre Annexe, Parel, Mumbai; [e] Homi Bhabha National Institute, Mumbai, India; [f] Department of Radiology, Hospital of the University of Pennsylvania, Philadelphia, PA, USA
* Corresponding author. Division of Diagnostic Nuclear Medicine, Department of Nuclear Medicine, All India Institute of Medical Sciences, Ansari Nagar, New Delhi 110029, India.
E-mail address: rkphulia@yahoo.com

PET Clin 17 (2022) 399–413
https://doi.org/10.1016/j.cpet.2022.04.001

therapy, whereas patients with HER2⁺ breast cancers are suitable to receive trastuzumab or other HER2-targeted therapies.[3] PET tracers targeting hormonal receptors, such as 16α-[18F]-fluoro-17β-estradiol (FES) for ER and [18F]-fluoro-furanyl-norprogesterone (FFNP) for PR imaging, can provide noninvasive receptor status assessment in patients with breast cancer. FES imaging has become a promising imaging tool in evaluating the ER status of primary as well as metastatic tumors and has recently been approved by the US Food and Drug Administration. In the current review, we have focused on the importance of PET-based molecular imaging in hormonally sensitive breast cancer.

## 2-[18F]-FLUORO-2-DEOXY-GLUCOSE-PET/computed TOMOGRAPHY SCANS

FDG has been the most popular PET tracer in oncology practice and has been used extensively in breast cancer. The metabolic information provided by FDG-PET is invaluable for staging in primary as well as recurrent breast cancer.[4–6] Although the detection of metastases across the whole of the body in a single examination is the most advocated advantage of PET, there are several other indications that can help physicians in the management of breast cancer.

### Indications

FDG-PET has a role in staging, prognostication, predicting response, and assessing response to treatment. Initial staging is critical in choosing appropriate management for breast cancer treatment. FDG has a proven role in detecting extra-axillary lymph nodal and distant metastases with high sensitivity.[7,8] FDG is useful for initial staging of breast cancer, regardless of tumor phenotype (triple negative, luminal/ER⁺ or HER2⁺) and tumor grade.[9] Along with initial staging, FDG has been proven useful in prognostication and intensity of FDG uptake has been correlated with poor prognosis.[10]

    FDG-PET can also predict response to neoadjuvant therapy and provides significant predictive value for disease recurrence, which might allow early risk stratification and may guide rational management.[11] Early response assessment is crucial in patient management in a metastatic setting. FDG-PET can detect metabolic changes that occur much earlier than change in tumor size and can provide early response assessment.[12] FDG has shown excellent performances in staging and assessing response to chemotherapy in triple negative breast cancer.[13] Although FDG uptake is lower in ER⁺/

PR⁺ tumors, FDG can still be beneficial in staging as well as in heterogeneity evaluation.[14] HER2⁺ breast tumors demonstrated upregulated glucose uptake owing to activation of the PI3K/AKT pathway. Effective HER2 blockade decreases glucose uptake and hence FDG can be useful in predicting response to anti-HER2 therapy.[15]

### Parameters Affecting 2-[18F]-Fluoro-2-Deoxy-Glucose Uptake in Breast Cancer Tumors

#### Tumor size
Smaller tumors (≤10 mm) can lead to false-negative FDG-PET results.[16]

#### Tumor grade
Low-grade tumors (grades 1 or 2) show lower FDG uptake than high-grade (grade 3) tumors.[10,16]

#### Proliferation index and markers
FDG uptake is higher in high-proliferative tumors as assessed by the Ki67 index, nuclear atypia, and mutated p53.[10]

#### Histologic subtype
FDG avidity is lower for invasive lobular carcinomas than invasive ductal carcinomas. Ductal carcinoma in situ usually shows a lower uptake compared with invasive carcinomas.[9]

#### Hormone receptor status
FDG uptake is lower in well-differentiated ER and PR–positive (ER⁺/PR⁺) tumors than ER⁻/PR⁻tumors.[10]

#### Tumor phenotype
Triple-negative tumors, that is, ER⁻/PR⁻ and having no overexpression of HER2 (ERBB2) show substantially higher standardized uptake values (SUVs) than other tumors.[17] Among luminal tumors, FDG uptake is lower in luminal A tumors than in luminal B tumors.[18]

### Limitations of 2-[18F]-Fluoro-2-Deoxy-Glucose-PET Scans

False positivity in benign inflammatory conditions is a major limitation of FDG-PET scanning, along with other false-positive results arising from invasive procedures or treatment.[7] In addition to small tumor size, the main factors limiting sensitivity of FDG in breast cancer imaging are low tumor grade, low proliferation, high expression of hormone receptors (ER⁺), and lobular histologic type.[7,11] The characterization of lung lesions and mediastinal lymph nodes on FDG alone is not easy, FES-PET scanning helps in the characterization of these lesions to a great extent (Fig. 1). FES-PET scans should be used along with FDG-PET scans in strongly ER-expressing patients for better

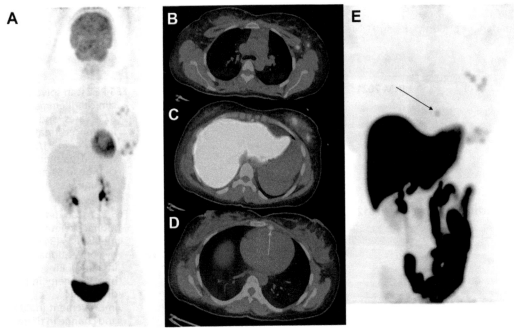

Fig. 1. A 32-year-old woman was diagnosed with left breast cancer cT2N1Mx, her left axillary lymph node biopsy revealed Invasive Ductal Carcinoma with hormonal status as ER$^+$/PR$^+$, HER2 negative. FDG and FES-PET/computed tomography (CT) scans were performed for staging and ER status evaluation. (A) An FDG maximum intensity projection (MIP) image reveals metabolically active multiple primary left breast lesions with left axillary lymph nodes metastases. ER positivity is seen in (B) left breast lesions, (C) left axillary lymph nodes, and (D) left internal mammary lymph node (marked with a *yellow arrow*). (E) Additional lesion (marked with a *black arrow*) is more noticeable on FES MIP image and seems advantageous in changing the overall stage.

specificity, evaluation of the disease extent, and impact on treatment.

## ESTROGEN RECEPTOR TRACER: 16α-[¹⁸F]-FLUORO-17β-ESTRADIOL-PET/ computed TOMOGRAPHY

Approximately 75% of breast tumors are ER$^+$, and these patients with ER$^+$ breast cancer have a better outcome with appropriate endocrine therapy. Knowledge of ER status can guide medical oncologists to individualize the management of patients with breast cancer individually.[19] The gold standard for ER status determination remains biopsy with immunohistochemical assays, and although primary breast tumors can be easily assessed, metastatic disease is often not amenable to immunohistochemical analysis. ¹⁸F-FES has a 60% to 100% relative binding affinity for the ER, which makes it suitable for noninvasive evaluation of ERs throughout the body.[20] FES uptake shows a good correlation with ER expression in primary as well as metastatic tumors, provides qualitative and quantitative assessment of multiple tumor sites simultaneously, and can predict response to endocrine therapies.[21]

The ER status of the primary tumor does not necessarily predict the ER status of metastatic lesions. The hormonal receptor heterogeneity can be seen within the primary tumor or between multiple lesions. The ability to predict a therapeutic response in distant lesions is critical in planning the treatment approach for metastatic disease. FES demonstrated a sensitivity of 0.78 (95% confidence interval, 0.65–0.88) and a specificity of 0.98 (95% confidence interval, 0.65–1.00) in a meta-analysis of metastatic lesions.[22]

### Indications for 16α-[¹⁸F]-Fluoro-17β-Estradiol Use in Breast Cancer

FES (CERIANNA)-PET tracer has been recently approved by the US Food and Drug Administration for the detection of ER$^+$ lesions as an adjunct to biopsy in patients with recurrent or metastatic breast cancer.[23] We have summarized the results of several studies published on FES-PET scans for evaluating ER status, solving clinical dilemmas, and guiding therapy in breast cancer management (**Table 1**).[24–32]

FES-PET scans can also evaluate potential receptor heterogeneity (**Fig. 2**). Yang and colleagues[28] showed that 37.5% of metastatic

**Table 1**
**Summary of publications on FES-PET/CT done for various indications**

| Author | Journal, year of Publication | Study Details | Study Purpose and Results |
|---|---|---|---|
| Boers J et al[24] | JNM 2021 | Retrospective study; 100 cases of suspected ER⁺ MBC | FES-PET scan solved the clinical dilemma in 87% cases, and influenced treatment decisions in 81/87 cases (treatment change in 51 and continuance in 30 cases) |
| van Kruchten et al[25] | JNM 2012 | Retrospective study; 33 women with MBC underwent FES and FDG-PET scan to solve clinical dilemma in standard workup | FES-PET scan detected higher skeletal metastases (341 vs 246 by conventional imaging), ER heterogeneity in 45%, diagnostic improvement in 88%, and change in therapy in 48% |
| Nienhuis H et al[26] | JNM 2018 | FES performed in 91 ER⁺ MBC patients to evaluate FES uptake heterogeneity based on anatomic sites | FES uptake in bone metastases was higher than in lymph node and lung metastases ($SUV_{max}$ 2.61 [95% CI, 2.31–2.94] vs 2.29 [95% CI, 2.00–2.61; $P < .001$] vs 2.23 [95% CI, 1.88–2.61; $P = .021$]), respectively. $SUV_{max}$ in surrounding normal tissue, highest in the bones, varied per patient (range, 0.7–3.3). |
| Peterson L et al[27] | Mol Imaging Biol 2014 | 19 women with newly diagnosed ER⁺ MBC were imaged before starting endocrine therapy. FES uptake was correlated with response and ER expression. | Low/absent FES uptake (4/5) correlates with lack of ER expression and progression within 6 mo. They concluded that FES could help identify patients with endocrine resistant disease and predict response in MBC. |
| Yang Z et al[28] | CNM 2017 | Retrospective study; 46 patients with invasive breast cancer | FES $SUV_{max}$ threshold of 1.82 to define ER ± lesions has sensitivity = 88.2%, specificity = 87.5% |

(continued on next page)

**Table 1**
*(continued)*

| Author | Journal, year of Publication | Study Details | Study Purpose and Results |
|---|---|---|---|
| Chae SY et al[29] | Lancet Oncology 2019 | Prospective study; 85 patients with recurrent or MBC | FES uptake correlated with ER status immunohistochemical with sensitivity = 76.6% (95% CI, 0.63–0.87) and specificity = 100% (95% CI, 0.9–1.0) |
| Van Kruchten et al[30] | EJNMMI 2015 | FES uptake correlated with prediction of hormone resistance in 19 MBC patients | PPV/NPV of FES-PET scan for response to treatment were 60% (95% CI: 31%–83%) and 80% (95% CI, 38%–96%), respectively, using $SUV_{max}$ of >1.5 |
| Hannah L et al[21] | JCO 2006 | Quantitative FES uptake correlated with treatment response in 47 patients. | 11/47 (23%) patients had objective response. Treatment selection using quantitative FES-PET scan would have increased the rate of response from 23% to 34% overall, and from 29% to 46% in the subset of patients lacking HER2/neu overexpression. |
| Evangelista et al[31] | CurrRadiopharm 2016 | Meta-analysis of nine selected studies with a total of 238 patients to correlate FES uptake and ER expression | A pooled sensitivity of 82% (95% CI, 74%–88%) and a pooled specificity of 95% (95% CI, 86%–99%) for the evaluation of ER functional status by FES-PET scans were found. |
| Mortimer JE et al[32] | Clin Cancer Res 1996 | 43 women with breast cancer underwent FDG and FES-PET scan before systemic therapy | Compared with in vitro assay of ER status, the FES-PET scan has an apparent sensitivity of 76% and specificity of 100%. |

*Abbreviations*: CI, confidence interval; FDG, 2-[18F]-Fluoro-2-deoxy-glucose; FES, 16α-[18F]-fluoro-17β-estradiol; MBC, metastatic breast cancer; NPV, negative predictive value; PET, positron emission tomography; PPV, positive predictive value.

patients with breast cancer had a heterogeneous pattern of both ER+ and ER− lesions. FES-PET imaging might reflect the ER expression better, especially in patients with metastatic disease after treatment, thus assisting in making individualized treatment decisions.[28]

The most impactful use of FES-PET imaging in the clinic will be the ability to predict the effectiveness of endocrine therapy (**Fig. 3**). The ability to

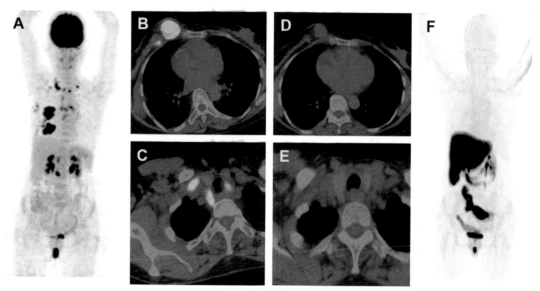

Fig. 2. 58-year-old woman with metabolically active right breast lesions, right axillary and extra-axillary medias-tinal lymph nodes on (A–C) FDG imaging but no ER expression on (D–F) FES imaging, which would predict resis-tance to endocrine therapy. The immunohistochemical assay revealed ER⁺/PR⁻, HER2⁺; and the discordance could be explained by weekly positive ER expression based on Allred score and intratumoral heterogeneity.

evaluate ER status in all tumor sites before endo-crine therapy can better guide patient manage-ment, especially if there is substantial heterogeneity between tumor sites.[33]

FES imaging could serve as a useful pharmaco-dynamic marker for evaluating the efficacy of ER antagonist therapies.[34] In a prospective study of 16 patients with metastatic ER⁺ breast cancer,

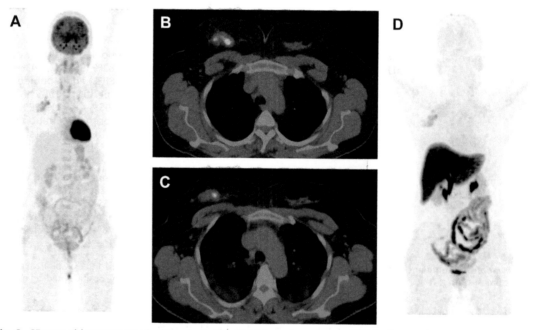

Fig. 3. 65-year-old woman newly diagnosed with right breast carcinoma (ER⁺/PR⁺, Her2⁻) underwent FDG and FES-PET/computed tomography (CT) scans for the initial workup. Metabolically active primary right breast lesions are seen on (A) maximum intensity projection (MIP) image and (B) a transaxial fused FDG-PET/CT image with same lesions showing positive ER expression on (C) transaxial fused and (D) FES MIP images, which would predict response to endocrine therapy.

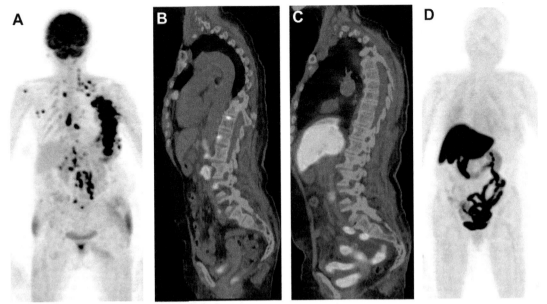

Fig. 4. An 83-year-old female patient has left carcinoma breast, multiple nodal and skeletal metastases showing increased uptake on an (A) FDG-PET maximum intensity projection (MIP) image. (B) Sagittal FDG-PET/computed tomography (CT) scan fused image shows increased uptake in mediastinal lymph nodes and multiple vertebral lesions but no ER expression in any of those lesions on (C) sagittal and (D) MIP FES-PET/CT images. Extensive metastases with high FDG positivity and no ER expression on FES-PET scans predicts a poor prognosis.

they tested whether the current standard dosing of fulvestrant optimally blocks tumor ER availability by performing FES-PET/computed tomography scans at baseline and during treatment. Incomplete blockade of ER was observed in 38% of patients and was associated with early disease progression.[35] In the clinical setting, FES-PET scans could be used to test ER blockade, both quantitatively and qualitatively, as an indicator that the drug is reaching the correct target. In addition, pharmacodynamic imaging of ER can be used to optimize drug dose and timing and whether or not complete blockade is necessary for drug effectiveness.[33]

### Factors Affecting 16α-[¹⁸F]-Fluoro-17β-Estradiol Uptake

Selective ER modulators (such as tamoxifen) block ERs, and selective ER downregulators (such as fulvestrant) block and damage ERs, which can diminish FES uptake in otherwise ER⁺ lesions. In contrast, the aromatase inhibitors such as anastrozole will not affect FES uptake because it does not affect receptor binding. Hence, FES imaging used to assess ER status is advisable to be performed before the initiation of endocrine therapy.

The decrease in FES avidity during or after endocrine therapy may be due to receptor

occupancy and/or other temporal molecular mechanisms such as loss of ER, emergence of PI3Kinase mutations, ESR1 genetic alterations, and others. Repeating FES imaging during the treatment course after withholding ER antagonists (approximately 8 weeks for selective ER modulators and approximately 28 weeks for ER downregulators) could indeed guide treatment choices.[36]

### Limitations of 16α-[¹⁸F]-Fluoro-17β-Estradiol Use

FES imaging can evaluate ER with high specificity, but a tissue biopsy should be used to confirm recurrence of breast cancer and to verify ER status by pathology, because FES has lower sensitivity and can miss lesions with no ER expression. Low estrogen levels in postmenopausal women and ongoing endocrine therapy blocking ERs will result in no or low uptake of FES. In addition, its ability to detect liver metastases is limited by high physiologic liver uptake owing to increased hepatic metabolism.

### Use of 16α-[¹⁸F]-Fluoro-17β-Estradiol-PET Scans in Conjunction with 2-[18F]-Fluoro-2-deoxy-Glucose-PET Scans

Combining FES with FDG is the basis of ER heterogeneity determination, which can also serve as a tool for prognostication (Fig. 4). FDG has

**Table 2**
Summary of studies comparing FDG-PET and FES-PET scans

| Author | Journal | Study Design | Results of FDG-PET scans | Results of FES-PET scans |
|---|---|---|---|---|
| Ulaner G et al[37] | JNM 2021 | Head-to-head comparison of FDG and FES in 7 metastatic invasive lobular patients with breast cancer (ER+), in 6 prospective clinical trials | 111 FDG-avid lesions (SUV$_{max}$: 3.3–9.9)<br>1/7 had liver metastases evident on FDG but not on FES. | 254 FES-avid lesions (SUV$_{max}$: 2.6–17.9)<br>5/7 patients: more lesions, more uptake on FES PET scan.<br>1/7 patient FES+/FDG− |
| Chae SY et al[38] | EJNMMI Res 2020 | 45 patients with recurrent breast cancer (ER+: 40, ER−: 4, unknown:1) enrolled in prospective study | Sensitivity of FDG: 80.0% (36/ 45; 95% CI, 65.4–90.4) | Sensitivity of FES: 71.1% (32/ 45; 95% CI, 55.7–83.6) |
| Gupta M et al[39] | World J Nucl Med 2017 | 12 female patients with breast cancer enrolled prospectively, 10 ER+ patients with 154 disease lesions were finally analyzed. | FDG picked-up 142 lesions (sensitivity 92.21%) | FES picked-up 116 lesions (sensitivity 75.32%) |
| Liu C et al[40] | Front Oncol 2020 | Retrospectively analyzed 35 HR+/HER2− MBC patients who underwent FES and FDG-PET scans before fulvestrant therapy | FDG++/FES+:12 patients demonstrated heterogeneity (both FES+ and FES− lesions); lowest median PFS = 5.5 mo (95% CI, 2.3–8.7) | All lesions FES++: 23<br>Low FES/FDG:11<br>PFS = 29.4 mo (95% CI, 2.3– 56.5)<br>High FES/FDG:12<br>PFS = 14.7 mo (95% CI, 10.9– 18.5) |
| Kurland B et al[41] | Clin Cancer Res 2017 | 90 patients with MBC from ER+/HER2− primary tumor underwent FES-PET and FDG-PET scans before endocrine therapy (PFS; n = 84) | FDG-PET scan identified 24 patients (29%) with low FDG uptake; median PFS = 26.1 mo (95% CI, 11.2– 49.7) | High FDG/high FES: 50 (59%)<br>PFS = 7.9 mo (5.6–11.8)<br>High FDG/low FES: 10 (12%)<br>PFS = 3.3 mo (1.4–not evaluable) |

Abbreviations: CI, confidence interval; FDG, 2-[18F]-Fluoro-2-deoxy-glucose; FES, 16α-[18F]-fluoro-17β-estradiol; MBC, metastatic breast cancer; PFS, progression-free survival.

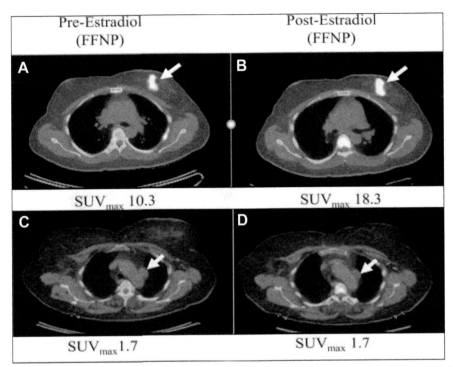

Fig. 5. (*Top*, responder) A woman with newly diagnosed ER⁺/PR⁺/HER2⁻ invasive ductal carcinoma with metastatic disease at diagnosis in left axillary lymph nodes and a rib. Fused transaxial FFNP-PET/computed tomography (CT) images at (*A*) baseline and (*B*) 1 day after estradiol show intense FFNP uptake in the primary left breast cancer (*arrows*). Tumor FFNP uptake was increased by 78% from baseline. She was treated with an aromatase inhibitor and palbociclib after the estradiol challenge test and showed excellent response. (*Bottom*, nonresponder) A woman with ER⁺/PR⁻/HER2⁻ invasive ductal carcinoma after neoadjuvant endocrine therapy and breast conserving surgery, developed metastatic disease to left prevascular and aortopulmonary lymph nodes. Fused transaxial FFNP-PET/CT images at (*C*) baseline and (*D*) 1 day after estradiol challenge show minimal FFNP uptake in the prevascular lymph node metastasis (*arrows*); tumor FFNP uptake remains unchanged. She was treated with an aromatase inhibitor after the estradiol challenge test but developed progressive disease. (*Adapted from*: Dehdashti F, Wu N, Ma CX, Naughton MJ, Katzenellenbogen JA, Siegel BA. Association of PET-based estradiol-challenge test for breast cancer progesterone receptors with response to endocrine therapy. Nat Commun. 2021;12(1):733.)

better sensitivity than FES in detection of ER⁺ lesions (**Table 2**).[37-39] Tumors with high FDG and low FES uptake have a poorer prognosis, whereas high FDG and high FES uptake is considered favorable.[40] The use of information from both FDG and FES-PET scans can predict endocrine therapy resistance in patients and may help guide the selection of other targeted and/or cytotoxic chemotherapy.[41]

## PROGESTERONE RECEPTOR TRACERS

The primary focus in hormonal receptor imaging in breast cancer has always been on the ER-targeting radiotracers, because PR expression is an estrogen-regulated process. However, several PR-targeting radiotracers have been investigated in preclinical and clinical studies. The most successful PR-targeted radiotracer is the progestin-analog (21-FFNP), which demonstrated higher

uptake in PR⁺ than PR⁻ breast cancers when compared with a normal tissue background.[42]

FFNP-PET imaging can be used as early response biomarker to predict response to antiestrogen treatment. The concept is based on the fact that the PR transcription is directly regulated by the action of estrogen through the ER, and the measurement of PR levels can identify ER⁺ tumors with functional ER capable of mediating response to endocrine therapy.[43] Given the importance of the ER ligand binding domain for FES binding, activating ESR1 mutations in patients with metastatic breast cancer leads to partial resistance to endocrine therapy and reduced binding affinity to estradiol (FES), which correlates to poor survival.[34,44] An estradiol-challenge test can monitor an increase in tumor PRs by FFNP-PET scans to predict response or resistance to endocrine therapy in patients with ER⁺ breast cancer. A study showed all subjects with a greater than

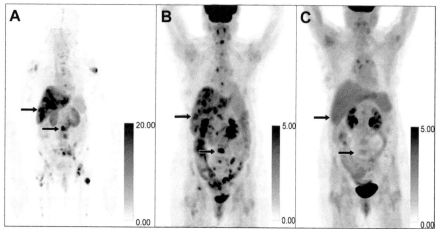

Fig. 6. In a 66-year-old woman with HER2-negative primary breast cancer. (*A*) Maximum intensity projection image from pretreatment HER2-targeted 89Zr-Pertuzumab-PET/CT identified multiple HER2-positive osseous and hepatic metastases (*arrows* show hepatic [maximum SUV ($SUV_{max}$) = 18.1] and osseous [$SUV_{max}$ = 16.5] reference lesions). Maximum intensity projection images from FDG-PET performed (*B*) before initiation of therapy and (*C*) after 2 months of anti-HER2 therapy demonstrate a substantial partial response (*arrows* in B and C indicate hepatic [$SUV_{max}$, 4.5 before therapy, decreased to background SUV after therapy] and osseous [$SUV_{max}$, 8.4 before therapy, equal to background after therapy] reference lesions). (*Adapted from*: Ulaner GA, Carrasquillo JA, Riedl CC, et al. Identification of HER2-Positive Metastases in Patients with HER2-Negative Primary Breast Cancer by Using HER2-targeted 89Zr-Pertuzumab PET/CT. *Radiology*. 2020;296(2):370 to 378.)

6.7% increase in FFNP uptake after estradiol challenge, classified as having functional ER, were identified as responders (100% positive predictive value and negative predictive value). They also had a significantly longer overall survival rate than non-responders, those with a decrease in FFNP or an increase of 6.7% or greater ($P<.0001$). FFNP-PET scans can distinguish likely responders from non-responders with high accuracy, thus allowing for risk stratification (Fig. 5).[43]

### Limitations of [18F]-Fluoro-Furanyl-Norprogesterone Use

A decrease in PR levels after a period of estrogen deprivation (eg, in postoophorectomy or menopausal women) or ER blockade can lead to false-negative results. Clinical studies of PR imaging significantly lag behind those of ER and considerable work is still required before FFNP is ready for translation into clinical practice.[45]

## HUMAN EPIDERMAL GROWTH FACTOR RECEPTOR-2 TRACERS

HER2 overexpression is associated with a highly aggressive infiltrating breast cancer prone to metastases and poor clinical outcomes. Molecular imaging targeting HER2 can determine in vivo HER2 status in primary as well as all the metastatic lesions at once during tumor progression and treatment response evaluation.[46] Radiolabeled

immunoglobulins (trastuzumab and pertuzumab), immunoglobulin fragments, F(ab')2, diabodies, nanobodies and nonimmunoglobulin scaffolds, affibody and designed ankyrin-repeat proteins might provide a reliable and quantitative method for detecting HER2-positive cancer using PET scanning.[47–49]

Radiolabeled trastuzumab and pertuzumab are promising tracers, because of their high accumulation in HER2-positive tumor tissue (Fig. 6).[50] However, they would be of limited effectiveness, because significant activity occurs 3 to 5 days after administration, too late for necessary treatment modification.[46] 89Zr (Zirconium-89) and 64Cu (Copper-64) labeled radiopharmaceuticals (89Zr-DFO-trastuzumab, 64Cu-DOTA-trastuzumab) are attractive option for antibody-based imaging agents owing to their comparatively longer half-life.[51–53] Biodistribution studies reported acceptable dosimetry and pharmacologic safety results with 64Cu-DOTA-trastuzumab in 6 patients with HER2-positive breast cancer.[54] It might predict the biologic effect of anti-HER2 antibodies, aiding in choosing treatment between anti-HER2 antibodies and HER2 tyrosine kinase inhibitors.[55] Additionally, radiolabeled HER2-targeting affibodies and nanobodies that can be labeled with different radionuclides (18F, 99mTc [technetium-99m], 68 Ga [gallium-68]) are being investigated for HER2 visualization in preclinical and clinical phases.[56,57]

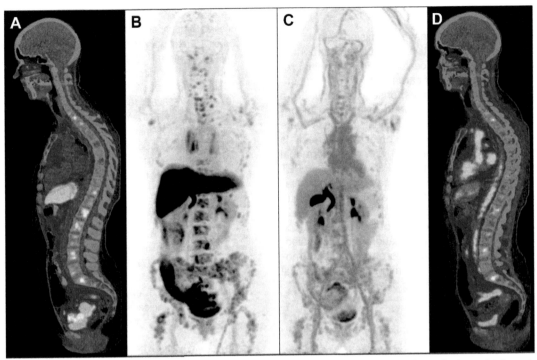

Fig. 7. (*A*) Sagittal FES-PET/computed tomography (CT) fusion image shows increased uptake in multiple verte-brae. (*B*) FES-PET maximum intensity projection (MIP) image reveals extensive skeletal metastases with positive ER expression. (*C*) MIP and (*D*) sagittal fusion images of FDHT-PET/CT imaging in the same patient show physio-logic uptake in blood vessels, heart, liver, urinary tracts and small intestines and pathologic uptake throughout multiple vertebrae, pelvic and femoral bones, which correlated with AR positivity on immunohistochemistry. (*Adapted from:* Venema CM, Mammatas LH, Schröder CP, et al. Androgen and Estrogen Receptor Imaging in Met-astatic Breast Cancer Patients as a Surrogate for Tissue Biopsies. *J Nucl Med Off Publ Soc Nucl Med.* 2017;58(12):1906-1912.)

## OTHER TRACERS

Molecular imaging offers the possibility to nonin-vasively determine the presence of relevant drug targets in all sites of metastatic spread throughout the body. Androgen receptors (AR) are not routinely determined in patients with breast can-cer, although they are present in 70% to 80% of them. Only ER+ patients benefit from antiestrogen endocrine therapy, because ER are functionally and structurally comparable with AR, but response to AR-targeting drugs may rely on AR expression as well.[58] AR expression in breast cancer could be assessed by 16β-[$^{18}$F]-fluoro-5α-dihydrotes-tosterone (FDHT)-PET (**Fig. 7**).[59] Antiandrogen therapy can be effective in negative patients with triple-negative breast cancer and FDHT-PET can determine the AR expression as relevant drug tar-gets in breast cancer.[59] The effectiveness of blocking AR can be imaged with FDHT-PET and can predict the treatment response. In a recent study, bicalutamide-induced reduction in FDHT

uptake (approximately 45%) was detected by follow-up FDHT-PET in patients with AR+/ER− breast cancer metastases.[60]

Similarly, PET with aromatase inhibitor tracer ($^{11}$C-vorozole)[61] has been used to measure intra-tumoral aromatase expression in individual pri-mary breast and metastatic lesions. The early response to neoadjuvant aromatase inhibitor (AI) therapy can also be evaluated by using baseline FDG and 18F-fluorothymidine PET imaging, in conjunction with tissue Ki-67 assay in early stage ER+ tumors.[62] Newer tracers targeting CXCR4 expression, DNA proliferation (18F-fluorothymi-dine), angiogenesis (radiolabeled RGD tracers binding to αvβ3-integrin receptor), apoptosis (radiolabeled Annexin V), and metabolism (18F-flu-orocholine) can also be used for better under-standing of changes in the microenvironment of breast tumors.[63,64] Future clinical studies might provide impactful information to include molecular imaging in the management of patients with breast cancer.

## SUMMARY

Molecular imaging has a promising role in the management of sensitive patients with hormonally sensitive breast cancer. FDG-PET imaging remains the standard of care for staging, prognostication, and predicting response to therapy. For a more personalized approach to the care of patients with breast cancer patient, because there is no single-target for all breast cancers, it is imperative to combine FDG with other hormonal receptor molecular imaging PET techniques. PET targeting ER, PR, and HER2 can provide noninvasive evaluation of receptor expression and can predict therapy response in patients with breast cancer. The early prediction of therapy resistance would provide useful information regarding selection of appropriate therapies on the basis of molecular imaging data and might improve survival in patients with metastatic breast cancer.

## CLINICS CARE POINTS

- Immunohistochemistry (IHC) remains the Gold Standard for confirmation of various receptor status in breast cancer.

- Receptor expression by on the tumour is hetergenous.IHC represent small area of tumour receptor expression.

- PET/CT using specific radiopharmaceuticals can demonstrate receptor status not only in the entire primary but also metastatic sites.

## DISCLOSURE

The authors have nothing to disclose. The authors have no conflict of interest. No financial aid was provided for this project.

## REFERENCES

1. Lebron L, Greenspan D, Pandit-Taskar N. PET imaging of breast cancer: role in patient management. PET Clin 2015;10:159–95. https://doi.org/10.1016/j.cpet.2014.12.004.

2. Kumar R, Alavi A. Fluorodeoxyglucose-PET in the management of breast cancer. Radiol Clin North Am 2004;42:1113–22. https://doi.org/10.1016/j.rcl.2004.08.005, ix.

3. NCCN Guidelines. NCCN: NCCN clinical practice guidelines in oncology (2021) breast cancer. version 7. 2021. Available at : http://www.nccn.org/professionals/physician_gls/f_guidelines.asp. Accessed September 10, 2021.

4. Caresia Aroztegui AP, García Vicente AM, Alvarez Ruiz S, et al. 18F-FDG PET/CT in breast cancer: evidence-based recommendations in initial staging. Tumor Biol 2017;39. https://doi.org/10.1177/1010428317728285. 1010428317728285.

5. Yararbas U, Avci NC, Yeniay L, et al. The value of 18F-FDG PET/CT imaging in breast cancer staging. Bosn J Basic Med Sci 2018;18:72–9. https://doi.org/10.17305/bjbms.2017.2179.

6. Groheux D, Cochet A, Humbert O, et al. 18F-FDG PET/CT for staging and restaging of breast cancer. J Nucl Med 2016;57:17S–26S. https://doi.org/10.2967/jnumed.115.157859.

7. Yadav D, Kumar R. Critical role of 2-[18F]-fluoro-2-deoxy-glucose in hormonally active malignancies. PET Clin 2021;16:177–89. https://doi.org/10.1016/j.cpet.2020.12.007.

8. Ulaner GA. PET/CT for patients with breast cancer: where is the clinical impact? Am J Roentgenol 2019;213:254–65. https://doi.org/10.2214/AJR.19.21177.

9. Groheux D, Hindie E. Breast cancer: initial workup and staging with FDG PET/CT. Clin Transl Imaging 2021;1–11. https://doi.org/10.1007/s40336-021-00426-z.

10. Groheux D, Giacchetti S, Moretti J-L, et al. Correlation of high 18F-FDG uptake to clinical, pathological and biological prognostic factors in breast cancer. Eur J Nucl Med Mol Imaging 2011;38:426–35. https://doi.org/10.1007/s00259-010-1640-9.

11. Han S, Choi JY. Prognostic value of 18F-FDG PET and PET/CT for assessment of treatment response to neoadjuvant chemotherapy in breast cancer: a systematic review and meta-analysis. Breast Cancer Res 2020;22:119. https://doi.org/10.1186/s13058-020-01350-2.

12. Groheux D. Role of fludeoxyglucose in breast cancer: treatment response. PET Clin 2018;13:395–414. https://doi.org/10.1016/j.cpet.2018.02.003.

13. Ulaner GA, Castillo R, Goldman DA, et al. 18)F-FDG-PET/CT for systemic staging of newly diagnosed triple-negative breast cancer. Eur J Nucl Med Mol Imaging 2016;43:1937–44. https://doi.org/10.1007/s00259-016-3402-9.

14. Ulaner GA, Castillo R, Wills J, et al. 18F-FDG-PET/CT for systemic staging of patients with newly diagnosed ER-positive and HER2-positive breast cancer. Eur J Nucl Med Mol Imaging 2017;44:1420–7. https://doi.org/10.1007/s00259-017-3709-1.

15. Lin NU, Guo H, Yap JT, et al. Phase II study of lapatinib in combination with trastuzumab in patients with human epidermal growth factor receptor 2-positive metastatic breast cancer: clinical outcomes and predictive value of early [18F]fluorodeoxyglucose positron emission tomography imaging (TBCRC

003). J Clin Oncol Off J Am Soc Clin Oncol 2015;33: 2623–31. https://doi.org/10.1200/JCO.2014.60. 0353.

16. Kumar R, Chauhan A, Zhuang H, et al. Clinicopathologic factors associated with false negative FDG-PET in primary breast cancer. Breast Cancer Res Treat 2006;98:267–74. https://doi.org/10.1007/s10549-006-9159-2.

17. Basu S, Chen W, Tchou J, et al. Comparison of triple-negative and estrogen receptor-positive/progesterone receptor-positive/HER2-negative breast carcinoma using quantitative fluorine-18 fluorodeoxyglucose/positron emission tomography imaging parameters: a potentially useful method for disease characterization. Cancer 2008;112: 995–1000. https://doi.org/10.1002/cncr.23226.

18. Humbert O, Berriolo-Riedinger A, Cochet A, et al. Prognostic relevance at 5 years of the early monitoring of neoadjuvant chemotherapy using (18)F-FDG PET in luminal HER2-negative breast cancer. Eur J Nucl Med Mol Imaging 2014;41:416–27. https://doi.org/10.1007/s00259-013-2616-3.

19. Grabher BJ. Breast cancer: evaluating tumor estrogen receptor status with molecular imaging to increase response to therapy and improve patient outcomes. J Nucl Med Technol 2020;48:191–201. https://doi.org/10.2967/jnmt.119.239020.

20. van Kruchten M, de Vries EGE, Brown M, et al. PET imaging of oestrogen receptors in patients with breast cancer. Lancet Oncol 2013;14:e465–75. https://doi.org/10.1016/S1470-2045(13)70292-4.

21. Linden HM, Stekhova SA, Link JM, et al. Quantitative fluoroestradiol positron emission tomography imaging predicts response to endocrine treatment in breast cancer. J Clin Oncol Off J Am Soc Clin Oncol 2006;24:2793–9. https://doi.org/10.1200/JCO.2005. 04.3810.

22. Kurland BF, Wiggins JR, Coche A, et al. Whole-body characterization of estrogen receptor status in metastatic breast cancer with 16α-18F-Fluoro-17β-Estradiol positron emission tomography: meta-analysis and recommendations for integration into clinical applications. Oncologist 2020;25:835–44. https://doi.org/10.1634/theoncologist.2019-0967.

23. Research C for DE. Drug trial snapshot: CERIANNA. FDA. Published online June 3, 2020. Available at: https://www.fda.gov/drugs/drug-approvals-and-databases/drug-trial-snapshot-cerianna. Accessed September 13, 2021.

24. Boers J, Loudini N, Brunsch CL, et al. Value of 18F-FES-PET to solve clinical dilemmas in breast cancer patients: a retrospective study. J Nucl Med 2021. https://doi.org/10.2967/jnumed.120.256826.

25. Kruchten M van, Glaudemans AWJM, Vries EFJ de, et al. PET imaging of estrogen receptors as a diagnostic tool for breast cancer patients presenting with a clinical dilemma. J Nucl Med 2012;53:182–90. https://doi.org/10.2967/jnumed.111.092734.

26. Nienhuis HH, Kruchten M van, Elias SG, et al. 18F-Fluoroestradiol tumor uptake is heterogeneous and influenced by site of metastasis in breast cancer patients. J Nucl Med 2018;59:1212–8. https://doi.org/10.2967/jnumed.117.198846.

27. Peterson LM, Kurland BF, Schubert EK, et al. A phase 2 study of 16α-[18F]-fluoro-17β-estradiol positron emission tomography (FES-PET) as a marker of hormone sensitivity in metastatic breast cancer (MBC). Mol Imaging Biol MIB Off Publ Acad Mol Imaging 2014;16:431–40. https://doi.org/10.1007/s11307-013-0699-7.

28. Yang Z, Sun Y, Xu X, et al. The assessment of estrogen receptor status and its intratumoral heterogeneity in patients with breast cancer by using 18F-fluoroestradiol PET/CT. Clin Nucl Med 2017;42: 421–7. https://doi.org/10.1097/RLU. 0000000000001587.

29. Chae SY, Ahn SH, Kim S-B, et al. Diagnostic accuracy and safety of 16α-[18F]fluoro-17β-oestradiol PET-CT for the assessment of oestrogen receptor status in recurrent or metastatic lesions in patients with breast cancer: a prospective cohort study. Lancet Oncol 2019;20:546–55. https://doi.org/10.1016/S1470-2045(18)30936-7.

30. van Kruchten M, Glaudemans AWJM, de Vries EFJ, et al. Positron emission tomography of tumour [(18) F]fluoroestradiol uptake in patients with acquired hormone-resistant metastatic breast cancer prior to oestradiol therapy. Eur J Nucl Med Mol Imaging 2015;42:1674–81. https://doi.org/10.1007/s00259-015-3107-5.

31. Evangelista L, Guarneri V, Conte PF. 18F-Fluoroestradiol positron emission tomography in breast cancer patients: systematic review of the literature & meta-analysis. Curr Radiopharm 2016;9:244–57. https://doi.org/10.2174/1874471009666161019144950.

32. Mortimer JE, Dehdashti F, Siegel BA, et al. Positron emission tomography with 2-[18F]Fluoro-2-deoxy-D-glucose and 16alpha-[18F]fluoro-17beta-estradiol in breast cancer: correlation with estrogen receptor status and response to systemic therapy. Clin Cancer Res Off J Am Assoc Cancer Res 1996;2:933–9.

33. Linden HM, Peterson LM, Fowler A. Clinical potential of estrogen and progesterone receptor imaging. PET Clin 2018;13:415–22. https://doi.org/10.1016/j.cpet.2018.02.005.

34. Kumar M, Salem K, Jeffery JJ, et al. Longitudinal molecular imaging of progesterone receptor reveals early differential response to endocrine therapy in breast cancer with an activating ESR1 mutation. J Nucl Med 2020. https://doi.org/10.2967/jnumed. 120.249508.

35. van Kruchten M, de Vries EG, Glaudemans AW, et al. Measuring residual estrogen receptor availability during fulvestrant therapy in patients with metastatic breast cancer. Cancer Discov 2015;5:72–81. https://doi.org/10.1158/2159-8290.CD-14-0697.

36. Zattarin E, Leporati R, Ligorio F, et al. Hormone receptor loss in breast cancer: molecular mechanisms, clinical settings, and therapeutic implications. Cells 2020;9:2644. https://doi.org/10.3390/cells9122644.

37. Ulaner GA, Jhaveri K, Chandarlapaty S, et al. Head-to-head evaluation of 18F-FES and 18F-FDG PET/CT in metastatic invasive lobular breast cancer. J Nucl Med Off Publ Soc Nucl Med 2021;62:326–31. https://doi.org/10.2967/jnumed.120.247882.

38. Chae SY, Son HJ, Lee DY, et al. Comparison of diagnostic sensitivity of [18F]fluoroestradiol and [18F]fluorodeoxyglucose positron emission tomography/computed tomography for breast cancer recurrence in patients with a history of estrogen receptor-positive primary breast cancer. EJNMMI Res 2020;10:54. https://doi.org/10.1186/s13550-020-00643-z.

39. Gupta M, Datta A, Choudhury PS, et al. Can 18F-fluoroestradiol positron emission tomography become a new imaging standard in the estrogen receptor-positive breast cancer patient: a prospective comparative study with 18F-fluorodeoxyglucose positron emission tomography? World J Nucl Med 2017;16:133–9. https://doi.org/10.4103/1450-1147.203071.

40. Liu C, Xu X, Yuan H, et al. Dual tracers of 16α-[18F]fluoro-17β-Estradiol and [18F]fluorodeoxyglucose for prediction of progression-free survival after fulvestrant therapy in patients with HR+/HER2- metastatic breast cancer. Front Oncol 2020;10:580277. https://doi.org/10.3389/fonc.2020.580277.

41. Kurland BF, Peterson LM, Lee JH, et al. Estrogen receptor binding (18F-FES PET) and Glycolytic activity ($^{18}$F-FDG PET) predict progression-free survival on endocrine therapy in patients with ER+ breast cancer. Clin Cancer Res 2017;23:407. https://doi.org/10.1158/1078-0432.CCR-16-0362.

42. Dehdashti F, Laforest R, Gao F, et al. Assessment of progesterone receptors in breast carcinoma by PET with 21-18F-fluoro-16α,17α-[(R)-(1'-α-furylmethylidene)dioxy]-19-norpregn-4-ene-3,20-dione. J Nucl Med Off Publ Soc Nucl Med 2012;53:363–70. https://doi.org/10.2967/jnumed.111.098319.

43. Dehdashti F, Wu N, Ma CX, et al. Association of PET-based estradiol-challenge test for breast cancer progesterone receptors with response to endocrine therapy. Nat Commun 2021;12:733. https://doi.org/10.1038/s41467-020-20814-9.

44. Paquette M, Lavallée É, Phoenix S, et al. Improved estrogen receptor assessment by PET using the novel radiotracer 18F-4FMFES in estrogen receptor-positive breast cancer patients: an ongoing phase II clinical trial. J Nucl Med Off Publ Soc Nucl Med 2018;59:197–203. https://doi.org/10.2967/jnumed.117.194654.

45. Fowler AM, Clark AS, Katzenellenbogen JA, et al. Imaging diagnostic and therapeutic targets: steroid receptors in breast cancer. J Nucl Med Off Publ Soc Nucl Med 2016;57:75S–80S. https://doi.org/10.2967/jnumed.115.157933.

46. Miladinova D. Molecular imaging in breast cancer. Nucl Med Mol Imaging 2019;53:313–9. https://doi.org/10.1007/s13139-019-00614-w.

47. Goldstein R, Sosabowski J, Vigor K, et al. Developments in single photon emission computed tomography and PET-based HER2 molecular imaging for breast cancer. Expert Rev Anticancer Ther 2013;13:359–73. https://doi.org/10.1586/era.13.11.

48. Baum RP, Prasad V, Müller D, et al. Molecular imaging of HER2-expressing malignant tumors in breast cancer patients using synthetic 111In- or 68Ga-labeled affibody molecules. J Nucl Med Off Publ Soc Nucl Med 2010;51:892–7. https://doi.org/10.2967/jnumed.109.073239.

49. Sörensen J, Sandberg D, Sandström M, et al. First-in-human molecular imaging of HER2 expression in breast cancer metastases using the 111In-ABY-025 affibody molecule. J Nucl Med Off Publ Soc Nucl Med 2014;55:730–5. https://doi.org/10.2967/jnumed.113.131243.

50. Ulaner GA, Carrasquillo JA, Riedl CC, et al. Identification of HER2-positive metastases in patients with HER2-negative primary breast cancer by using HER2-targeted 89Zr-pertuzumab PET/CT. Radiology 2020;296:370–8. https://doi.org/10.1148/radiol.2020192828.

51. Henry KE, Ulaner GA, Lewis JS. Human epidermal growth factor receptor 2-targeted PET/single-photon emission computed tomography imaging of breast cancer: noninvasive measurement of a biomarker integral to tumor treatment and prognosis. PET Clin 2017;12:269–88. https://doi.org/10.1016/j.cpet.2017.02.001.

52. Mortimer JE, Bading JR, Colcher DM, et al. Functional imaging of human epidermal growth factor receptor 2-positive metastatic breast cancer using (64)Cu-DOTA-trastuzumab PET. J Nucl Med Off Publ Soc Nucl Med 2014;55:23–9. https://doi.org/10.2967/jnumed.113.122630.

53. Paquette M, Phoenix S, Lawson C, et al. A preclinical PET dual-tracer imaging protocol for ER and HER2 phenotyping in breast cancer xenografts. EJNMMI Res 2020;10:69. https://doi.org/10.1186/s13550-020-00656-8.

54. Tamura A, Yamamoto N, Nino N, et al. Pazopanib maintenance therapy after tandem high-dose chemotherapy for disseminated Ewing sarcoma. Int Cancer Conf J 2019;8:95–100. https://doi.org/10.1007/s13691-019-00362-w.

55. Mortimer JE, Bading JR, Park JM, et al. Tumor uptake of 64Cu-DOTA-Trastuzumab in patients with metastatic breast cancer. J Nucl Med Off Publ Soc Nucl Med 2018;59:38–43. https://doi.org/10.2967/jnumed.117.193888.

56. Xu Y, Wang L, Pan D, et al. Synthesis of a novel 89Zr-labeled HER2 affibody and its application study in tumor PET imaging. EJNMMI Res 2020;10:58. https://doi.org/10.1186/s13550-020-00649-7.

57. Xu Y, Wang L, Pan D, et al. PET imaging of a 68Ga labeled modified HER2 affibody in breast cancers: from xenografts to patients. Br J Radiol 2019;92:20190425. https://doi.org/10.1259/bjr.20190425.

58. Venema CM, Mammatas LH, Schröder CP, et al. Androgen and estrogen receptor imaging in metastatic breast cancer patients as a surrogate for tissue biopsies. J Nucl Med Off Publ Soc Nucl Med 2017;58:1906–12. https://doi.org/10.2967/jnumed.117.193649.

59. Jacene HA, Liu M, Cheng S-C, et al. Imaging androgen receptors in breast cancer with 18F-fluoro-5α-dihydrotestosterone-PET: a pilot study. J Nucl Med 2021. https://doi.org/10.2967/jnumed.121.262068.

60. Boers J, Venema CM, Vries EFJ de, et al. Serial [18F]-FDHT-PET to predict bicalutamide efficacy in patients with androgen receptor positive metastatic breast cancer. Eur J Cancer 2021;144:151–61. https://doi.org/10.1016/j.ejca.2020.11.008.

61. Biegon A, Shroyer KR, Franceschi D, et al. Initial studies with 11C-vorozole PET detect overexpression of intratumoral aromatase in breast cancer. J Nucl Med 2020;61:807–13. https://doi.org/10.2967/jnumed.119.231589.

62. Romine PE, Peterson LM, Kurland BF, et al. 18F-fluorodeoxyglucose (FDG) PET or 18F-fluorothymidine (FLT) PET to assess early response to aromatase inhibitors (AI) in women with ER+ operable breast cancer in a window-of-opportunity study. Breast Cancer Res 2021;23:88. https://doi.org/10.1186/s13058-021-01464-1.

63. Iakovou I, Giannoula E, Gkantaifi A, et al. Positron emission tomography in breast cancer: 18F- FDG and other radiopharmaceuticals. Eur J Hybrid Imaging 2018;2:20. https://doi.org/10.1186/s41824-018-0039-x.

64. Dalm SU, Verzijlbergen JF, De Jong M. Review: receptor targeted nuclear imaging of breast cancer. Int J Mol Sci 2017;18:260. https://doi.org/10.3390/ijms18020260.

# $^{18}$F-FDG Versus Non-FDG PET Tracers in Multiple Myeloma

Angel Hemrom, MD[a], Avinash Tupalli, MD, DM[a], Abass Alavi, MD[b],
Rakesh Kumar, MBBS, DRM, DNB, MNAMS, PhD[c],*

## KEYWORDS

- Multiple myeloma • $^{18}$F-FDG PET-CT • $^{11}$C-choline • $^{68}$Ga-FAPI • $^{68}$Ga-pentixafor

## KEY POINTS

- Multiple myeloma (MM) accounts for 0.9% of all cancer diagnoses, and its incidence and mortality rate have increased in previous years.
- $^{18}$F-fluorodeoxyglucose (FDG) PET–computed tomography (CT) is already an established modality for evaluation of MM.
- MR imaging is helpful in certain conditions where $^{18}$F-FDG PET-CT may be lacking, as in diffuse bone marrow involvement.
- To standardize PET reporting, methods like the Italian Myeloma Criteria for PET Use (IMPeTUs) and Deauville criteria have been studied for its feasibility in clinical practice.
- Tracers like $^{11}$C-acetate and $^{11}$C-choline/$^{18}$F-fluoromethylcholine (FCH) have shown higher sensitivity and detected more focal lesions and diffuse involvement than $^{18}$F-FDG PET-CT. $^{18}$F-FCH also showed higher maximum standardized uptake value than $^{18}$FDG.
- $^{11}$C-methionine (MET) appears to be the best radiopharmaceutical currently, apart from $^{18}$F-FDG, for evaluating MM, with higher sensitivity in detecting focal lesions and extramedullary disease and better correlation with tumor burden.
- $^{68}$Ga–fibroblast-activation-protein inhibitor, $^{68}$Ga-pentixafor, and $^{68}$Ga-prostate-specific membrane antigen have also shown promising result with potential of therapeutic implications.

## INTRODUCTION

Multiple myeloma (MM) is a neoplastic disease associated with monoclonal proliferation of plasma cells, producing a protein referred to as M or myeloma protein (usually IgG or IgA) in the bone marrow. It comes under a group of disorders known as monoclonal gammopathies. The other disorders in the group are monoclonal gammopathy of undetermined significance (MGUS), smoldering MM, nonsecretory myeloma, solitary plasmacytoma, extramedullary plasmacytoma, immunoglobulin amyloid light chain amyloidosis, and the polyneuropathy, organomegaly, endocrinopathy, monoclonal gammopathy, and skin changes (POEMS) syndrome.

Conflicts of interest: Angel Hemrom, Avinash Tupalli, Abass Alavi, and Rakesh Kumar declare that they have no competing financial interest and no conflict of interest.
Ethical approval statement: All procedures performed in studies involving human participants were in accordance with the ethical standards of the institutional and/or national research committee and with the 1964 Helsinki declaration and its later amendments or comparable ethical standards.
Informed consent: Informed consent from the patients was obtained to be included in the study.
[a] Department of Nuclear Medicine, All India Institute of Medical Sciences, New Delhi 110029, India; [b] Hospital of the University of Pennsylvania, Philadelphia, PA, USA; [c] Diagnostic Nuclear Medicine Division, Department of Nuclear Medicine, All India Institute of Medical Sciences, New Delhi 110029, India
* Corresponding author.
E-mail address: rkphulia@hotmail.com

PET Clin 17 (2022) 415–430
https://doi.org/10.1016/j.cpet.2022.03.001
1556-8598/22/© 2022 Elsevier Inc. All rights reserved.

## MULTIPLE MYELOMA DEFINITION

The current definition of MM requires 10% or more clonal plasma cells on bone marrow examination (or biopsy-proved bony or extramedullary plasmacytoma) and any one or more of myeloma-defining events.

Myeloma-defining events

1. Evidence of end organ damage, manifested by hypercalcemia (C), renal insufficiency (R), anemia (A), or bone lesions (B) in x-ray/CT/PET-CT (CRAB) attributed to the plasma cell proliferative process
2. Any/more biomarkers of malignancy
   - Clonal bone marrow plasma cell percentage greater than or equal to 60%
   - Involved:uninvolved serum free light chain ratio greater than or equal to 100
   - Greater than one focal lesion in MR imaging studies.

The requirement for monoclonal protein presence as part of the diagnostic criteria is not mandatory. Its presence or absence is used to subdivide MM into secretory and nonsecretory types.[1–3]

## EPIDEMIOLOGY

MM accounts for 0.9% of all cancer diagnoses. The disease is approximately 1.5-times more likely in men. It is more common in developed countries, with highest incidence in Australia, Western Europe, and the United States. The global incidence of MM increased by 126% from 1990 to 2016, although the global mortality rate increased by 94%. Median age at diagnosis is 69 years. Risk factors include age, race, sex, gender, and family history. Survival depends on the stage at diagnosis, with a 74.8% 5-year survival with localized disease (which accounts for only 5% of all cases) and 52.9% for systemic MM (95% of diagnoses).[4–6]

Approximately 80% of MMs originates from non-IgM immunoglobulin MGUS (non-IgM MGUS) and 20% from light chain immunoglobulin MGUS. The rate of progression of MGUS to MM is 0.5% to 1% per year. Smoldering MM is the intermediate stage between MGUS and MM. For smoldering myeloma diagnosis, 2 criteria must be met, that is, serum monoclonal protein (IgG or IgA) should be greater than or equal to 30 g/L or urinary monoclonal protein greater than or equal 500 mg/24 h and/or clonal bone marrow plasma cells 10% to 60% and absence of myeloma-defining events or amyloidosis.[2] With smoldering MM, the overall risk of progression is 10% per year for the first

5 years, 3% per year in the next 5 years, and 1% per year afterward; the cumulative probability of progression is 73% after 15 years.[7]

## STAGING

MM has been classically classified via 2 staging systems: Durie-Salmon staging system (DSS) and International Staging System (ISS). The original DSS, introduced in 1975, based the staging on extent of bone lesion, hemoglobin level, serum calcium level, and M component level.[8] Later, with the availability of more sensitive imaging modalities like PET-CT and MR imaging, the staging system was refined and DSS plus was introduced. The DSS plus classified patients on the basis of tumor burden in imaging modality (MR imaging and/or PET-CT): stage I (0–4 lytic lesions), stage II (5–20 lytic lesions), and stage III (>20 lytic lesions).[9]

Problems of reproducibility, however, were there due to interobserver variation. On the other hand, ISS used serum $\beta_2$-microglobulin and serum albumin for staging.[8,10] Neither system included disease biology, which was a key determinant of overall survival. Presence or absence of high-risk cytogenetics [t(14;4), t(14;16), or del(17p)] and normal/elevated levels of lactate dehydrogenase were added in the Revised ISS (RISS) to create a unified prognostic index. A study showed that the 5-year survival rates of patients with stages I, II, and III RISS were 82%, 62%, and 40%, respectively.[11]

## IMAGING MODALITIES
### X-ray

During initial work-up in patients with MM, skeletal survey may be used. It can show localized lytic lesion, fracture, or diffuse osteopenia. Diffuse osteopenia also may be due to other etiology, which x-rays are not able to differentiate. It is of low cost and wider availability. Early MM may not show any change, however, in x-ray. A false-negative rate is seen in 30% to 70% of cases, leading to significant underestimation in diagnosing and staging.[12]

### Computed Tomography

Computed tomography (CT) can detect early bone destruction and can detect extramedullary lesions, unlike x-rays. The false-negative rate is high in diffuse bone marrow infiltration. Myeloma lesions frequently do not heal, despite eradication of the disease. It cannot assess continued activity of myeloma, in areas of prior bone destruction, and can show persistent bone lesions even after treatment, leading to false interpretation. In MM, evaluation of entire skeleton is required; thus, whole-body (WB) multidetector CT (MDCT) is helpful. High radiation dose to the patient is an important drawback with MDCT. To overcome this problem, low-dose CT (LDCT) was introduced. It operates at lower radiation dose and is superior in detecting skeletal lesions compared with conventional radiography.[9,12,13]

## Bone Scan

Bone scan has limited use in the evaluation of MM. Disease is characterized by multiple mechanisms of osteoblastic inhibition, including inhibition of differentiation. Bone scan uses technetium Tc 99m–labeled diphosphonates, which are taken up by osteoblastic lesions in the bone. Thus, it is less sensitive in detecting MM lesions.[9]

## MR Imaging

MR imaging is useful in identifying in marrow infiltration and is especially helpful in evaluation of axial skeleton. Infiltration at the site of osteopenia or at the site of lytic lesion is diagnostically important. The number of lesions detected in MR imaging has a good correlation with treatment outcome and overall survival. Thus, MR imaging is one of the modalities included in DSS to evaluate tumor burden. For screening purposes, spine and pelvis are scanned, and symptomatic areas can be included. WB–MR imaging was introduced to overcome the disadvantage of partial field of view; however, it is not widely employed and is less available. WB–MR imaging has superior sensitivity than WB–MDCT, for both diffuse and focal pattern of bone marrow involvement. Longer time to perform the study, cost, and patient factors, such as claustrophobia and metal devices in the body, are certain drawbacks. In disease monitoring, it has a limited role, because it takes 9 to 12 months for lesions evident on MR imaging to disappear.[9,12,13]

## PET–Computed Tomography

PET-CT is a WB imaging technique which uses functional information obtained from PET and anatomic information obtained from CT. It is an advanced, noninvasive imaging tool that allows identification of metabolic and physiologic alterations in tumors. The most used PET tracer is [18]F-FDG, which is a biomarker of intracellular glucose metabolism. Malignant tumor cells have increased glycolytic activity and are characterized by increase in membrane glucose transporters and modification in enzymes responsible for phosphorylation and glucose metabolism. It leads to preferential concentration of glucose in malignant cells. FDG, a glucose analog, is transported into cells via glucose transporter proteins, undergoes phosphorylation by hexokinase, and is converted to FDG-6-phosphate. But, FDG-6-phosphate is not further metabolized and becomes metabolically trapped in cancer cells. The ability of cancer cells to trap the FDG metabolite forms the basis for imaging the in vivo distribution of the tracer with [18]F-FDG PET.[14,15]

## National Comprehensive Cancer Network® (NCCN®)

In the 2017 NCCN Clinical Practice Guidelines In Oncology (NCCN Guidelines®) for MM (Table 1), skeletal survey was recommended for initial diagnostic work-up. WB PET-CT was recommended to be useful only under certain circumstances.[16] In the 2021 recommendations, however, skeletal survey was replaced by CT or PET-CT since skeletal survey is acceptable in a low-resource setting, where advanced imaging techniques are not available (Box 1).[17] All recommendations are category 2A, unless otherwise noted. For initial diagnostic work-up of patients suspected of having MM, either WB LDCT or [18]F-FDG PET-CT is recommended. Contrast agents are not necessary and should be avoided whenever possible. WB MR imaging can be considered for differentiating smoldering myeloma from MM, when WB LDCT and [18]F-FDG PET-CT are negative.[17]

## ROLE OF PET–COMPUTED TOMOGRAPHY IN MONOCLONAL GAMMOPATHY OF UNDETERMINED SIGNIFICANCE

MGUS is defined by the presence of less than 10% of monoclonal plasma cells in the bone marrow, along with the presence of monoclonal protein in serum or urine, or both. Risk factors for progression of MGUS to active myeloma include M protein greater than or equal to 1.5 g/dL and an abnormal free light chain ratio in patients with non-IgM MGUS. WB MR imaging previously has been studied for assessing MGUS. Studies showed that approximately 3.5% to 23.4% of the patients showed focal lesions in MR imaging. Presence of focal lesions in bone and value of M protein were independently predictive of progression to systemic disease.[18,19] Despite the lack of evidence regarding imaging assessment, the International Myeloma Working Group (IMWG) recommended WB CT in high-risk MGUS. In cases of equivocal findings in CT, WB MR imaging can be done, whereas, in positive CT scans, a PET-CT needs to be done to rule out myeloma or any other malignant disease.[20]

**Table 1**
**NCCN categories of evidence and consensus**

| | |
|---|---|
| Category 1 | Based on high-level evidence, there is uniform NCCN consensus that the intervention is appropriate. |
| Category 2A | Based on lower-level evidence, there is uniform NCCN consensus that the intervention is appropriate. |
| Category 2B | Based on lower-level evidence, there is NCCN consensus that the intervention is appropriate. |
| Category 3 | Based on any level of evidence, there is major NCCN disagreement that the intervention is appropriate. |

## ROLE OF PET–COMPUTED TOMOGRAPHY IN SMOLDERING MULTIPLE MYELOMA

Presence of more than 10% of monoclonal plasma cells in the bone marrow, along with monoclonal protein in serum or urine or both, without CRAB symptoms is defined as smoldering MM. Low-risk smoldering MM can take years to progress to active MM, whereas high-risk patients can become symptomatic MM within 2 years. One or more lesions in MR imaging in a patient is a strong indicator of progression to symptomatic MM, approximately more than 60% in 2 years. Thus,

**Box 1**
**Indications for PET–computed tomography in multiple myeloma**

1. Diagnosis and staging
2. Prognostication
3. Treatment response evaluation
4. MRD detection
5. Surveillance

this is one of the myeloma-defining events.[21] [18]F-FDG PET-CT has also shown prognostic value. A positive [18]F-FDG PET-CT is defined as presence of focal lesion with/without underlying osteolytic lesions. Studies found a patient with positive PET-CT has 58% to 75% probability of progressing to symptomatic MM at 2 years, compared with PET-negative patients. Also, PET-positive patients with underlying osteolysis have a higher progression probability than PET-positive patients without underlying osteolysis.[22,23] According to recent IMWG recommendations WB CT or PET-CT is the first imaging of choice to exclude osteolytic lesions. If it is negative, then WB MR imaging or MR imaging of spine and pelvis is done. It should be done at yearly intervals for at least 5 years.[20]

## ROLE OF PET–COMPUTED TOMOGRAPHY IN SOLITARY PLASMACYTOMA

Solitary plasmacytoma can occur as either solitary bone lesion or extramedullary lesion, where solitary bone plasmacytoma is more prevalent and has a higher risk of progression to MM (35%) than extramedullary lesion (7%) within 2 years.[24] The role of imaging is to exclude any other osteolytic or soft tissue lesion to exclude systemic MM. WB MR imaging is the preferred modality for solitary plasmacytoma, and PET-CT can be done if MR imaging not available. MR imaging has higher sensitivity to detect diffuse infiltration, which, although not a myeloma-defining event, should warrant additional examinations to rule out reasons for higher bone marrow cellularity, including MM. PET-CT is the preferred modality for imaging extramedullary lesions.[20] In a study of 62 patients with solitary plasmacytoma, it was found that [18]F-FDG uptake was seen in most of the cases and was associated independently with tumor size. [18]F-FDG–avid plasmacytoma, body surface area standardized uptake value (SUV) greater than 1.7, and lean body mass SUV greater than 5.2 correlated with shorter time to transformation in MM.[25]

## ROLE OF PET–COMPUTED TOMOGRAPHY IN MULTIPLE MYELOMA

WB CT or PET-CT is the first choice of imaging to identify and assess the extent of osteolytic lesions. In cases of negative CT, WB MR imaging can be used. PET-CT is the preferred modality to get baseline for response assessment.[20] Relying solely on PET without the CT component may lead to underestimation of overall disease burden, especially while evaluating osseous structures

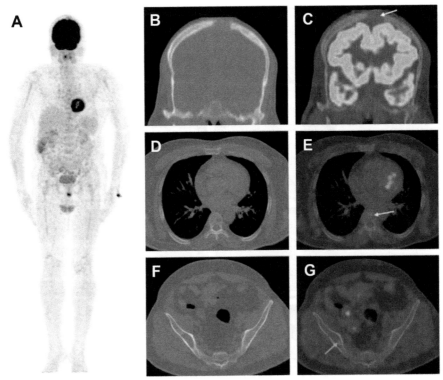

Fig. 1. A 59-year-old man with presentation of swelling in frontal region was suspected of having MM. Head-to-toe PET-CT acquisition was done 60 minutes after injection of 10-mCi $^{18}$F-FDG by intravenous route. Maximum intensity projection image (*A*) shows abnormal along focal uptake in left frontal bone region. Coronal images of skull (*B*, *C*) and axial images (*D–G*) of chest and pelvic region show lytic lesions in left frontal bone, D7 vertebral body, and right iliac bone with increased FDG uptake (*arrows*).

near area of high metabolic activity, such as brain.[26] $^{18}$F-FDG PET-CT has an overall sensitivity of 80% to 100% in evaluation of osseous lesions. It is superior to skeletal survey in detecting additional osseous lesion as well as extramedullary lesions, having an impact on their management[27] (Fig. 1).

$^{18}$F-FDG PET-CT and MR imaging are similar in detecting focal lesions; however, MR imaging is superior in detecting diffuse infiltration.[28–30] Moreau and colleagues (2017) found that, compared with clinico-biologic findings, higher marrow plasmacytosis was observed in patients with abnormal MR imaging and PET-CT findings. They also found that PET-CT findings had a higher clinical impact on clinical decisions, that is, clinician did not make new therapeutic decisions if PET-CT was negative; however, they changed the management in positive PET-CT.[31]

MR imaging is ineffective during follow-up to assess prognosis. There was no difference in the detection of bone lesions when comparing PET-CT and MR imaging at the time of diagnosis. However, a low number of MR imaging normalizations was seen after 3 cycles of lenalidomide,

bortezomib, and dexamethasone (RVD) and before maintenance. This did not allow for prognostic information. Resolution of focal lesions takes several months. PET-CT was better for evaluation of prognosis and showed strong relation to progression-free survival (PFS) and overall survival.[31] (Fig. 2).

For detection of minimal residual disease (MRD), IMWG proposed that flow cytometry and PET-CT may be complementary to each other.[32] A study done by Moreau and colleagues (2017)[31] found the same, PFS was higher in patients with both normalized PET-CT and negative MRD (flow cytometry) versus patients with either PET positivity and/or MRD positivity before mainatenance[31] (Figs. 3 and 4).

In a recent meta-analysis comparing MR imaging and 18F-FDG PET-CT for treatment assessment in MM, the study found that performance of $^{18}$F-FDG PET-CT was satisfactory in assessment of treatment effect and had higher sensitivity for the detecting early treatment response. Also, those who showed good response in $^{18}$F-FDG PET-CT can be expected to achieve good remission rate.[33]

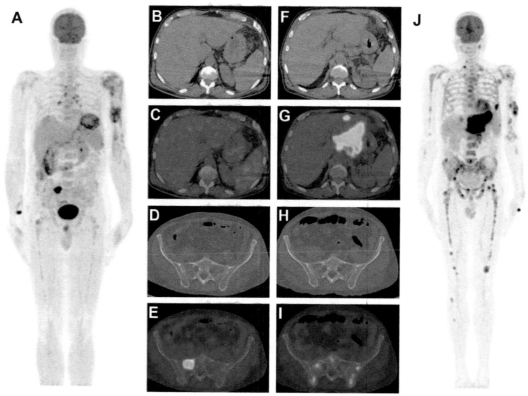

Fig. 2. A 60-year-old man with a known case of MM post-VRd (Bortezomib, Lenalidomide, Dexamethasone) regimen. Head-to-toe PET-CT acquisition was done 60 minutes after injection of 10-mCi $^{18}$F-FDG by intravenous route. Pretreatment maximum intensity projection (MIP) image (A) shows abnormal focal increased uptake in lumbar vertebra, sacrum, and right femur and periprosthetic uptake in left humeral region. Multiple FDG-avid mediastinal lymph nodes are seen, which are likely are infective. Axial images (B, C) show normal physiologic uptake in liver with no focal lesion in CT and in pelvic sections (D, E) show focal uptake in right ala of sacrum, whereas post-treatment images (F, G) show appearance of new discrete and confluent FDG-avid lesions in left lobe of liver. Also, the pelvic sections (H, I) show multiple foci of FDG uptake in pelvis and sacrum. New lesions can be visualized clearly in MIP image (J). Findings suggested disease progression.

## ITALIAN MYELOMA CRITERIA FOR PET USE

To standardize $^{18}$F-FDG PET-CT in MM evaluation, a group of nuclear medicine physicians and hematologists proposed a new criterion for visual interpretation of $^{18}$F-FDG PET-CT and tested its reproducibility. This multicenter protocol was agreed at multidisciplinary consensus meeting and was set up as a subprotocol of the European Myeloma Network. This protocol included description of bone marrow metabolic state, site, and number of PET-positive focal lesions; number of osteolytic lesions; and presence and site of extramedullary disease, paramedullary disease, and fractures (Table 2).

In this study, MM patients who had undergone baseline $^{18}$F-FDG PET-CT (PET-0), after induction (PET-AI), and at the end of treatment (PET-EoT) were prospectively enrolled and studies were interpreted by 5 independent nuclear medicine physicians. For initial evaluation, 17 patients were enrolled, and results showed the new interpretation using the Italian Myeloma Criteria for PET Use (IMPeTUs) appeared to be feasible in clinical practice.[34]

The same group published final results[35] in 86 patients and, in patient-based analysis, concordance among the reviewers were tested by threshold of positivity using a Deauville score (DS 1, 2, 3, 4, or 5). The percentage agreement was superior to 75% for all the time points, reaching 100% of agreement in assessing the presence skull lesions after therapy and also comparable results were obtained when using Krippendorff's alpha coefficient for agreement analysis, either in every single time point of scanning (PET-0, PET-AI, or PET-EoT) or overall for all the scans together and concluded that IMPeTUs proved simple and highly reproducible and can be considered as a base for harmonizing PET interpretation in MM.

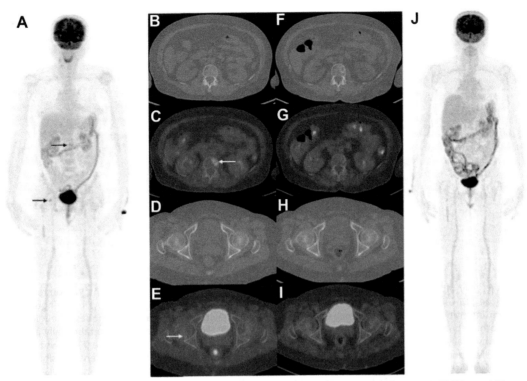

Fig. 3. A 60-year-old woman with known case of MM post-chemotherapy. Head-to-toe PET-CT acquisition was done 60 minutes after injection of 10-mCi $^{18}$F-FDG by intravenous route. Pretreatment maximum intensity projection (MIP) image (A) shows focal increased FDG uptake in L2 vertebra and head of right femur (black arrows). Axial images of abdomen (B, C) show FDG-avid lytic lesion in L2 vertebra, and pelvic regions (D, E) show focal FDG uptake in head of right femur with no significant change in CT (white arrows). Post-therapy axial images (F–I) show metabolic resolution of lesions. MIP image (J) shows no abnormal FDG uptake in the body. Findings suggested complete metabolic response.

## DEAUVILLE 5-POINT SCALE

After the usefulness of the Deauville 5-point scale in routine clinical reporting and in prognostication in lymphoma,[36,37] the role of Deauville has been evaluated in several different cancers, including MM.

As discussed previously, Deauville 5-point scoring was used to interpret focal lesions, bone marrow metabolic state, and osteolytic lesions in IMPeTUs criteria[34,35] and opined that the Deauville 5-point scale is simple and easily reproducible in standardizing reporting of $^{18}$F-FDG PET-CT scans in MM.

In further continuation, to evaluate the usefulness of the Deauville 5-point scale, a few other studies showed that it has prognostic significance, whereby, in multivariate analysis, it was shown that DS greater than or equal to 4 was an independent prognostic factor (hazard ratio [HR] 3.487; P = .03) associated with overall survival.[38] Another study, found that,[39] prior to maintenance therapy, focal lesions DS (FS) and bone marrow

DS (BMS) greater than 3 (higher than the liver) were the strongest predictor for prolonged PFS (FS ≤3 vs >3: median 40 vs 26.6 months; HR 0.6; 95% CI 0.39–0.98; P = .0019; and BMS ≤3 vs >3: median 39.8 vs 26.6 months; HR 0.47; 95% CI 0.24–0.91; P = .024, respectively). Also, another study, showed after 100 days after autologous stem cell transplantation, DS calculated by liver cutoff was statistically significant for PFS, although not statistically significant for overall survival.[40]

## OTHER PET TRACERS
### $^{11}$C-acetate

Cancer cells can metabolize exogenous acetate for de novo membrane biosynthesis by utilizing fatty acid synthase through tricarboxylic acid cycle, and MM cells are not an exception.[41,42] With initial cell line studies using plasma cells[43] and clinical case reports showing $^{11}$C-acetate accumulation in MM,[44] it was assumed to be useful in evaluation. In a head-to-head comparative

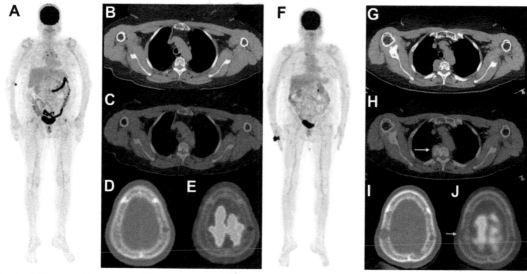

**Fig. 4.** A 61-year-old woman with known case of MM post-chemotherapy and post-transplant, was on follow-up. Head-to-toe PET-CT acquisition was done 60 minutes after injection of 10-mCi [18]F-FDG by intravenous route. Maximum intensity projection (MIP) image (*A*) shows few FDG-avid mediastinal lymph nodes, likely infective with no other abnormal FDG uptake in the body. Axial images (*B–E*) show no abnormal metabolically active lesions; however, a lytic lesion in skull is seen with no significant FDG uptake. A later MIP image (*F*) shows focal FDG uptake in skull and mediastinal region. Axial images (*G, H*) show new FDG-avid soft tissue density lesion in right paravertebral location with erosion of D3 vertebra (*white arrow*). Axial images (*I, J*) show new FDG-avid lytic lesion in skull (*yellow arrow*). Findings suggested recurrent disease.

study using [11]C-acetate and [18]F-FDG PET-CT in 15 patients, in evaluating diffuse MM involvement, [11]C-acetate detected all, whereas 18F-FDG detected only in six patients. Also, focal lesions were detected in 13 patients by [11]C-acetate compared with 10 patients by [18]F-FDG which demonstrated significantly high maximum SUV (SUVmax) (11.4 ± 3.3 compared with 6.6 ± 3.1).[45] Similar results have been published with another study, with a sample size of 35, which showed higher sensitivity of 84.6% with [11]C-acetate versus 57.5% with [18]F-FDG.[46]

**Table 2**
**Summary of Italian Myeloma Criteria for PET Use**

| Lesion Type | Site | Number of Lesions | Grading |
|---|---|---|---|
| Diffuse | Bone marrow[a] | | Deauville 5-point scale |
| Focal | Skull<br>Spine<br>Extraspinal | x = 1 (no lesion)<br>x = 2 (1–3 lesions)<br>x = 3 (4–10 lesions)<br>x = 4 (>10 lesions) | Deauville 5-point scale |
| Lytic | | x = 1 (no lesion)<br>x = 2 (1–3 lesions)<br>x = 3 (4–10 lesions)<br>x = 4 (>10 lesions) | |
| Fracture | At least 1 | | |
| Paramedullary | At least 1 | | |
| Extramedullary | At least 1 | Nodal/extranodal[b] | Deauville 5-point scale |

[a] "A" if hypermetabolism in limbs and ribs.
[b] For nodal disease: cervical, supraclavicular, mediastinal, axillary retroperitoneal, mesenteric, or inguinal; for extranodal disease: liver, muscle, spleen, skin, or other.
*From* Nanni C, Zamagni E, Versari A, Chauvie S, Bianchi A, Rensi M, Bellò M, Rambaldi I, Gallamini A, Patriarca F, Gay F, Gamberi B, Cavo M, Fanti S. Image interpretation criteria for FDG PET/CT in multiple myeloma: a new proposal from an Italian expert panel. IMPeTUs (Italian Myeloma criteria for PET USe). Eur J Nucl Med Mol Imaging. 2016 Mar;43(3):414-21.

## $^{11}$C-choline and $^{18}$F–fluoromethylcholine

Choline, a small molecule precursor of phospho-lipids, which are part of the cell wall membrane, and proliferating cells exhibit increased cell wall membrane synthesis and increased choline kinase activity, leading to increased choline uptake.[47,48] It has been approved by the Food and Drug Administration (FDA) for PET imaging in recurrent prostate cancer.[49]

Solitary plasmacytoma was detected incidentally by $^{11}$C-choline in a case of MGUS, and it led to a hypothesis that MM cells can exhibit increased choline uptake.[50] A prospective comparative study on 10 patients, evaluated with $^{11}$C-choline and $^{18}$F-FDG, showed that the former appears to be more specific, and also the SUVmax was found to be significantly higher for $^{11}$C-choline–positive lesions compared with $^{18}$F-FDG–positive lesions.[51] A main disadvantage with $^{11}$C-choline is high physiologic liver uptake that may obscure hepatic lesions that rarely may present in MM patients.

Another prospective study,[52] comparing $^{18}$F-FDG and $^{18}$F-fluoromethylcholine (FCH) imaging in 21 MM patients found 75% to 76% more lesions on $^{18}$F-FCH compared with $^{18}$F-FDG, and matched foci that took up both the tracers revealed a significantly higher median SUVmax for $^{18}$F-FCH (Fig. 5).

In conclusion, $^{11}$C-choline/$^{18}$F-FCH appears to be more sensitive in MM evaluation with detection of significantly more lesions compared with $^{18}$F-FDG.

## $^{11}$C-methionine

After the usefulness of $^{18}$F-FDG PET-CT in evaluating MM patients, the next best radiotracer with promising results is $^{11}$C-methionine (MET) PET-CT. Uptake of amino acids by tumor cells represents the mechanism and rate of uptake[53] and can be detected by $^{11}$C-MET. MM is characterized by excessive production of monoclonal immuno-globulin, which is detected in serum and/or urine; it is reasonable to think that an amino acid-based tracer, such as $^{11}$C-MET, might be useful in MM. Initial data have reported and this approach appears promising.[54] Initial myeloma cell line and patient-derived plasma cell studies showed higher relative uptake of methionine in these cells in comparison to $^{18}$F-FDG by 1.5- to 5-fold and also showed correlation of increasing $^{11}$C-MET uptake with poor prognosis.[55]

Nakamoto and colleagues[53] compared $^{11}$C-MET PET-CT with $^{18}$F-FDG PET-CT in 20 patients. Lesion-based semiquantitative analysis was done on a 5-point scale (0, negative; 1, probably negative; 2, equivocal; 3, probably positive, and 4, positive). Uptake of $^{11}$C-MET appeared to be higher (SUVmax, mean ± SD, 10.3 ± 5.6) than that of $^{18}$F-FDG (3.4 ± 2.7; $P< .001$), and more lesions of grade 3 or 4 were depicted by $^{11}$C-MET (156 lesions vs 58 lesions on $^{18}$F-FDG). Also, the patient-based sensitivity and specificity were 89% and 100% for $^{11}$C-MET compared with 78% and 100% for $^{18}$F-FDG, indicating higher sensitivity.

Lapa and colleagues[56] compared $^{11}$C-MET PET-CT with $^{18}$F-FDG PET-CT in 43 proved MM patients, wherein patient-based analysis showed $^{11}$C-MET detected lesions in 39/43 (90.7%) compared with 33/43 (76.7%) patients detected on $^{18}$F-FDG. Even in lesion-based analysis, $^{11}$C-MET detected more focal lesions in 28/43 patients (65.1%; $P<.001$), and, in remaining cases, an equal number of lesions was detected by both tracers. Even in patients with extramedullary disease, $^{11}$C-MET performed better compared with $^{18}$F-FDG.

In an extension to that study, Lapa and colleagues[57] conducted a study in two different institutions on 78 patients and, along similar lines to the previous studies, found that $^{11}$C-MET PET-CT detected focal lesions in more patients (59 vs 47; $P<.01$) with higher in compared with $^{18}$F-FDG methionine PET-CT and concluded that $^{11}$C-MET PET-CT is superior in comparison to the latter.

Two other recently published studies,[58,59] with low sample sizes of n = 10 and n = 22, also showed similar results, with $^{11}$C-MET PET-CT showing higher sensitivity than $^{18}$F-FDG PET-CT in detecting bone marrow involvement also in smoldering MM and also showed $^{11}$C-MET PET biomarkers had a better correlation with tumor burden (bone marrow plasma cell infiltration, and M component).

In conclusion, $^{11}$C-MET PET-CT appears to be the best radiopharmaceutical currently in evaluating MM with higher patient-based and lesion-based detection, with higher sensitivity compared with $^{18}$F-FDG PET-CT and having prognostic implication with higher uptake proportional to poorer prognosis.

## $^{18}$F–sodium fluoride

Although $^{18}$F-sodium fluoride (NaF) has a theoretic advantage, with its high sensitivity and uptake reflecting bone remodeling,[60] few previously conducted studies concluded otherwise and reported that $^{18}$F-NaF does not add much significant information compared with $^{18}$F-FDG.

In a prospective study conducted by Sachpeki-dis and colleagues,[61] comparing $^{18}$F-FDG PET-CT

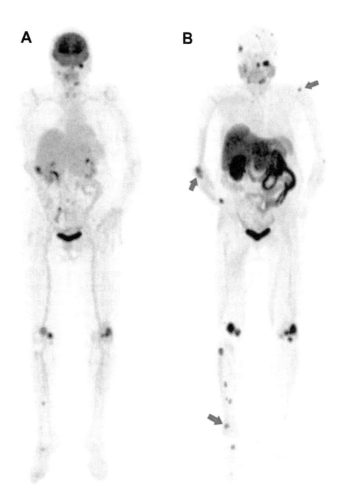

**Fig. 5.** Maximum intensity projection images of $^{18}$F-FDG (*A*) and $^{18}$F-FCH (*B*) of an MM patient show much more bone foci in $^{18}$F-FCH (*blue arrows*). (*From* Cassou-Mounat T, Balogova S, Nataf V, Calzada M, Huchet V, Kerrou K, Devaux JY, Mohty M, Talbot JN, Garderet L. 18F-fluorocholine versus 18F-fluorodeoxyglucose for PET-CT imaging in patients with suspected relapsing or progressive multiple myeloma: a pilot study. Eur J Nucl Med Mol Imaging. 2016 Oct;43(11):1995-2004.)

head on with $^{18}$F-NaF PET-CT in an initial evaluation of 60 MM patients diagnosed according to standard criteria, $^{18}$F-FDG PET-CT revealed 343 focal lesions compared with 132 lesions on $^{18}$F-NaF PET-CT, with 39% correlation. The overall conclusion was that $^{18}$F-FDG PET-CT is more specific in comparison to $^{18}$F-NaF PET-CT.

In another published prospective study, comparing $^{18}$F-PET-CT with $^{18}$F-NaF PET-CT[62] in 26 proved cases of MM, $^{18}$F-NaF PET-CT could detect only 57 lesions in comparison to 128 lesions on $^{18}$F-FDG PET-CT.

In conclusion, $^{18}$F-FDG PET-CT is superior to $^{18}$F-NaF PET-CT in evaluation of MM cases and no significant advantage can be expected from $^{18}$F-NaF PET-CT.

### $^{89}$Zr-daratumumab

CD38 is a 45-kDa type II membrane surface glycoprotein that is expressed on plasma cells in high numbers and is implicated in cell signaling.[63] It represents an ideal target for the treatment of MM, with anti-CD38 monoclonal antibodies (mAbs) like daratumumab, and several studies already have shown the benefit, and it has been approved by the FDA.[64,65]

CD38 antibody labeled with 89Zr appears to show high radiochemical purity and show saturable binding to CD38, and small animal PET-CT imaging showed high radiotracer uptake in variable size tumors, with good tumor-to-background contrast.[66] A first-in-human study using 89Zr-DFO-daratumumab in 6 MM patients showed successful visualization of myeloma in all patients.[67] The main advantage of this tracer is, in image-positive cases, it can be useful for personalized management and help in predicting effectiveness of therapy.[68]

### $^{68}$Ga–fibroblast activation protein inhibitor

Neoplastic tumors are composed of tumor cells (approximately 10% of mass) and stroma (remaining 90%). Fibroblasts are constituents of stroma and in tumors and are called cancer-associated fibroblasts (CAFs), which predominantly help in tumor growth, migration, and progression. These

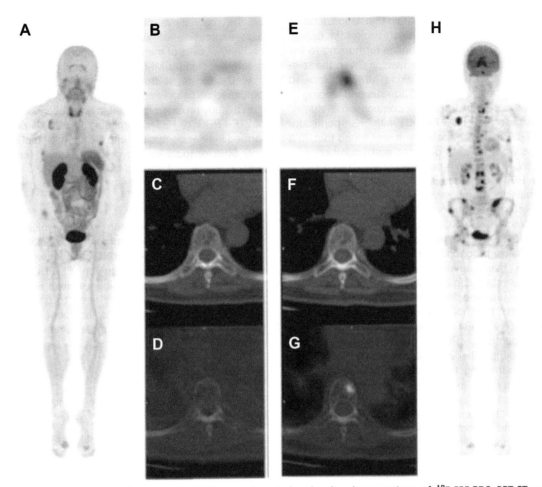

**Fig. 6.** Relapsed case of MM, 4 years after treatment; head-to-head comparison of [18F]-FPRGD2 PET-CT and [18F]-NaF[18F]-FDG PET-CT and maximum intensity projection of the former (*A*) show significantly fewer numbers ($n_1$ = 28 compared with $n_2$ = 40) compared with the latter (*H*); also, axial PET (*B*), axial CT (*C*), and axial PET-CT (*D*) of [18F]-FPRGD2 showed no uptake in the vertebra, in which the [18F]-NaF/[18F]-FDG (*E-G*) showed relatively good tracer uptake. (*From* Withofs N, Cousin F, De Prijck B, Bonnet C, Hustinx R, Gambhir SS, Beguin Y, Caers J. A First Report on [18F]FPRGD2 PET-CT Imaging in Multiple Myeloma. Contrast Media Mol Imaging. 2017 Jul 27;2017:6162845. Article available under open access CC-BY 4.0 license. https://creativecommons.org/licenses/by/4.0/)

CAFs also are involved in immunosuppression and angiogenesis. Because CAFs are most stable than tumor cells and less susceptible to therapy resistance, these are suitable targets for tumor imaging and therapy. They differ from normal fibroblasts in terms of markers expressed, the most significant being fibroblast activation protein (FAP).[69] FAP is a membrane-bound glycoprotein of dipeptidyl peptidase-4 family and is a suitable target for tumor imaging.[70] FAP inhibitors (FAPIs) like FAPI-04 labeled with [68]Ga currently are in use for imaging multiple tumors, including MM.

Tang and colleagues[71] published an interesting image in which they showed increased [68]Ga-FAPI activity in a case of plasmacytoma of ribs.

A head-to-head [68]Ga -FAPI versus [18F]-FDG PET-CT comparison study on different tumors, done by Lan and colleagues,[72] in which they included 3 MM cases, demonstrated that [68]Ga FAPI PET-CT had a lower activity (SUVmax 6.84 ± 4.67 vs 13.09 ± 7.29; $P<.001$) and lower detection rate ($\chi2$ = 5.166; $P<.001$) in comparison with [18F]-FDG.

### C-X-C chemokine receptor 4 receptor imaging

C-X-C chemokine receptor 4 (CXCR4) is G protein–coupled receptor, implicated in cell migration, homing process, angiogenesis, and cell proliferation. Binding of CXCL12 to CXCR4 receptor leads to downstream signaling pathways, resulting in gene expression and protein translation, leading to tumor growth and metastasis.[73] MM cancer cells use the same mechanism for homing to the bone marrow and homeostasis.[74] Given the relevance of CXCR4/CXCL12 axis in MM, radiolabeled analogs can be used for diagnosis and staging.

In a head-to-head comparison study[75] comparing [18]F-FDG PET-CT with [68]Ga-pentixafor PET-CT in 19 MM patients, it was found that, in 8 cases, both tracers detected equal number of lesions, whereas in 4 patients (21%), [68]Ga-pentixafor PET-CT detected more lesions and in the remaining 7 patients (37%) [18]F-FDG PET-CT detected more lesions. This study also provides that increased CXCR4 expression frequently occurs in advanced stages of MM, thus representing a negative prognostic factor.

The main advantage of evaluating CXCR4 uptake in MM can be in its theragnostic approach using [177]Lu- and [90]Y-labeled pentixather. In a first-in-human proof-of-principle study[76] in 3 patients, in which CXCR4 expression was confirmed by [68]Ga-pentixafor PET-CT and later treated with [177]Lu-pentixather in 2 patients and [90]Y-pentixather in the remaining 1 patient and biodistribution and dosimetry was evaluated by post-therapy scans, 2 of these 3 patients who had response evaluation scans were found to have partial response in one case and complete metabolic response in the other, thereby showing promising future for MM treatment with CXCR- based theragnostic.

### [68]Ga–Prostate Specific Membrane Antigen

[68]Ga–prostate specific membrane antigen (PSMA) is already an established modality for imaging in prostate cancer.[77–79] In contrast to the name, PSMA expression is not exclusive to prostate cancer cells, and many studies have been published the role of [68]Ga PSMA in nonprostatic malignancies[80–83] and infection/inflammation in which [68]Ga-PSMA uptake is due mainly to neovascular tissue binding.[84] Neovascularization promoted by endothelial progenitor cells appears to be the mechanism of evolution/progression from asymptomatic stage of MGUS to MM[85] and so it can be a potential target for [68]Ga-PSMA PET-CT imaging.

Sasikumar and colleagues[86] published a case report in which they showed increased [68]Ga-PSMA uptake in lytic skeletal lesions in a histologically proved case of MM and also signifies that there is potential possibility in treating MM patients with [177]Lu-PSMA.

### RGD

As discussed previously, neovascularization promoted by endothelial progenitor cells appears to be the mechanism of progression in MM and high expression of αVβ3 integrin by activated endothelial cells of many tumors have been documented, including MM.[87] RGD-based radiopharmaceuticals target the αVβ3 integrin and were proposed as useful in detection of MM.[88]

In a study reported by Withofs and colleagues[89] of [18]F-FPRGD2 PET-CT imaging in MM, it performed inferior compared with CT scan, detecting only 50% of focal lesions detected by CT, suggesting the clinical utility is limited (Fig. 6).

### SUMMARY

[18]F-FDG traditionally has been used for evaluation of MM. With development of newer tracers, their potential use in MM needs to be researched and studied. Initial results for some non–[18]F-FDG PET tracers have shown promising results. Further studies with large populations need to be done to find a suitable and better replacement of [18]F-FDG and a possibility of theragnostic implications of tracers.

### ACKNOWLEDGMENTS

There are no more people to be acknowledged regarding this article.

### REFERENCES

1. International Myeloma Working Group. Criteria for the classification of monoclonal gammopathies, multiple myeloma and related disorders: a report of the International Myeloma Working Group. Br J Haematol 2003;121(5):749–57.
2. Rajkumar SV, Dimopoulos MA, Palumbo A, et al. International Myeloma Working Group updated criteria for the diagnosis of multiple myeloma. Lancet Oncol 2014;15(12):e538–48.
3. Rajkumar SV, Dispenzieri A, Kyle RA. Monoclonal gammopathy of undetermined significance, Waldenström macroglobulinemia, AL amyloidosis, and related plasma cell disorders: diagnosis and treatment. Mayo Clin Proc 2006;81(5):693–703.
4. Bray F, Ferlay J, Soerjomataram I, et al. Global cancer statistics 2018: GLOBOCAN estimates of incidence and mortality worldwide for 36 cancers in 185 countries. CA Cancer J Clin 2018;68(6):394–424.
5. Cowan AJ, Allen C, Barac A, et al. Global burden of multiple myeloma: a systematic analysis for the global burden of disease study 2016. JAMA Oncol 2018;4(9):1221–7.
6. Padala SA, Barsouk A, Barsouk A, et al. Epidemiology, staging, and management of multiple myeloma. Med Sci (Basel) 2021;9(1):3.

7. Kyle RA, Remstein ED, Therneau TM, et al. Clinical course and prognosis of smoldering (asymptomatic) multiple myeloma. N Engl J Med 2007;356(25): 2582–90.

8. Durie BG, Salmon SE. A clinical staging system for multiple myeloma. Correlation of measured myeloma cell mass with presenting clinical features, response to treatment, and survival. Cancer 1975; 36(3):842–54.

9. Durie BGM. The role of anatomic and functional staging in myeloma: description of Durie/Salmon plus staging system. Eur J Cancer 2006;42(11): 1539–43.

10. Greipp PR, San Miguel J, Durie BGM, et al. International staging system for multiple myeloma. J Clin Oncol 2005;23(15):3412–20.

11. Rajkumar SV. Updated diagnostic criteria and staging system for multiple myeloma. Am Soc Clin Oncol Educ Book 2016;35:e418–23.

12. Lütje S, de Rooy JWJ, Croockewit S, et al. Role of radiography, MRI and FDG-PET/CT in diagnosing, staging and therapeutical evaluation of patients with multiple myeloma. Ann Hematol 2009;88(12): 1161–8.

13. Gleeson TG, Moriarty J, Shortt CP, et al. Accuracy of whole-body low-dose multidetector CT (WBLDCT) versus skeletal survey in the detection of myelomatous lesions, and correlation of disease distribution with whole-body MRI (WBMRI). Skeletal Radiol 2009;38(3):225–36.

14. Abouzied MM, Crawford ES, Nabi HA. 18F-FDG imaging: pitfalls and artifacts. J Nucl Med Technol 2005;33(3):145–55. quiz 162-163.

15. Kostakoglu L, Agress H, Goldsmith SJ. Clinical role of FDG PET in evaluation of cancer patients. Radiographics 2003;23(2):315–40 [quiz: 533].

16. Referenced with permission from the NCCN Clinical Practice Guidelines in Oncology (NCCN Guidelines®) for Guideline Name V.X.201X. © National Comprehensive Cancer Network, Inc. 201X. All rights reserved. To view the most recent and complete version of the guideline, go online to NCCN.org. NCCN makes no warranties of any kind whatsoever regarding their content, use or application and disclaims any responsibility for their application or use in any way.

17. Kumar SK, Callander NS, Adekola K, et al. Multiple myeloma, version 3.2021, NCCN clinical practice guidelines in oncology. J Natl Compr Canc Netw 2020;18(12):1685–717.

18. Hillengass J, Weber MA, Kilk K, et al. Prognostic significance of whole-body MRI in patients with monoclonal gammopathy of undetermined significance. Leukemia 2014;28(1):174–8.

19. Minarik J, Krhovska P, Hrbek J, et al. Prospective comparison of conventional radiography, low-dose computed tomography and magnetic resonance imaging in monoclonal gammopathies. Biomed Pap Med Fac Univ Palacky Olomouc Czech Repub 2016;160(2):305–9.

20. Hillengass J, Usmani S, Rajkumar SV, et al. International myeloma working group consensus recommendations on imaging in monoclonal plasma cell disorders. Lancet Oncol 2019;20(6): e302–12.

21. Hillengass J, Fechtner K, Weber MA, et al. Prognostic significance of focal lesions in whole-body magnetic resonance imaging in patients with asymptomatic multiple myeloma. J Clin Oncol 2010;28(9):1606–10.

22. Siontis B, Kumar S, Dispenzieri A, et al. Positron emission tomography-computed tomography in the diagnostic evaluation of smoldering multiple myeloma: identification of patients needing therapy. Blood Cancer J 2015;5:e364.

23. Zamagni E, Nanni C, Gay F, et al. 18F-FDG PET/CT focal, but not osteolytic, lesions predict the progression of smoldering myeloma to active disease. Leukemia 2016;30(2):417–22.

24. Nahi H, Genell A, Wålinder G, et al. Incidence, characteristics, and outcome of solitary plasmacytoma and plasma cell leukemia. Population-based data from the Swedish Myeloma Register. Eur J Haematol 2017;99(3):216–22.

25. Albano D, Bosio G, Treglia G, et al. 18F-FDG PET/CT in solitary plasmacytoma: metabolic behavior and progression to multiple myeloma. Eur J Nucl Med Mol Imaging 2018;45(1):77–84.

26. Regelink JC, Minnema MC, Terpos E, et al. Comparison of modern and conventional imaging techniques in establishing multiple myeloma-related bone disease: a systematic review. Br J Haematol 2013;162(1):50–61.

27. Vicentini JRT, Bredella MA. Role of FDG PET in the staging of multiple myeloma. Skeletal Radiol 2021. https://doi.org/10.1007/s00256-021-03771-2.

28. Nanni C, Zamagni E, Farsad M, et al. Role of 18F-FDG PET/CT in the assessment of bone involvement in newly diagnosed multiple myeloma: preliminary results. Eur J Nucl Med Mol Imaging 2006;33(5): 525–31.

29. Zamagni E, Nanni C, Patriarca F, et al. A prospective comparison of 18F-fluorodeoxyglucose positron emission tomography-computed tomography, magnetic resonance imaging and whole-body planar radiographs in the assessment of bone disease in newly diagnosed multiple myeloma. Haematologica 2007;92(1):50–5.

30. Hur J, Yoon CS, Ryu YH, et al. Comparative study of fluorodeoxyglucose positron emission tomography and magnetic resonance imaging for the detection of spinal bone marrow infiltration in untreated patients with multiple myeloma. Acta Radiol 2008; 49(4):427–35.

31. Moreau P, Attal M, Caillot D, et al. Prospective evaluation of magnetic resonance imaging and [18F]fluorodeoxy-glucose positron emission tomographycomputed tomography at diagnosis and before maintenance therapy in symptomatic patients with multiple myeloma included in the IFM/DFCI 2009 trial: results of the IMA-JEM study. J Clin Oncol 2017;35(25):2911–8.

32. Kumar S, Paiva B, Anderson KC, et al. International Myeloma Working Group consensus criteria for response and minimal residual disease assessment in multiple myeloma. Lancet Oncol 2016;17(8): e328–46.

33. Yokoyama K, Tsuchiya J, Tateishi U. Comparison of [18F]FDG PET/CT and MRI for treatment response assessment in multiple myeloma: a meta-analysis. Diagnostics (Basel) 2021;11(4):706.

34. Nanni C, Zamagni E, Versari A, et al. Image interpretation criteria for FDG PET/CT in multiple myeloma: a new proposal from an Italian expert panel. IMPeTUs (Italian Myeloma criteria for PET USe). Eur J Nucl Med Mol Imaging 2016;43(3):414–21.

35. Nanni C, Versari A, Chauvie S, et al. Interpretation criteria for FDG PET/CT in multiple myeloma (IMPeTUs): final results. IMPeTUs (Italian myeloma criteria for PET USe). Eur J Nucl Med Mol Imaging 2018;45(5):712–9.

36. Cheson BD, Fisher RI, Barrington SF, et al. Recommendations for initial evaluation, staging, and response assessment of Hodgkin and non-Hodgkin lymphoma: the Lugano classification. J Clin Oncol 2014;32(27):3059–68.

37. Gallamini A, Barrington SF, Biggi A, et al. The predictive role of interim positron emission tomography for Hodgkin lymphoma treatment outcome is confirmed using the interpretation criteria of the Deauville five-point scale. Haematologica 2014;99(6):1107–13.

38. Deng S, Zhang B, Zhou Y, et al. The role of 18F-FDG PET/CT in multiple myeloma staging according to IMPeTUs: comparison of the Durie-Salmon plus and other staging systems. Contrast Media Mol Imaging 2018;2018:4198673.

39. Zamagni E, Nanni C, Dozza L, et al. Standardization of 18F-FDG-PET/CT according to Deauville criteria for metabolic complete response definition in newly diagnosed multiple myeloma. J Clin Oncol 2021; 39(2):116–25.

40. Tuglular T, Şahin E, Öneş T, et al. The effect of PET/CT Deauville criteria on progression free survival and overall survival in multiple myeloma patients following autologous stem cell transplantation. Clin Lymphoma Myeloma Leuk 2019;19(10):e302.

41. Lyssiotis CA, Cantley LC. Acetate fuels the cancer engine. Cell 2014;159(7):1492–4.

42. qin Wang W, ying Zhao X, yan Wang H, et al. Increased fatty acid synthase as a potential therapeutic target in multiple myeloma. J Zhejiang Univ Sci B 2008;9(6):441–7.

43. Stjernholm RL. Carbohydrate metabolism in leukocytes. VII. Metabolism of glucose, acetate, and propionate by human plasma cells. J Bacteriol 1967; 93(5):1657–61.

44. Lee SM, Kim TS, Lee JW, et al. Incidental finding of an 11C-acetate PET-positive multiple myeloma. Ann Nucl Med 2010;24(1):41–4.

45. Lin C, Ho CL, Ng SH, et al. 11)C-acetate as a new biomarker for PET/CT in patients with multiple myeloma: initial staging and postinduction response assessment. Eur J Nucl Med Mol Imaging 2014; 41(1):41–9.

46. Iai Ho C, Chen S, Leung YL, et al. 11C-acetate PET/CT for metabolic characterization of multiple myeloma: a comparative study with 18F-FDG PET/CT. J Nucl Med 2014;55(5):749–52.

47. Gibellini F, Smith TK. The Kennedy pathway–De novo synthesis of phosphatidylethanolamine and phosphatidylcholine. IUBMB Life 2010;62(6): 414–28.

48. Bouchelouche K, Tagawa ST, Goldsmith SJ, et al. PET/CT imaging and Radioimmunotherapy of prostate cancer. Semin Nucl Med 2011;41(1):29–44.

49. FDA approves 11C-choline for PET in prostate cancer. J Nucl Med 2012;53(12):11N.

50. Ambrosini V, Farsad M, Nanni C, et al. Incidental finding of an (11)C-choline PET-positive solitary plasmacytoma lesion. Eur J Nucl Med Mol Imaging 2006;33(12):1522.

51. Nanni C, Zamagni E, Cavo M, et al. 11C-choline vs. 18F-FDG PET/CT in assessing bone involvement in patients with multiple myeloma. World J Surg Oncol 2007;5:68.

52. Cassou-Mounat T, Balogova S, Nataf V, et al. 18F-fluorocholine versus 18F-fluorodeoxyglucose for PET/CT imaging in patients with suspected relapsing or progressive multiple myeloma: a pilot study. Eur J Nucl Med Mol Imaging 2016;43(11):1995–2004.

53. Nakamoto Y, Kurihara K, Nishizawa M, et al. Clinical value of 11C-methionine PET/CT in patients with plasma cell malignancy: comparison with 18F-FDG PET/CT. Eur J Nucl Med Mol Imaging 2013;40(5): 708–15.

54. Dankerl A, Liebisch P, Glatting G, et al. Multiple myeloma: molecular imaging with 11C-methionine PET/CT–Initial experience. Radiology 2007;242(2): 498–508.

55. Lückerath K, Lapa C, Spahmann A, et al. Targeting paraprotein biosynthesis for non-invasive characterization of myeloma biology. PLoS One 2013;8(12): e84840.

56. Lapa C, Knop S, Schreder M, et al. 11C-Methionine-PET in multiple myeloma: correlation with clinical parameters and bone marrow involvement. Theranostics 2016;6(2):254–61.

57. Lapa C, Garcia-Velloso MJ, Lückerath K, et al. 11C-Methionine-PET in multiple myeloma: a combined

study from two different institutions. Theranostics 2017;7(11):2956–64.

58. Morales-Lozano MI, Viering O, Samnick S, et al. 18 F-FDG and 11 C-methionine PET/CT in newly diagnosed multiple myeloma patients: comparison of volume-based PET biomarkers. Cancers 2020; 12(4). https://doi.org/10.3390/cancers12041042.

59. Zhou X, Dierks A, Kertels O, et al. 18F-FDG, 11C-methionine, and 68Ga-pentixafor PET/CT in patients with smoldering multiple myeloma: imaging pattern and clinical features. Cancers (Basel) 2020;12(8): E2333.

60. Czernin J, Satyamurthy N, Schiepers C. Molecular mechanisms of bone 18F-NaF deposition. J Nucl Med 2010;51(12):1826–9.

61. Sachpekidis C, Goldschmidt H, Hose D, et al. PET/ CT studies of multiple myeloma using (18) F-FDG and (18) F-NaF: comparison of distribution patterns and tracers' pharmacokinetics. Eur J Nucl Med Mol Imaging 2014;41(7):1343–53.

62. Ak İ, Onner H, Akay OM. Is there any complimentary role of F-18 NaF PET/CT in detecting of osseous involvement of multiple myeloma? A comparative study for F-18 FDG PET/CT and F-18 FDG NaF PET/CT. Ann Hematol 2015;94(9):1567–75.

63. Funaro A, Spagnoli GC, Ausiello CM, et al. Involvement of the multilineage CD38 molecule in a unique pathway of cell activation and proliferation. J Immunol 1990;145(8):2390–6.

64. Facon T, Kumar S, Plesner T, et al. Daratumumab plus lenalidomide and dexamethasone for untreated myeloma. N Engl J Med 2019;380(22):2104–15.

65. Moreau P, Attal M, Hulin C, et al. Bortezomib, thalidomide, and dexamethasone with or without daratumumab before and after autologous stem-cell transplantation for newly diagnosed multiple myeloma (CASSIOPEIA): a randomised, open-label, phase 3 study. Lancet 2019;394(10192):29–38.

66. Ghai A, Maji D, Cho N, et al. Preclinical development of CD38-targeted [89Zr]Zr-DFO-Daratumumab for imaging multiple myeloma. J Nucl Med 2018;59(2): 216–22.

67. Ulaner G, Sobol N, O'Donoghue J, et al. Preclinical development and First-in-human imaging of 89Zr-Daratumumab for CD38 targeted imaging of myeloma. J Nucl Med 2019;60(supplement 1): 203.

68. Sachpekidis C, Goldschmidt H, Dimitrakopoulou-Strauss A. Positron emission tomography (PET) radiopharmaceuticals in multiple myeloma. Molecules 2019;25(1):134.

69. Lindner T, Loktev A, Giesel F, et al. Targeting of activated fibroblasts for imaging and therapy. EJNMMI Radiopharm Chem 2019;4:16.

70. Hamson EJ, Keane FM, Tholen S, et al. Understanding fibroblast activation protein (FAP): substrates, activities, expression and targeting for cancer therapy. Proteomics Clin Appl 2014;8(5–6):454–63.

71. Tang W, Wang Q, Yang S, et al. Elevated 68Ga-FAPI activity in the plasmacytoma of the ribs. Clin Nucl Med 2021;46(6):523–4.

72. Lan L, Liu H, Wang Y, et al. The potential utility of [68 Ga]Ga-DOTA-FAPI-04 as a novel broad-spectrum oncological and non-oncological imaging agent-comparison with [18F]FDG. Eur J Nucl Med Mol Imaging 2021. https://doi.org/10.1007/s00259-021-05522-w.

73. Domanska UM, Kruizinga RC, Nagengast WB, et al. A review on CXCR4/CXCL12 axis in oncology: no place to hide. Eur J Cancer 2013;49(1):219–30.

74. Alsayed Y, Ngo H, Runnels J, et al. Mechanisms of regulation of CXCR4/SDF-1 (CXCL12)-dependent migration and homing in multiple myeloma. Blood 2007;109(7):2708–17.

75. Lapa C, Schreder M, Schirbel A, et al. [68Ga]Pentixafor-PET/CT for imaging of chemokine receptor CXCR4 expression in multiple myeloma - comparison to [18F]FDG and laboratory values. Theranostics 2017;7(1):205–12.

76. Herrmann K, Schottelius M, Lapa C, et al. First-in-Human experience of CXCR4-Directed endoradiotherapy with 177Lu- and 90Y-labeled pentixather in advanced-stage multiple myeloma with extensive Intra- and extramedullary disease. J Nucl Med 2016;57(2):248–51.

77. Hofman MS, Hicks RJ, Maurer T, et al. Prostate-specific membrane antigen PET: clinical utility in prostate cancer, normal patterns, pearls, and pitfalls. Radiographics 2018;38(1):200–17.

78. Afshar-Oromieh A, Avtzi E, Giesel FL, et al. The diagnostic value of PET/CT imaging with the (68)Ga-labelled PSMA ligand HBED-CC in the diagnosis of recurrent prostate cancer. Eur J Nucl Med Mol Imaging 2015;42(2):197–209.

79. Sterzing F, Kratochwil C, Fiedler H, et al. 68)Ga-PSMA-11 PET/CT: a new technique with high potential for the radiotherapeutic management of prostate cancer patients. Eur J Nucl Med Mol Imaging 2016; 43(1):34–41.

80. de Galiza Barbosa F, Queiroz MA, Nunes RF, et al. Nonprostatic diseases on PSMA PET imaging: a spectrum of benign and malignant findings. Cancer Imaging 2020;20(1):23.

81. Kumar A, ArunRaj ST, Bhullar K, et al. Ga-68 PSMA PET/CT in recurrent high-grade gliomas: evaluating PSMA expression in vivo. Neuroradiology 2021. https://doi.org/10.1007/s00234-021-02828-2.

82. Taywade SK, Damle NA, Bal C. PSMA expression in papillary thyroid carcinoma: Opening a new horizon in management of thyroid cancer? Clin Nucl Med 2016;41(5):e263–5.

83. Backhaus P, Noto B, Avramovic N, et al. Targeting PSMA by radioligands in non-prostate disease-

current status and future perspectives. Eur J Nucl Med Mol Imaging 2018;45(5):860–77.

84. Chang SS, O'Keefe DS, Bacich DJ, et al. Prostate-specific membrane antigen is produced in tumor-associated neovasculature. Clin Cancer Res 1999; 5(10):2674–81.

85. Tenreiro MM, Correia ML, Brito MA. Endothelial progenitor cells in multiple myeloma neovascularization: a brick to the wall. Angiogenesis 2017;20(4):443–62.

86. Sasikumar A, Joy A, Pillai MRA, et al. 68Ga-PSMA PET/CT imaging in multiple myeloma. Clin Nucl Med 2017;42(2):e126–7.

87. Wu Z, Li ZB, Cai W, et al. 18F-labeled mini-PEG spacered RGD dimer (18F-FPRGD2): synthesis and microPET imaging of alphavbeta3 integrin expression. Eur J Nucl Med Mol Imaging 2007; 34(11):1823–31.

88. Weis SM, Cheresh DA. αV integrins in angiogenesis and cancer. Cold Spring Harb Perspect Med 2011; 1(1):a006478.

89. Withofs N, Cousin F, De Prijck B, et al. A first report on [18F]FPRGD2 PET/CT imaging in multiple myeloma. Contrast Media Mol Imaging 2017;2017: 6162845.

# Role of Molecular Imaging with PET/MR Imaging in the Diagnosis and Management of Brain Tumors

Austin J. Borja, BA[a], Jitender Saini, DM[b], William Y. Raynor, MD[a],
Cyrus Ayubcha, MSc[c], Thomas J. Werner, MS[a], Abass Alavi, MD[a],
Mona-Elisabeth Revheim, MD, PhD, MHA[d,e], Chandana Nagaraj, DNB[b,*]

## KEYWORDS

- PET • [18]F-FDG • Glioma • Brain tumor • Amino acid

## KEY POINTS

- Genetic/epigenetic molecular and imaging evidence determine diagnosis, prognosis, and individualized treatment of gliomas.
- [18]F-fluorodeoxyglucose (FDG)–PET is the most widely used molecular imaging modality to assess gliomas; non–[18]F-FDG radiotracers have been employed but several require further investigations in large, prospective trials to define their role in glioma imaging.
- Multiparametric simultaneous PET/MR imaging may improve diagnosis, treatment planning, and response assessment of glial neoplasms.

## INTRODUCTION

Gliomas are the most common primary brain tumors, constituting 25% of primary central nervous system (CNS) tumors and 80% of malignant CNS tumors.[1] Neuroimaging with MR imaging plays a critical role in initial screening but may not fully characterize the tumor.[2] Although histopathology remains the gold standard in the diagnosis and grading of gliomas, the World Health Organization (WHO) 2021 classification of CNS tumors combines both histologic and molecular findings into its four-grade classification.[3,4] This integrated approach aims to improve objectivity, diagnostic accuracy, and prognostication to better guide medical treatment and management. In addition, the Response Assessment in Neuro-Oncology (RANO) criteria recently were updated to include molecular imaging parameters to supplement MR imaging in the clinical management of glioma, differentiate between treatment-related responsivity and true tumor progression.[5–11] As such, clinicians must incorporate such molecular insights into the consideration of CNS neoplasms.

The blood-brain barrier (BBB) restricts which substances are allowed to pass from the blood to the brain.[12] With disruption of the BBB (eg, from primary CNS tumors), substances, such as metastatic cells and radiotracers, can penetrate

[a] Department of Radiology, Hospital of the University of Pennsylvania, 3400 Spruce Street, Philadelphia, PA 19104, USA; [b] Department of Neuro Imaging and Interventional Radiology, National Institute of Mental Health and Neurosciences, Hosur Road, Bengaluru, Karnataka 560-029, India; [c] Harvard Medical School, 25 Shattuck Street, Boston, MA 02115, USA; [d] Division of Radiology and Nuclear Medicine, Oslo University Hospital, Sognsvannsveien 20, Oslo 0372, Norway; [e] Institute of Clinical Medicine, Faculty of Medicine, University of Oslo, Problemveien 7, Oslo 0315, Norway
* Corresponding author: Department of Neuro Imaging and Interventional Radiology, National Institute of Mental Health and Neurosciences, Hosur Road, Bengaluru, Karnataka 560-029, India.
E-mail address: chandana@nimhans.ac.in

PET Clin 17 (2022) 431–451
https://doi.org/10.1016/j.cpet.2022.03.002
1556-8598/22/© 2022 Elsevier Inc. All rights reserved.

and readily affect the brain.[13] Nonetheless, this remains a late-stage complication of brain neoplasms.[13] Hence, attention has turned toward the development and evaluation of PET radiotracers, such as [18]F-fluorodeoxyglucose ([18]F-FDG) and labeled amino acid (AA) analogs, which are readily transferred across even an intact BBB by large-capacity specific transporters (Table 1). Furthermore, the introduction of hybrid PET/MR imaging has revolutionized brain tumor imaging, allowing for noninvasive, simultaneous assessment of morphologic, functional, metabolic, and molecular parameters within the brain. This article reviews the role of molecular imaging with [18]F-FDG, the most used PET radiopharmaceutical; AA tracers, including [11]C-methionine ([11]C-MET), [18]F-fluoroethyltyrosine ([18]F-FET), [18]F-dihydroxyphenylalanine ([18]F-FDOPA), and [18]F-fluciclovine ([18]F-FACBC); and non–[18]F-FDG, non-AA brain tumor radiotracers, [13]N-ammonia ([13]N-NH$_3$), [11]C-choline ([11]C-CHO), and [18]F-fluorocholine ([18]F-FCH), as well as the use of PET/MR imaging in brain tumors.

## IMAGING TECHNIQUE AND PROTOCOLS

[18]F-FDG and AA radiotracers are transferred across the BBB in both physiologic and pathologic states, enabling the depiction of the tumor mass in response to the radioactive molecules and complementing contrast enhancement on MR imaging. Multiparametric PET and MR imaging has increased the accuracy in determining brain tumor grade, extent, and other biological/molecular metrics.[2] Hybrid PET/MR imaging is an emerging technology that aims to capitalize on the inherent advantages of MR imaging (eg, increased soft tissue contrast, lack of ionizing radiation exposure, and functional imaging) and PET (eg, noninvasive and traces physiologic and pathophysiological processes at molecular level).[14–17] This is particularly relevant toward challenging determinations, such as differentiating between tumor recurrence and treatment-induced changes.

Anatomic considerations (Table 2) and multiple static and dynamic acquisition protocols that exist in hybrid PET/MR imaging are relevant when performing brain tumor imaging (Table 3). Both [18]F-FDG–PET and AA-PET scans are acquired after a 4- to 6-hour fast. Patients are positioned in the scanner, such that slices parallel to the orbitomeatal line are obtained with appropriate attenuation correction for reconstruction and quantification. Standard interpretation involves the comparison of tracer uptake within a suspect lesion to a reference value, typically determined by measuring uptake in the corresponding region of the contralateral hemisphere (Table 4). Nevertheless, tracers may show false-positive uptake in many benign conditions that need to be evaluated further with multiparametric imaging for differential diagnosis.

## TUMOR DETECTION AND GRADING

Accurate tumor grading plays a critical role in treatment planning and prognostication. Reliance

---

**Table 1**
**Indications for PET imaging of brain tumors**

| Indication | Justification |
|---|---|
| Initial diagnosis | Differentiate neoplastic vs benign lesion<br>Delineate tumor extent<br>Biopsy planning<br>Prognostication |
| Postsurgery | To assess the completion of resection<br>Radiotherapy planning, if indicated<br>Crucial for monitoring future response to treatment<br>Prognostication |
| Post-chemoradiation therapy | Differentiate recurrence vs radiation injury<br>Differentiate pseudo-progression vs pseudo-response<br>Adjuvant therapy planning, if indicated |
| Continued follow-up | Differentiate recurrence vs necrosis<br>Differentiate pseudo-progression vs pseudo-response<br>Adjuvant therapy planning, if indicated<br>Addition surgical resection, if indicated |

*Adapted from* Albert NL, Weller M, Suchorska B, et al. Response Assessment in Neuro-Oncology working group and European Association for Neuro-Oncology recommendations for the clinical use of PET imaging in gliomas. *Neuro Oncol.* 2016;18(9):1199-1208.

**Table 2**
Anatomic considerations in PET/MR imaging brain tumor imaging

| | Tumor Biological or Anatomic Characteristic | MR Imaging Sequence | Amino Acid–PET | [18F]-Fluorodeoxyglucose–PET |
|---|---|---|---|---|
| 1 | Vascularity and integrity of BBB | ASL<br>DCE perfusion–T1 perfusion<br>PWI/DSC-enhanced perfusion–T2 perfusion<br>APTw | Dynamic AA-PET imaging, especially $^{18}$F-FET and $^{18}$F-FDOPA | Its current role in presurgical diagnosis, tumor grading, and post-treatment assessment is limited. |
| 2 | Cellular density/grading | DWI for ADC maps | TAC, TTP, and slope, especially $^{18}$F-FET and $^{18}$F-FDOPA<br>Kinetic modeling<br>Uptake by LAT reflects cell proliferation, related to increased molecular synthesis, transamination, and transmethylation[10,96] | Delayed $^{18}$F-FDG–PET imaging at 3–8 h postinjection[27]<br>$^{18}$F-FDG uptake in tumors T/WM ratio 1.5 or T/GM ratio 0.6) were able to identify and distinguish benign tumors (grades I and II) from malignant tumors (grades III and IV)[26] |
| 3 | Cell proliferation and metabolites | Uni- and multivoxel MRS for prediction of IDH mutation status | Pattern and intensity of tracer uptake<br>Semiquantitative and quantitative analysis with cutoff values | SUVmax in primary brain tumor correlates with histologic tumor grade, cell density, and survival[97–101] |
| 4 | Tumor volume | Postcontrast MP-RAGE<br>T2/FLAIR | Cutoff thresholds for definition of biological tumor volume<br>$^{18}$F-FET: SUV >1.6–1.8 of the mean value in healthy-appearing brain<br>$^{11}$C-MET: SUV >1.3 of the mean value in healthy-appearing brain<br>$^{18}$F-FDOPA: SUV more than the mean value in healthy striatum[102] | Cutoff thresholds for definition of biological tumor volume<br>$^{18}$F-FDG: not available |
| 5 | Recurrence vs necrosis | DTI to delineate margins of primary brain tumors better than conventional MR imaging alone<br>Diffusion tensor tractography | Quantitative analysis of AA PET data with pattern uptake<br>Low, homogenous uptake around the resection cavity: likely postsurgical changes<br>High, focal uptake: likely recurrence | Evaluate T/N ratio<br>High FDG uptake in a previously diagnosed LGG with low FDG uptake is diagnostic of anaplastic transformation |

(continued on next page)

**Table 2**
**(continued)**

| Tumor Biological or Anatomic Characteristic | MR Imaging Sequence | Amino Acid–PET | $^{18}$F-Fluorodeoxyglucose–PET |
|---|---|---|---|
| 6  Intratumoral hemorrhage | SWI Sensitivity for microhemorrhages and microvasculature itself, correlates with tumor grade and neoangiogenesis[103] | False-positive uptake | False-positive uptake |
| 7  Eloquent areas/neuronal activation | Functional MR imaging to localize regions of motor/language activation nearby or within a brain tumor | | Task-specific changes in glucose metabolism, functional connectivity, and corresponding white matter fiber tracts |

*Abbreviations:* ADC, apparent diffusion coefficient; APTw, amide proton transfer–weighted; ASL, arterial spin labeling; DCE, dynamic contrast–enhanced; DSC, dynamic susceptibility contrast; DTI, diffusion tensor imaging; DWI, diffusion-weighted imaging; MP-RAGE, magnetization prepared–rapid gradient echo; MRS, magnetic resonance spectroscopy; PWI, perfusion-weighted imaging; SUV, standardized uptake value; SWI, susceptibility-weighted imaging; T/GM, tumor-to-gray matter ratio; T/N, tumor–to–normal ratio. T/WM, tumor–to–white matter ratio; TAC, time activity curve.

**Table 3**
**PET acquisition protocols**

| Tracer | Dose To Be Injected (MBq) | Static Imaging | Dynamic Imaging |
|---|---|---|---|
| $^{18}$F-FDG | 185–200 | 10- to 20-min image acquisition beginning 45+ min after tracer injection | Not recommended |
| $^{11}$C-MET | 370–555 | 20-min image acquisition beginning 10 min after tracer injection | 40-min image acquisition at tracer injection |
| $^{18}$F-FET | 185–200 | 20-min image acquisition beginning 20 min after tracer injection | 40- to 50-min image acquisition at tracer injection |
| $^{18}$F-FDOPA | 185–200 | 0 to 20-min image acquisition beginning 10–30 min after tracer injection | 75-min image acquisition at tracer injection |
| $^{13}$N-NH$_3$ | 444–592 | 10-min image acquisition beginning 5 min after tracer injection | 15-min image acquisition at tracer injection |
| $^{11}$C-CHO/$^{18}$F-FCH | 370–444 | 10–20 min image acquisition ($^{18}$F-FCH) | 2–5 min after tracer injection ($^{11}$C-CHO) |
| $^{18}$F-FACBC | 185–399 | 45- to 65-min after tracer injection | 0–60 min after tracer injection |

*Adapted from* Law I, Albert NL, Arbizu J, et al. Joint EANM/EANO/RANO practice guidelines/SNMMI procedure standards for imaging of gliomas using PET with radiolabeled amino acids and [(18)F]FDG: version 1.0. *Eur J Nucl Med Mol Imaging.* 2019;46(3):540-557.

solely on structural imaging modalities, however, presents multiple limitations. MR imaging enhancement, a byproduct of BBB disruption, is neither sensitive nor specific for gliomas. Most low-grade gliomas (LGGs)—and as many as one-third of high-grade gliomas (HGGs)—do not enhance on MR imaging.[18–20] Meanwhile, other conditions, including infections, demyelinating diseases, and radiation necrosis, may contrast enhance. Therefore, strategies to mitigate these challenges, such as augmentation of structural imaging with molecular parameters, are of significant interest.

$^{18}$F-FDG–PET has long been utilized in the imaging of brain tumors. Glucose hypermetabolism among gliomas is likely a combined effect of increased energetic demand secondary to proliferative processes, overexpression of glucose transporters in response to oncogene expression, and dysregulation of the hexokinase enzymatic activity (**Fig. 1**).[21,22] As such, $^{18}$F-FDG can help to characterize brain tumors as well as differentiate between LGGs and HGGs, on the basis of differential glucose metabolism. In addition, $^{18}$F-FDG–PET appears uniquely useful in the differentiation of primary CNS lymphoma from glioblastoma (GBM) by means of semiquantitative parameters,

serving as a strong confirmatory tool among high-risk patients.[23] Despite its demonstrated clinical utility, standard $^{18}$F-FDG–PET is subject to a handful of limitations. First, high–normal cortical brain uptake at baseline may make the detection of LGG) challenging.[24] Additionally, it may be equally difficult to distinguish between inflammatory and neoplastic lesions. In response, several techniques have been employed to enhance the performance of $^{18}$F-FDG–PET imaging in brain tumors, namely hybrid PET/MR imaging and delayed PET imaging.[25–28] Other strategies, such as coregistration with rubidium-82 (a PET tracer related to BBB dysregulation), may improve delineation of lesions with indeterminate boundaries further.[29,30] Finally, introduction of total-body PET instrumentation may be applied to more readily detect brain neoplasms, particularly metastases (see **Fig. 1E**).[31] As such, it seems likely that $^{18}$F-FDG–PET will remain a mainstay of CNS tumor imaging.

$^{11}$C-MET represents the first AA radiopharmaceutical to gain widespread traction in glioma imaging (**Fig. 2**).[32] Unlike $^{18}$F-FDG, $^{11}$C-MET exhibits a low–normal cortical background with a high tumoral uptake. $^{11}$C-MET transport is facilitated by an increased number of microvessels

**Table 4**
**PET interpretation criteria**

| Parameter | 11C-MET | 18F-FET | 18F-FDOPA | 13N-NH3 | 11C-CHO/18F-FCH | 18F-FACBC |
|---|---|---|---|---|---|---|
| Neoplastic vs non-neoplastic | TBRmax 1.3–1.5[90,104] | TBRmax 2.5 TBRmax 1.9[105,106] | T/N 2.16[107] | T/WM 1.2 ± 1.0 T/GM 0.5±0.4[108,109] | 18F-FCH: T/WM 1.89 ± 0.78 T/N 5.54 ± 2.43 (inflammation), 15.29 ± 5.32 (GBM)[67] | SUVmax 1.5–10.5[87] |
| WHO grade I/II vs III/IV | N/A | TBRmax 1.9–2.0 TBRmean 2.5–2.7 TTP <35 min TAC pattern II or III[106,110,111] | SUVmax 2.1–2.72 | T/WM 1.76 ± 0.51 (LGG), 2.59 ± 0.54 (HGG)[108,109] | 18F-FCH: TBR >2.55 11C-CHO: T/N 0.6 ± 0.6 (LGG), 1.4 ± 0.9 (HGG)[112–114] | SUVmax 1.5–0.8 (grade II/III) SUVmax 0.7–0.4 (grade II)[58] |
| Delineation | TBR 1.3[115] | TBR 1.6[36] | TBR 2.0[63] | N/A | N/A | TBR 2.0[58] |
| Recurrence | TBRmax 1.6[116] | TBRmean 2.0 TTP <45 min[105] | TSRmax 2.1 TSRmean 1.8[117] | T/W 2.9 ± 1.9 T/G 1.3±0.8[108,109] | T/N 5.5 ± 2.4 (acute inflammatory demyelination)[114] | SUVmax 5.2 TBR 7.4[58] |
| Malignant transformation | N/A | TBRmax >33% increase TBRmean >13% increase TTP 6 min decrease[118] | T/N 1.33–1.7 | N/A | 11C-CHO: SUVmax 1.0–2.5 (WHO II), 2.6–4.2 (WHO III)[68] | T/N 2.15 TBR 2.8[59] |
| Pseudo-progression vs true progression | N/A | Early: TBRmax 2.3[119,120] Late: TBRmax and TBRmean 1.9[119,120] | Early: T/N 1.33–1.7 Late: SUVmean 2.5 (threshold 1.8)[105,121] | N/A | N/A | Early: TBR 2.8[58] |
| Treatment response | Temozolomide: TBRmax stable or decreasing[34,122] | Radiotherapy (7–10d): TBRmax >20% decrease TBRmean >5% decrease Bevacizumab/irinotecan (4–12 wk): BTV >45% decrease[123–126] | Bevacizumab (2 wk): BTV >35% decrease or <18 mL[102] | N/A | N/A | N/A |

*Abbreviations:* BTV, biological tumor volume; TBRmax, maximum target-to-background ratio; TBRmean, mean target-to-background ratio; TSRmax, maximum T/s ratio; TSRmean, mean T/s ratio; SUVmean, mean standardized uptake value; TAC, time activity curve; T/N, tumor-to-normal ratio; T/GM, tumor-to-gray matter ratio; T/WM, tumor-to-white matter ratio.

*Adapted from* Law I, Albert NL, Arbizu J, et al. Joint EANM/EANO/RANO practice guidelines/SNMMI procedure standards for imaging of gliomas using PET with radiolabeled amino acids and [(18)F]FDG: version 1.0. *Eur J Nucl Med Mol Imaging.* 2019;46(3):540-557.

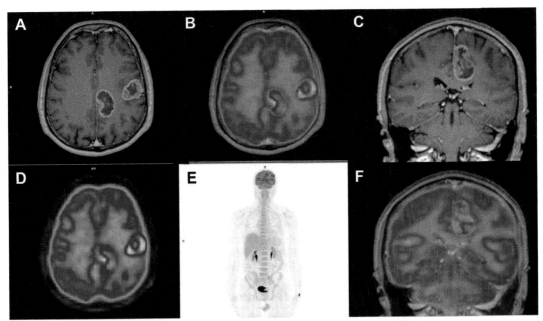

Fig. 1. A 58-year-old man patient presenting with headache and seizures. MR imaging (*A, C*) showed two ring-enhancing lesions in the left posterior parasagittal and left parietal lobe, concerning for a primary brain neoplasm or metastatic disease. [18]F-FDG–PET redemonstrated the ring-enhancing lesions and abnormal peripheral(*B*) [18]F-FDG uptake (SUVmax 10 and 13, respectively). Whole-body maximum intensity projection (*E*) shows no other focal abnormal [18]F-FDG uptake to suggest a primary non-CNS malignancy(*D*). The lesion subsequently was found to be multicentric GBM(*F*) (IDH–wild-type).

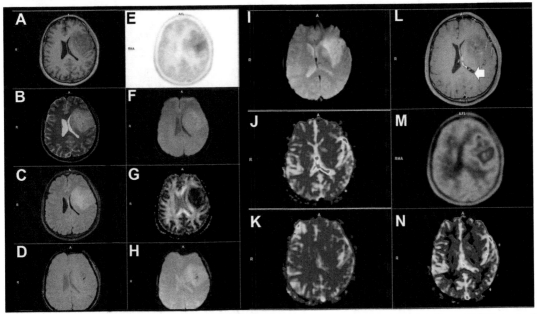

Fig. 2. A patient with 10-year seizure, found to have HGG, likely anaplastic oligodendroglioma (WHO grade III, IDH-mutant, 1p/9q deleted). T1 magnetization prepared–rapid gradient echo and T2 FLAIR (*A–C*) show an ill-defined heterogeneous mass in left frontal lobe with hyperintense signal changes. Susceptibility-weighted imaging (*D*) demonstrates foci of blooming consistent with calcification. Patchy foci are seen on diffusion-weighted imaging restriction (*F–I*). Postcontrast images (*L*) demonstrate subtle ill-defined enhancement within the lesion and mass effect (*white arrow*). MR spectroscopy demonstrates a large choline peak with reduced *N*-acetylaspartate. Cerebral blood volume and cerebral blood flow maps (*J, K, N*) show increased perfusion within the lesion. [11]C-MET–PET/MR imaging (*E, M*) shows heterogenous tracer uptake (SUVmax 3.90, TBR 3.64). (*Courtesy of* P.K. Singh, MD, and J. Saini, MD, Bengaluru, Karnataka, India.)

combined with higher L-AA transporter (LAT)-1 expression in tumor endothelial cells, aiding tumor delineation and grading.[33,34] Saito and colleagues[35] concluded that these factors may account for higher [11]C-MET uptake in higher-grade lesions. In addition, Kim and colleagues[36] demonstrated [11]C-MET may help differentiate between LGGs and HGGs. They observed that isocitrate dehydrogenese (IDH)–wild-type (a high-grade phenotype) gliomas demonstrated higher [11]C-MET uptake than IDH-mutant (low-grade) tumors and similar uptake to oligodendrogliomas with 1p/19q codeletion (high-grade).

[18]F-FET–PET has also been utilized to detect brain tumors (**Fig. 3**) as well as differentiate LGGs from HGGs.[5,37–40] Vettermann and colleagues[41] used both static and dynamic [18]F-FET–PET to develop a threshold for prediction of IDH–wild-type genotype in glioma, and they identified the time to peak (TTP) parameter as a useful prognostic marker, even in non–contrast-enhancing gliomas. Similarly, Lohmann and colleagues[42] found that a combination of a dynamic parameter (slope) with textural analysis provided

the high accuracy (81%) for prediction of an IDH-mutation genotype. Taken together, these studies point toward dynamic [18]F-FET–PET as a biologically and clinically relevant imaging modality in the context of molecular glioma diagnosis. [18]F-FET–PET, however, is not without its limitations. Although studies have found that FET-PET may add information on glioma biology beyond MR imaging alone, the spatial congruence of both methods was poor, and the localization of tumor hot spots led to conflicting results.[43,44] In addition, Lohmann and colleagues[42] showed that, in neuropathologically confirmed GBM, the metabolically active tumor volume delineated by [18]F-FET–PET is significantly larger than that delineated by contrast-enhanced MR imaging. Other studies have called into question the reliability of [18]F-FET–PET to consistently diagnose gliomas, with up to 50% of nonglioma brain tumors and nonneoplastic lesions also exhibiting uptake.[45–47]

[18]F-FDOPA, an AA radiotracer labeled with [18]F and with a longer half-life than [11]C-MET, also has been employed in the setting of brain tumors (**Fig. 4**) and initially displayed promise. Chen and

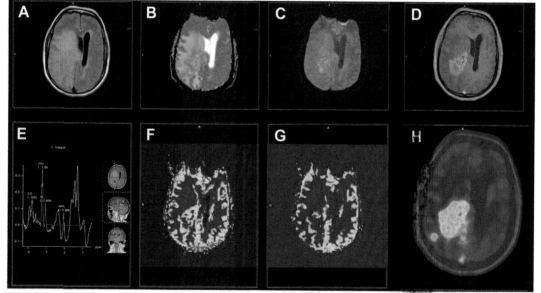

**Fig. 3.** A patient with a history of right parietal GBM, status–post resection and chemoradiation in 2011, complicated by seizure and treated with stereotactic radiosurgery in 2014. Postprocedural MR imaging showed enhancing lesion. In 2016, [18]F-FET–PET shows avid tumor. Axial T2 FLAIR (*A*), postcontrast magnetization prepared–rapid gradient echo (*B*), and diffusion-weighted imaging with reduced apparent diffusion coefficient (*C*) and contrast enhancement (*D*) demonstrate evidence of right parietal craniotomy with resection cavity and encephalomalacic changes in the parasagittal parietal region with a bulky rim enhancing mass lesion measuring 3.7 cm × 4.99 cm × 5.23 cm. MR spectroscopy (*E*) demonstrates increased choline-to-creatinine ratio (3.12) and choline–to–N-acetylaspartate ratio (8.13), with prominent lactate peak. Cerebral blood volume and cerebral blood flow maps (*F, G*) reveal increased relative blood volume and increased perfusion. [18]F-FET–PET (*H*) reveals increased uptake within the mass (SUVmax 3.97, TBR 1.93), concerning for recurrence. (*Courtesy of* A. Jena, MD, New Delhi, Delhi, India.)

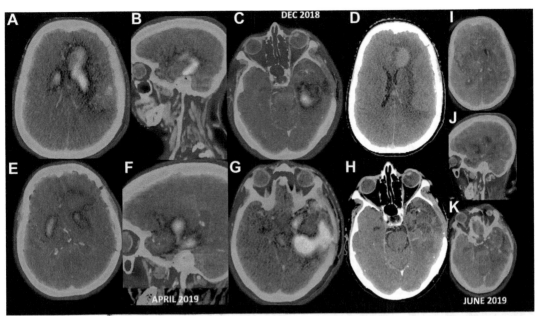

**Fig. 4.** A 64-year male patient with history of left posterior temporal GBM. Serial [18]F-FDOPA–PET/CT was performed to guide delineation, grading, biopsy, surgery, and postoperative radiation therapy. Imaging at diagnosis (*A–D*) shows a large, ill-defined infiltrative lesion in the left frontoparietotemporal lobe with abnormal increase in uptake (SUVmax 4.7). Postcontrast CT (*D*) demonstrates a hyperdense lesion in the left frontal parasagittal region with extensive hypodensity involving the left frontoparietotemporal lobe. Imaging performed 3 months postoperatively (*E–H*) shows left parietotemporal craniotomy defect, resection cavity in the left temporal lobe measuring 3.7 cm × 4.3 cm, and persistent abnormal tracer uptake predominantly in the temporal lobe (SUVmax 3.8). Imaging performed 6 months postoperatively (*I–K*) shows faint tracer uptake in the lesion (SUV$_{max}$ 2.9). (*Courtesy of* K. Kallur, MD, Bengaluru, Karnataka, India.)

colleagues[48] found that [18]F-FDOPA exhibited a sensitivity of 100% and specificity of 86%, at a tumor-to-striatum (T/s) ratio threshold of 0.75, potentially able to detect LGGs and recurrent tumors with greater sensitivity than [18]F-FDG–PET. Cicone and colleagues,[49] however, raised concern in using T/s ratio for thresholding, because most LGG tumors demonstrate threshold lesser than the striatum. In addition, Verger and colleagues[50] found that IDH-mutant WHO II/III lesions showed higher [18]F-FDOPA tumor-to-normal (T/N) ratios and T/s than patients without IDH mutation (*P* < .05), in direct contrast to other published literature. Therefore, the utility of [18]F-FDOPA remains uncertain.

Other, lesser-used tracers have also been studied in brain tumor imaging. Choline analogs were introduced to evaluate prostate and brain neoplasms. Hara and colleagues[51] compared the performance of [11]C-CHO–PET and [18]F-FCH–PET among 12 patients with untreated gliomas. Both tracers showed higher uptake in HGGs versus LGGs, and the investigators concluded that both were adequate for the delineation and characterization of primary brain tumors.[51] Mertens and colleagues[52] examined [18]F-FCH–PET in 25 space-occupying brain lesions and demonstrated the feasibility of a dynamic acquisition protocol to ascertain uptake kinetics, offering improved accuracy in the differential diagnosis. Originally used as a tracer for myocardial perfusion imaging, [13]N-NH$_3$ has emerged as a potential tracer in evaluating gliomas, meningiomas, and primary CNS lymphomas.[53–56] Further studies have suggested that [13]N-NH$_3$ can distinguish HGGs from either LGGs and inflammatory lesions—however, [13]N-NH$_3$ was unable to differentiate the latter two pathologies.[57] Similarly, Herholz and colleagues[58] compared [13]N-NH$_3$, [11]C-MET, and [18]F-FDG and concluded that [13]N-NH$_3$–PET has remarkably high specificity but low sensitivity for the detection of LGGs and a limited role in tumor grading. Widely used in prostate imaging, [18]F-FACBC has recently been applied to glioma imaging. HGGs have been demonstrated to exhibit significantly greater [18]F-FACBC uptake than LGGs by both visual and semiquantitative analyses.[59,60] Parent and colleagues[61] proposed a maximum standardized uptake value (SUVmax) threshold of 4.3 to differentiate between LGG and HGG, observing a sensitivity of 90.9% and specificity of 97.5% in evaluating tumor extent and regional involvement;

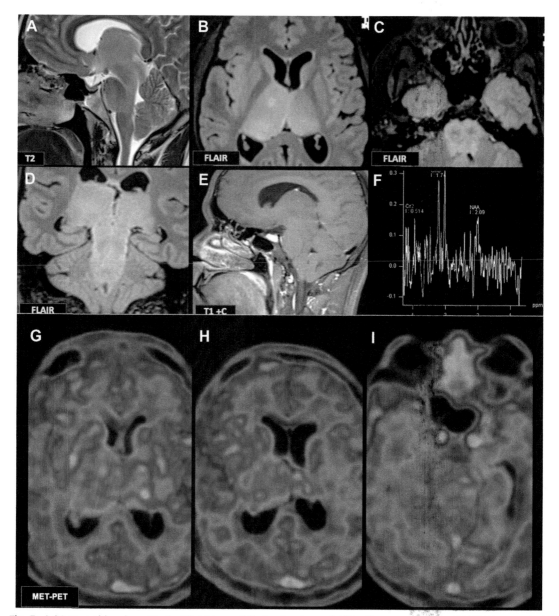

**Fig. 5.** A 21-year-old male patient with history of thalamic glioma (infiltrating zone glioma, H3K27 M negative), status–post stereotactic biopsy and chemoradiation, currently on maintenance temozolomide therapy. Follow-up MR imaging indicated stable disease; however, $^{11}$C-MET–PET/MR imaging revealed findings concerning for residual active disease. T2/FLAIR images (A–E) demonstrate an ill-defined expansile, infiltrative hyperintense lesion involving the bilateral thalami, pons, tectum, midbrain, and medulla. Susceptibility-weighted imaging (D) focus of blooming in right thalamus. Sagittal T1 magnetization prepared–rapid gradient echo (E) shows tiny focus of postcontrast enhancement. MR spectroscopy (F) reveals elevated choline-to-creatinine ratio. Axial $^{11}$C-MET–PET/ MR imaging (G–I) shows tracer uptake within bilateral thalami and brainstem (SUVmax 1.6, TBR 1.2). (Courtesy of P.K. Singh, MD, and J. Saini, MD, Bengaluru, Karnataka, India. )

there was particular value in cases where MR imaging was not diagnostic. There is a paucity of literature, however, comparting $^{18}$F-FACBC to established brain tumor tracers.

Several studies suggest that the use of hybrid PET/MR imaging is superior to MR imaging alone in the differentiation of LGGs from HGGs and the detection of malignant transformation within LGGs.[62] In a retrospective study by Shaw and colleagues,[62] the combined $^{18}$F-FDG–PET and MR imaging information provided an increased accuracy in the detection of HGG regions with

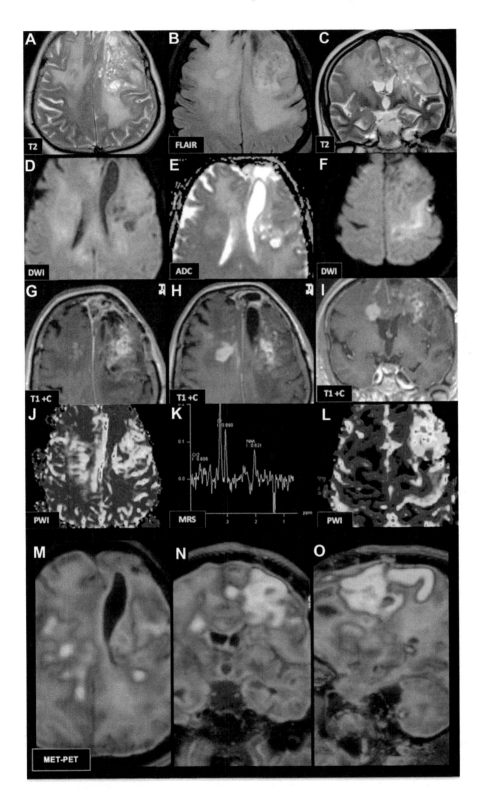

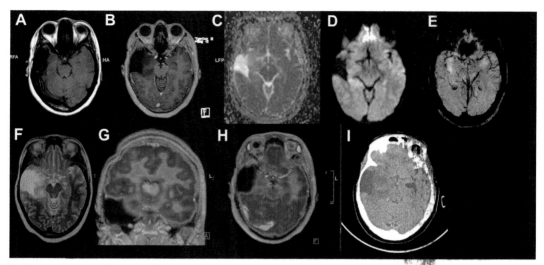

**Fig. 7.** A patient with history of right temporal lobe GBM, status–post resection and chemoradiation(*A*). Follow-up scans demonstrated an interval increase in an area of nodular enhancement in the lateral aspect of the temporal horn of right lateral ventricle(*B*). [11]C-MET–PET dynamic images raised suspicion of recurrence. Axial T2 (*F*) shows expansile hyperintense lesion involving the medial aspect of the right temporal pole, amygdala, uncus, piriform cortex, temporal stem, insular/subinsular regions, right orbitofrontal gyrus, hippocampus, and posterior aspect of parahippocampal gyrus. Diffusion-weighted imaging (*C, D*) images show areas of diffusion restriction. Susceptibility-weighted imaging (*E*) images show no areas of blooming suggestive of hemorrhage. [11]C-MET–PET/ MR imaging (*G, H*) shows no significant increase in metabolic activity. Follow-up CT at 3 months (*I*) shows areas of hypodensity adjacent to the resection cavity.

histopathology as reference standard. Increased accuracy also was achieved when performing simultaneous [18]F-FET–PET/diffusion-weighted MR imaging in the detection of glioma infiltration compared with T1-wighted MR imaging with gadolinium, and a possible benefit in the differentiation of HGG and LGG was reported in a small study consisting of 11 patients using hybrid [18]F-FACBC–PET/MR imaging.[60,63]

In summary, although numerous studies have demonstrated feasibility of these non–18F-FDG tracers toward glioma detection grading[36,48,50,51] and the use of hybrid PET/MR imaging,[60,62,63]

future large-scale research is warranted to corroborate these findings.

## TUMOR EXTENT

Accurate delineation of the tumor is critical for decision making regarding surgery or stereotactic biopsy of these lesions.[64] [18]F-FDG–PET routinely is utilized to detect abnormal metabolic areas in heterogeneous tumors and is recommended as part of stereotactic biopsy guidance.[21,22] Because of its low background uptake, [18]F-FET provide clear borders of lesions and is the preferred AA tracer

**Fig. 6.** A 30-year-old female patient with history of left frontal diffuse astrocytoma (WHO grade II), status–post resection in 2009, presenting with tumor recurrence and progression to anaplastic astrocytoma (WHO grade III, IDH-1[R132H]-positive, α-thalassemia/mental retardation syndrome X-linked [ATRX] loss of expression, p53 positive, MIB-1 labeling 10% to 12%). T2-weighted MR imaging (*A, C*) shows heterogeneous signal intensity lesion in the left frontal region with diffuse confluent hyperintensity in the bilateral hemispheric white matter, left greater than right. FLAIR (*B*) demonstrates a predominantly hyperintense lesion with areas of suppression. Diffusion-weighted imaging (*D–F*) show patchy areas of restriction within the lesion. Postcontrast T1 (*G–I*) shows heterogeneous enhancement in both cerebral hemispheres with a well-defined nodular enhancing focus in the right anterior periventricular region. T2 perfusion maps (*J, L*) demonstrate elevated relative cerebral blood volume values within the lesion in the left frontal region, with patchy areas of increased perfusion in the right centrum semiovale. MR spectroscopy (*K*) from the left frontal lobe lesion reveals a markedly elevated choline peak with reduced creatine and *N*-acetylaspartate peaks and a prominent, inverted lactate peak. Fused [11]C-MET–PET/MR imaging (*M–O*) shows heterogeneous increased tracer uptake involving the bilateral frontoparietal regions in the setting of extensive recurrence. (*Courtesy of* P.K. Singh, MD, and J. Saini, MD, Bengaluru, Karnataka, India. )

for glioma imaging. Song and colleagues[65] found that the metabolically active biodistribution of gliomas delineated with 18F-FET–PET significantly exceeds tumor volume on contrast-enhanced MR imaging, suggesting a clinical value for delineating tumor extent with 18F-FET–PET before treatment planning. 18F-FET–PET and fluid-attenuated inversion recovery (FLAIR) images show different tumor volume, and both play an important role in the evaluating prognosis in glioma; hence, a combination of multimodality imaging to tumor spatial delineation may be valuable to optimize treatment planning.

Non–18F-FDG tracers—including 11C-MET, 18F-FDOPA, and choline analogs—may have comparable potential. Voges and colleagues[66] demonstrated that 11C-MET–PET outlines tumor volume more accurately than structural imaging in as many as two-thirds of cases. Meanwhile, 18F-FDOPA–PET has demonstrated highly sensitive for gliomas, irrespective of tumor grade, labeling both enhancing and nonenhancing tumors equally well.[67–69] Pafundi and colleagues[67] correlated 18F-FDOPA uptake to postresection pathology and found that high 18F-FDOPA uptake was associated with tumor grade and cellularity better

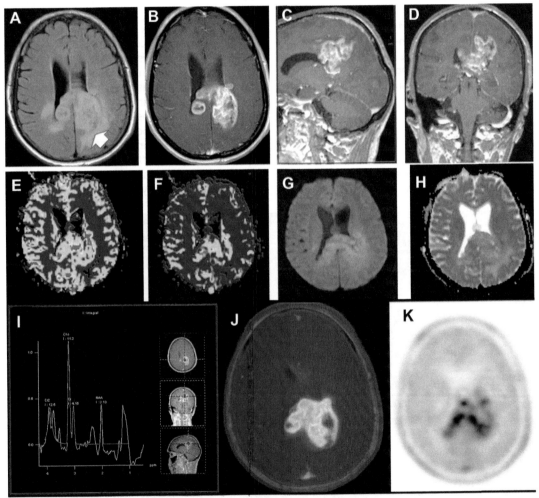

Fig. 8. A 60-year-old female patient presenting with headache and left parietal biopsy demonstrated anaplastic astrocytoma. Axial T2 FLAIR and postcontrast T1 magnetization prepared–rapid gradient echo images (A–D) show a heterogeneously enhancing lesion, measuring 4.3 cm × 5.2 cm × 5.2 cm in the left posterior parietal region infiltrating the splenium and posterior body of the corpus callosum, with a discrete rim enhancing cystic/necrotic lesion involving the fornix. Nonenhancing white matter hyperintensity is visualized in bilateral periventricular regions (white arrow). PWI (E, F) shows increased perfusion. Diffusion-weighted imaging (G, H) shows low apparent diffusion coefficient (0.90). MR spectroscopy (I) shows increased choline-to-creatine ratio (2.71) and choline–to–N-acetylaspartate ratio (3.53). 18F-FET–PET/MR imaging (J, K) demonstrates increased 18F-FET uptake (SUVmax 3.34, T/s ratio 2.83) concerning for recurrent tumor. (Courtesy of A. Jena, MD, New Delhi, Delhi, India.)

predicted HGG than contrast-enhanced MR imaging alone. [18]F-FDOPA uptake extended well beyond MR imaging–defined borders. Fraioli and colleagues[70] used [18]F-FDOPA–PET and MR imaging to estimate tumor volumes and during post-therapy assessment. They also found significantly higher glioma volumes calculated using [18]F-FDOPA–PET than MR imaging. Finally, choline analogs correspondingly exhibit a characteristic uptake of choline tracers outside the margins of the contrast-enhanced HGGs.[71] Hara and colleagues[51] showed that both [11]C-CHO– and [18]F-FCH–PET are useful to determine the appropriate subjects for surgical sampling. Further, Li and colleagues[72] concluded that [11]C-CHO–PET might complement MR imaging for more accurate delineation of target volumes prior to radiation therapy. Taken together, these non–[18]F-FDG tracers may serve as useful adjuvants for risk stratification, treatment planning, and biopsy guidance, although prospective confirmatory is still research needed.

## TREATMENT RESPONSE, PROGNOSTICATION, AND FOLLOW-UP

Glioma treatment is guided by histopathologic classification and baseline health characteristics and may include a combination of surgical resection, chemotherapy, and radiation therapy.[73] Differentiation of glioma recurrence from post-treatment changes and other pseudo-progression changes are key challenges faced during long-term brain tumor management. Historically, the screening for post-treatment residual typically has required serial MR imaging and computed tomography (CT). These structural imaging modalities, however, only detect changes once they reach macroscopic proportions.[74] In contrast, any area of focal uptake on PET may represent pathology, potentially suggesting a need for therapy initiation or augmentation. As such, PET imaging has displayed an important role in detecting and managing pseudo-progression in clinical trials for glioma therapies. With the advent of combined PET/MR imaging technology, the acquisition of molecular parameters during post-treatment monitoring may better track residual disease or complications and improve clinical outcomes.

[18]F-FDG–PET represents an excellent modality for identification of post-treatment inflammatory changes.[75] In addition, [18]F-FDG–PET has been demonstrated to differentiate between tumor recurrence and radiation-induced necrosis with acceptable sensitivity and specificity.[76–78] [18]F-

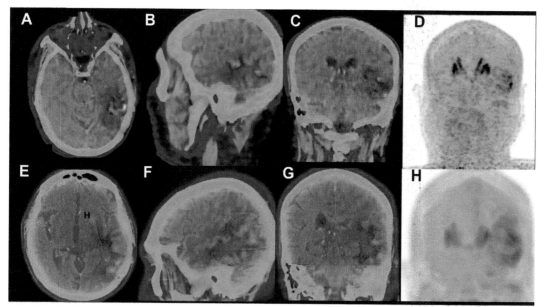

Fig. 9. A 60-year-old male patient with history of GBM, status–post resection and chemoradiation. [18]F-FDOPA-PET was performed for evaluation of response assessment. Serial images show favorable response. Fused [18]F-FDOPA–PET/CT images obtained in May 2019 (A–D) and August 2019 (E–H) show left posterior temporo-parietal craniotomy postoperative changes. There is mild progression of large area of ill-defined hypodensity involving the left temporal lobe and left posterior parietal lobe with nodular cortical and subcortical hypermetabolism in the left posterior temporo-parietal lobe. There is increased [18]F-FDOPA uptake in the periphery of the resection cavity in left temporal and posterior parietal lobe (standardized uptake value 3.1, previously 3.9; T/s ratio 1.5). (Courtesy of K. Kallur, MD, Bengaluru, Karnataka, India.)

FDG also may be helpful for prognostic purposes. Pretreatment [18]F-FDG–PET has been reported to correlate with survival in patients with newly diagnosed GBM or recurrent HGGs receiving bevacizumab.[79,80] Similarly, Di Chiro[81] found, among patients with proved HGG who underwent surgery, radiation, and chemotherapy, that poorly differentiated tumors exhibited significantly higher glucose metabolism than well differentiated ones. Moreover, patients with target-to-background ratio (TBR) greater than 1.4 were found to have an average survival of only 5 months versus 19 months in patients with a TBR less than 1.4. Finally, a meta-analysis by Quartuccio and colleagues[82] showed that [18]F-FDG–PET and MR imaging enhance the accuracy in predicting

**Table 5**
**Strengths and weaknesses of PET brain tumor imaging tracers**

| | Strengths | Weaknesses |
|---|---|---|
| [11]C-MET[127] | <ul><li>Grading</li><li>Delineating extent of tumor</li><li>Biopsy guidance</li><li>Radiotherapy</li><li>Prognostication</li></ul> | <ul><li>Challenging to interpret normal brain uptake</li><li>Requires on-site cyclotron</li><li>Poor differentiation between reactive gliosis and radiation injury</li><li>Poor differentiation between LGGs and non-neoplastic lesions</li></ul> |
| [18]F-FET[128–130] | <ul><li>Grading</li><li>Biopsy guidance</li><li>Radiotherapy</li><li>Differentiation between radiation injury and tumor recurrence</li><li>Prognostication</li></ul> | <ul><li>Not widely available</li></ul> |
| [18]F-FDOPA[131] | <ul><li>Grading</li><li>Biopsy guidance</li><li>Radiotherapy</li><li>Differentiation between radiation injury and tumor recurrence</li><li>Prognostication</li></ul> | <ul><li>Poor utility in radiotherapy</li><li>Low yield</li><li>Not widely available</li></ul> |
| [13]N-NH$_3$[93,108,109] | <ul><li>Differentiation between brain tumors and non-neoplastic lesions</li></ul> | <ul><li>Grading</li><li>Low sensitivity for LGG</li><li>Poor differentiation between reactive gliosis and radiation injury</li><li>Low expression of glutamine synthetase enzyme in oligodendroglial tumors could be responsible for the negative findings in these tumors.</li><li>Short half life</li><li>Requires on-site cyclotron</li></ul> |
| [11]C-CHO/[18]F-FCH[112–114,132] | <ul><li>Grading</li><li>Differentiation between radiation injury and tumor recurrence</li></ul> | <ul><li>Poor differentiation between LGGs and non-neoplastic lesions</li></ul> |
| [18]F-FACBC[58,59,133–138] | <ul><li>Grading</li><li>Delineating extent of tumor</li><li>Biopsy guidance</li></ul> | <ul><li>N/A</li></ul> |

*Adapted from* Moreau A, Febvey O, Mognetti T, Frappaz D, Kryza D. Contribution of Different Positron Emission Tomography Tracers in Glioma Management: Focus on Glioblastoma. *Front Oncol.* 2019;9:1134.

prognosis and detecting recurrence in patients with HGG. Expected pathophysiologic phenomena must be considered when reading post-treatment [18]F-FDG–PET images. Edema may result in mass effect upon adjacent structures and reversible hypometabolism, which may be confused on [18]F-FDG–PET for radiation-induced necrosis.[83,84]

Several studies have demonstrated that AA-PET assesses response to treatment better than structural imaging alone (Figs. 5–9).[85–91] [18]F-FET–PET–defined tumor volume has been demonstrated to be an independent prognostic factor for overall and progression-free survival among GBM patients treated with surgery and radiochemotherapy.[92,93] Likewise, Werner and colleagues[87] found that an [18]F-FET–PET TBR less than 1.95 predicted significantly longer survival among glioma patients. In addition, others have proposed uptake thresholds that may differentiate recurrence from stable disease, with acceptable accuracy and precision.[94] Tripathi and colleagues[95] utilized TBR threshold of greater than 1.9 to differentiate recurrence from stable disease, with a sensitivity of 95% and specificity of 89%.

The utility of other non–18F-FDG radiotracers has not been similarly established. Li and colleagues[96] evaluated the utility [11]C-CHO–PET/CT in detecting HGG (WHO III/IV) recurrence. They determined that [11]C-CHO–PET/CT demonstrated superior sensitivity (100%) and specificity (70%) compared with gadolinium-enhanced MR imaging. Moreover, Khangembam and colleagues[97] found tumor–to–white matter ratio cutoff of 2.16 for [13]N-NH$_3$ demonstrated a high specificity (98%) but low sensitivity of only 64%. Therefore, clinicians should remain cautious while interpreting non–18F-FDG–PET images. In addition, AA tracers may be subject to additional practical challenges. For example, Geisler and colleagues[98] studied [11]C-MET– and [18]F-FET–PET in rats that underwent glioma resection and observed focal uptake around the resection cavity up to a week postoperatively. Clinically, postoperative imaging routinely is performed rapidly following surgery, during which time these tracers may reflect off-target binding and unintended processes.

## SUMMARY

Imaging protocols and classifications of CNS tumors have been changing at a torrid pace. Brain PET imaging increasingly is used to supplement MR imaging in the clinical management of glioma. The recently proposed RANO guidelines recommend PET imaging as the standard of care in evaluation of primary brain tumors. [18]F-FDG–PET has

been the workhorse of nuclear medicine and has been employed in brain tumor imaging for nearly 50 years, representing the true intertumoral metabolism. Although AA tracers have been developed directly with tumor imaging in mind, many were originally employed for malignancies of other organ systems, with variable success.[99] Despite the many proposed advantages of various non–18F-FDG tracers, there still exist limitations (Table 5). Additionally, their uptake may reflect BBB dysregulation but not necessarily other clinically significant pathophysiological parameters beyond what can be ascertained from MR imaging. Although studies in these novel tracers provide valuable initial guidance, further validation from large, prospective trials is required. Hybrid PET/MR imaging is a unique imaging modality that has the potential to improve both the diagnostic accuracy and the follow-up of patients with brain tumors.

## CLINICS CARE POINTS

- Simultaneous PET/MR imaging will be instrumental in determining grade, treatment, and prognosis for primary brain tumors.

- [18]F-FDG has been widely used in the setting of brain tumor imaging. Delayed [18]F-FDG–PET may improve discrimination between tumor and healthy background tissue.

- Several AA and other non–18F-FDG–PET radiotracers have been developed for brain imaging. Although they show promise, more extensive research is warranted to identify their role in clinical routine.

## DISCLOSURE

The authors have nothing to disclose.

## REFERENCES

1. Herholz K, Langen KJ, Schiepers C, et al. Brain tumors. Semin Nucl Med 2012;42(6):356–70.
2. Heiss WD, Raab P, Lanfermann H. Multimodality assessment of brain tumors and tumor recurrence. J Nucl Med 2011;52(10):1585–600.
3. Louis DN, Perry A, Reifenberger G, et al. The 2016 world health organization classification of tumors of the central nervous system: a summary. Acta Neuropathol 2016;131(6):803–20.

4. Louis DN, Perry A, Wesseling P, et al. The 2021 WHO classification of tumors of the central nervous system: a summary. Neuro Oncol 2021;23(8): 1231–51.

5. Albert NL, Weller M, Suchorska B, et al. Response assessment in neuro-oncology working group and european association for neuro-oncology recommendations for the clinical use of PET imaging in gliomas. Neuro Oncol 2016;18(9):1199–208.

6. Law I, Albert NL, Arbizu J, et al. Joint EANM/EANO/RANO practice guidelines/SNMMI procedure standards for imaging of gliomas using PET with radiolabelled amino acids and [(18)F]FDG: version 1.0. Eur J Nucl Med Mol Imaging 2019; 46(3):540–57.

7. Choi YS, Ahn SS, Lee SK, et al. Amide proton transfer imaging to discriminate between low- and high-grade gliomas: added value to apparent diffusion coefficient and relative cerebral blood volume. Eur Radiol 2017;27(8):3181–9.

8. Zhou J, Tryggestad E, Wen Z, et al. Differentiation between glioma and radiation necrosis using molecular magnetic resonance imaging of endogenous proteins and peptides. Nat Med 2011;17(1): 130–4.

9. Jiang S, Eberhart CG, Lim M, et al. Identifying recurrent malignant glioma after treatment using amide proton transfer-weighted mr imaging: a validation study with image-guided stereotactic biopsy. Clin Cancer Res 2019;25(2):552–61.

10. Abrol S, Kotrotsou A, Salem A, et al. Radiomic phenotyping in brain cancer to unravel hidden information in medical images. Top Magn Reson Imaging 2017;26(1):43–53.

11. Jager PL, Vaalburg W, Pruim J, et al. Radiolabeled amino acids: basic aspects and clinical applications in oncology. J Nucl Med 2001;42(3):432–45.

12. Daneman R, Prat A. The blood-brain barrier. Cold Spring Harb Perspect Biol 2015;7(1):a020412.

13. Arvanitis CD, Ferraro GB, Jain RK. The blood-brain barrier and blood-tumour barrier in brain tumours and metastases. Nat Rev Cancer 2020;20(1): 26–41.

14. Boss A, Bisdas S, Kolb A, et al. Hybrid PET/MRI of intracranial masses: initial experiences and comparison to PET/CT. J Nucl Med 2010;51(8): 1198–205.

15. Fink JR, Muzi M, Peck M, et al. Multimodality brain tumor imaging: MR imaging, PET, and PET/MR imaging. J Nucl Med 2015;56(10):1554–61.

16. Holdsworth SJ, Bammer R. Magnetic resonance imaging techniques: fMRI, DWI, and PWI. Semin Neurol 2008;28(4):395–406.

17. Brendle C, Hempel JM, Schittenhelm J, et al. Glioma grading and determination of IDH mutation status and ATRX loss by DCE and ASL perfusion. Clin Neuroradiol 2018;28(3):421–8.

18. Sharma A, McConathy J. Overview of PET tracers for brain tumor imaging. PET Clin 2013;8(2): 129–46.

19. Borja AJ, Hancin EC, Raynor WY, et al. A critical review of pet tracers used for brain tumor imaging. PET Clin 2021;16(2):219–31.

20. Scott JN, Brasher PM, Sevick RJ, et al. How often are nonenhancing supratentorial gliomas malignant? A population study. Neurology 2002;59(6): 947–9.

21. Herholz K, Rudolf J, Heiss WD. FDG transport and phosphorylation in human gliomas measured with dynamic PET. J Neurooncol 1992;12(2):159–65.

22. Fischman AJ, Alpert NM. FDG-PET in oncology: there's more to it than looking at pictures. J Nucl Med 1993;34(1):6–11.

23. Coope DJ, Cízek J, Eggers C, et al. Evaluation of primary brain tumors using 11C-methionine PET with reference to a normal methionine uptake map. J Nucl Med 2007;48(12):1971–80.

24. Jung JH, Ahn BC. Current radiopharmaceuticals for positron emission tomography of brain tumors. Brain Tumor Res Treat 2018;6(2):47–53.

25. Basu S, Alavi A. Molecular imaging (PET) of brain tumors. Neuroimaging Clin N Am 2009;19(4): 625–46.

26. Janus TJ, Kim EE, Tilbury R, et al. Use of [18F]fluorodeoxyglucose positron emission tomography in patients with primary malignant brain tumors. Ann Neurol 1993;33(5):540–8.

27. Delbeke D, Meyerowitz C, Lapidus RL, et al. Optimal cutoff levels of F-18 fluorodeoxyglucose uptake in the differentiation of low-grade from high-grade brain tumors with PET. Radiology 1995;195(1):47–52.

28. Spence AM, Muzi M, Mankoff DA, et al. 18F-FDG PET of gliomas at delayed intervals: improved distinction between tumor and normal gray matter. J Nucl Med 2004;45(10):1653–9.

29. Valk PE, Budinger TF, Levin VA, et al. PET of malignant cerebral tumors after interstitial brachytherapy. demonstration of metabolic activity and correlation with clinical outcome. J Neurosurg 1988;69(6):830–8.

30. Roelcke U, Radü EW, von Ammon K, et al. Alteration of blood-brain barrier in human brain tumors: comparison of [18F]fluorodeoxyglucose, [11C]methionine and rubidium-82 using PET. J Neurol Sci 1995;132(1):20–7.

31. Vandenberghe S, Moskal P, Karp JS. State of the art in total body PET. EJNMMI Phys 2020;7(1):35.

32. Bergström M, Collins VP, Ehrin E, et al. Discrepancies in brain tumor extent as shown by computed tomography and positron emission tomography using [68Ga]EDTA, [11C]glucose, and [11C]methionine. J Comput Assist Tomogr 1983; 7(6):1062–6.

33. Dandois V, Rommel D, Renard L, et al. Substitution of 11C-methionine PET by perfusion MRI during the follow-up of treated high-grade gliomas: preliminary results in clinical practice. J Neuroradiol 2010;37(2):89–97.

34. Sadeghi N, Salmon I, Decaestecker C, et al. Stereotactic comparison among cerebral blood volume, methionine uptake, and histopathology in brain glioma. AJNR Am J Neuroradiol 2007;28(3): 455–61.

35. Saito T, Maruyama T, Muragaki Y, et al. 11C-methionine uptake correlates with combined 1p and 19q loss of heterozygosity in oligodendroglial tumors. AJNR Am J Neuroradiol 2013;34(1):85–91.

36. Kim D, Chun JH, Kim SH, et al. Re-evaluation of the diagnostic performance of (11)C-methionine PET/CT according to the 2016 WHO classification of cerebral gliomas. Eur J Nucl Med Mol Imaging 2019; 46(8):1678–84.

37. Pauleit D, Floeth F, Hamacher K, et al. O-(2-[18F] fluoroethyl)-L-tyrosine PET combined with MRI improves the diagnostic assessment of cerebral gliomas. Brain 2005;128(Pt 3):678–87.

38. Jansen NL, Suchorska B, Wenter V, et al. Dynamic 18F-FET PET in newly diagnosed astrocytic low-grade glioma identifies high-risk patients. J Nucl Med 2014;55(2):198–203.

39. Jansen NL, Suchorska B, Wenter V, et al. Prognostic significance of dynamic 18F-FET PET in newly diagnosed astrocytic high-grade glioma. J Nucl Med 2015;56(1):9–15.

40. Röhrich M, Huang K, Schrimpf D, et al. Integrated analysis of dynamic FET PET/CT parameters, histology, and methylation profiling of 44 gliomas. Eur J Nucl Med Mol Imaging 2018;45(9):1573–84.

41. Vettermann F, Suchorska B, Unterrainer M, et al. Non-invasive prediction of IDH-wildtype genotype in gliomas using dynamic (18)F-FET PET. Eur J Nucl Med Mol Imaging 2019;46(12):2581–9.

42. Lohmann P, Stavrinou P, Lipke K, et al. FET PET reveals considerable spatial differences in tumour burden compared to conventional MRI in newly diagnosed glioblastoma. Eur J Nucl Med Mol Imaging 2019;46(3):591–602.

43. Filss CP, Galldiks N, Stoffels G, et al. Comparison of 18F-FET PET and perfusion-weighted MR imaging: a PET/MR imaging hybrid study in patients with brain tumors. J Nucl Med 2014;55(4):540–5.

44. Göttler J, Lukas M, Kluge A, et al. Intra-lesional spatial correlation of static and dynamic FET-PET parameters with MRI-based cerebral blood volume in patients with untreated glioma. Eur J Nucl Med Mol Imaging 2017;44(3):392–7.

45. Jansen NL, Graute V, Armbruster L, et al. MRI-suspected low-grade glioma: is there a need to perform dynamic FET PET? Eur J Nucl Med Mol Imaging 2012;39(6):1021–9.

46. Hutterer M, Nowosielski M, Putzer D, et al. [18F]-fluoro-ethyl-L-tyrosine PET: a valuable diagnostic tool in neuro-oncology, but not all that glitters is glioma. Neuro Oncol 2013;15(3):341–51.

47. Pichler R, Dunzinger A, Wurm G, et al. Is there a place for FET PET in the initial evaluation of brain lesions with unknown significance? Eur J Nucl Med Mol Imaging 2010;37(8):1521–8.

48. Chen W, Silverman DH, Delaloye S, et al. 18F-FDOPA PET imaging of brain tumors: comparison study with 18F-FDG PET and evaluation of diagnostic accuracy. J Nucl Med 2006;47(6): 904–11.

49. Cicone F, Carideo L, Minniti G, et al. The mean striatal (18)F-DOPA uptake is not a reliable cut-off threshold for biological tumour volume definition of glioma. Eur J Nucl Med Mol Imaging 2019; 46(5):1051–3.

50. Verger A, Metellus P, Sala Q, et al. IDH mutation is paradoxically associated with higher (18)F-FDOPA PET uptake in diffuse grade II and grade III gliomas. Eur J Nucl Med Mol Imaging 2017;44(8): 1306–11.

51. Hara T, Kondo T, Hara T, et al. Use of 18F-choline and 11C-choline as contrast agents in positron emission tomography imaging-guided stereotactic biopsy sampling of gliomas. J Neurosurg 2003; 99(3):474–9.

52. Mertens K, Bolcaen J, Ham H, et al. The optimal timing for imaging brain tumours and other brain lesions with 18F-labelled fluoromethylcholine: a dynamic positron emission tomography study. Nucl Med Commun 2012;33(9):954–9.

53. Shi X, Yi C, Wang X, et al. 13N-ammonia combined with 18F-FDG could discriminate between necrotic high-grade gliomas and brain abscess. Clin Nucl Med 2015;40(3):195–9.

54. Xiangsong Z, Changhong L, Weian C, et al. PET Imaging of cerebral astrocytoma with 13N-ammonia. J Neurooncol 2006;78(2):145–51.

55. Xiangsong Z, Xingchong S, Chang Y, et al. 13N-NH3 versus F-18 FDG in detection of intracranial meningioma: initial report. Clin Nucl Med 2011; 36(11):1003–6.

56. Yi C, Shi X, Zhang X, et al. The role of (13)N-ammonia in the differential diagnosis of gliomas and brain inflammatory lesions. Ann Nucl Med 2019;33(1):61–7.

57. Oka S, Hattori R, Kurosaki F, et al. A preliminary study of anti-1-amino-3-18F-fluorocyclobutyl-1-carboxylic acid for the detection of prostate cancer. J Nucl Med 2007;48(1):46–55.

58. He Q, Zhang L, Zhang B, et al. Diagnostic accuracy of (13)N-ammonia PET, (11)C-methionine PET and (18)F-fluorodeoxyglucose PET: a comparative study in patients with suspected cerebral glioma. BMC Cancer 2019;19(1):332.

59. Shoup TM, Olson J, Hoffman JM, et al. Synthesis and evaluation of [18F]1-amino-3-fluorocyclobutane-1-carboxylic acid to image brain tumors. J Nucl Med 1999;40(2):331–8.

60. Karlberg A, Berntsen EM, Johansen H, et al. 18F-FACBC PET/MRI in diagnostic assessment and neurosurgery of gliomas. Clin Nucl Med 2019; 44(7):550–9.

61. Parent EE, Benayoun M, Ibeanu I, et al. [(18)F]Fluciclovine PET discrimination between high- and low-grade gliomas. EJNMMI Res 2018;8(1):67.

62. Shaw TB, Jeffree RL, Thomas P, et al. Diagnostic performance of 18F-fluorodeoxyglucose positron emission tomography in the evaluation of glioma. J Med Imaging Radiat Oncol 2019;63(5):650–6.

63. Verburg N, Koopman T, Yaqub MM, et al. Improved detection of diffuse glioma infiltration with imaging combinations: a diagnostic accuracy study. Neuro Oncol 2020;22(3):412–22.

64. Gumprecht H, Grosu AL, Souvatsoglou M, et al. 11C-Methionine positron emission tomography for preoperative evaluation of suggestive low-grade gliomas. Zentralbl Neurochir 2007;68(1):19–23.

65. Song S, Cheng Y, Ma J, et al. Simultaneous FET-PET and contrast-enhanced MRI based on hybrid PET/MR improves delineation of tumor spatial biodistribution in gliomas: a biopsy validation study. Eur J Nucl Med Mol Imaging 2020;47(6):1458–67.

66. Voges J, Herholz K, Hölzer T, et al. 11C-methionine and 18F-2-fluorodeoxyglucose positron emission tomography: a tool for diagnosis of cerebral glioma and monitoring after brachytherapy with 125I seeds. Stereotact Funct Neurosurg 1997;69(1–4 Pt 2):129–35.

67. Pafundi DH, Laack NN, Youland RS, et al. Biopsy validation of 18F-DOPA PET and biodistribution in gliomas for neurosurgical planning and radiotherapy target delineation: results of a prospective pilot study. Neuro Oncol 2013;15(8):1058–67.

68. Kosztyla R, Chan EK, Hsu F, et al. High-grade glioma radiation therapy target volumes and patterns of failure obtained from magnetic resonance imaging and 18F-FDOPA positron emission tomography delineations from multiple observers. Int J Radiat Oncol Biol Phys 2013;87(5):1100–6.

69. Weber MA, Henze M, Tüttenberg J, et al. Biopsy targeting gliomas: do functional imaging techniques identify similar target areas? Invest Radiol 2010;45(12):755–68.

70. Fraioli F, Shankar A, Hyare H, et al. The use of multiparametric 18F-fluoro-L-3,4-dihydroxy-phenylalanine PET/MRI in post-therapy assessment of patients with gliomas. Nucl Med Commun 2020;41(6):517–25.

71. Kwee SA, Ko JP, Jiang CS, et al. Solitary brain lesions enhancing at MR imaging: evaluation with fluorine 18 fluorocholine PET. Radiology 2007; 244(2):557–65.

72. Li FM, Nie Q, Wang RM, et al. 11C-CHO PET in optimization of target volume delineation and treatment regimens in postoperative radiotherapy for brain gliomas. Nucl Med Biol 2012;39(3):437–42.

73. McFaline-Figueroa JR, Lee EQ. Brain tumors. Am J Med 2018;131(8):874–82.

74. Nandu H, Wen PY, Huang RY. Imaging in neuro-oncology. Ther Adv Neurol Disord 2018;11. 1756286418759865.

75. Patronas NJ, Di Chiro G, Brooks RA, et al. Work in progress: [18F] fluorodeoxyglucose and positron emission tomography in the evaluation of radiation necrosis of the brain. Radiology 1982;144(4): 885–9.

76. Di Chiro G, Oldfield E, Wright DC, et al. Cerebral necrosis after radiotherapy and/or intraarterial chemotherapy for brain tumors: PET and neuropathologic studies. AJR Am J Roentgenol 1988; 150(1):189–97.

77. Doyle WK, Budinger TF, Valk PE, et al. Differentiation of cerebral radiation necrosis from tumor recurrence by [18F]FDG and 82Rb positron emission tomography. J Comput Assist Tomogr 1987;11(4): 563–70.

78. Davis WK, Boyko OB, Hoffman JM, et al. [18F]2-fluoro-2-deoxyglucose-positron emission tomography correlation of gadolinium-enhanced MR imaging of central nervous system neoplasia. AJNR Am J Neuroradiol 1993;14(3):515–23.

79. Omuro A, Beal K, Gutin P, et al. Phase II study of bevacizumab, temozolomide, and hypofractionated stereotactic radiotherapy for newly diagnosed glioblastoma. Clin Cancer Res 2014; 20(19):5023–31.

80. Colavolpe C, Chinot O, Metellus P, et al. FDG-PET predicts survival in recurrent high-grade gliomas treated with bevacizumab and irinotecan. Neuro Oncol 2012;14(5):649–57.

81. Di Chiro G. Positron emission tomography using [18F] fluorodeoxyglucose in brain tumors. A powerful diagnostic and prognostic tool. Invest Radiol 1987;22(5):360–71.

82. Quartuccio N, Laudicella R, Vento A, et al. The additional value of (18)F-FDG PET and MRI in patients with glioma: a review of the literature from 2015 to 2020. Diagnostics (Basel) 2020;10(6).

83. Hustinx R, Pourdehnad M, Kaschten B, et al. PET imaging for differentiating recurrent brain tumor from radiation necrosis. Radiol Clin North Am 2005;43(1):35–47.

84. Pourdehnad M, Basu S, Duarte P, et al. Reduced grey matter metabolism due to white matter edema allows optimal assessment of brain tumors on 18F-FDG-PET. Hell J Nucl Med 2011;14(3):219–23.

85. Deuschl C, Kirchner J, Poeppel TD, et al. 11)C-MET PET/MRI for detection of recurrent glioma. Eur J Nucl Med Mol Imaging 2018;45(4):593–601.

86. Ribom D, Schoenmaekers M, Engler H, et al. Evaluation of 11C-methionine PET as a surrogate endpoint after treatment of grade 2 gliomas. J Neurooncol 2005;71(3):325–32.

87. Werner JM, Stoffels G, Lichtenstein T, et al. Differentiation of treatment-related changes from tumour progression: a direct comparison between dynamic FET PET and ADC values obtained from DWI MRI. Eur J Nucl Med Mol Imaging 2019; 46(9):1889–901.

88. Kondo A, Ishii H, Aoki S, et al. Phase IIa clinical study of [(18)F]fluciclovine: efficacy and safety of a new PET tracer for brain tumors. Ann Nucl Med 2016;30(9):608–18.

89. Fraioli F, Shankar A, Hargrave D, et al. 18F-fluoroethylcholine (18F-Cho) PET/MRI functional parameters in pediatric astrocytic brain tumors. Clin Nucl Med 2015;40(1):e40–5.

90. Gómez-Río M, Testart Dardel N, Santiago Chinchilla A, et al. 18F-Fluorocholine PET/CT as a complementary tool in the follow-up of low-grade glioma: diagnostic accuracy and clinical utility. Eur J Nucl Med Mol Imaging 2015;42(6):886–95.

91. Michaud L, Beattie BJ, Akhurst T, et al. 18)F-Fluciclovine ((18)F-FACBC) PET imaging of recurrent brain tumors. Eur J Nucl Med Mol Imaging 2020; 47(6):1353–67.

92. Poulsen SH, Urup T, Grunnet K, et al. The prognostic value of FET PET at radiotherapy planning in newly diagnosed glioblastoma. Eur J Nucl Med Mol Imaging 2017;44(3):373–81.

93. Piroth MD, Holy R, Pinkawa M, et al. Prognostic impact of postoperative, pre-irradiation (18)F-fluoroethyl-l-tyrosine uptake in glioblastoma patients treated with radiochemotherapy. Radiother Oncol 2011;99(2):218–24.

94. Herholz K, Hölzer T, Bauer B, et al. 11C-methionine PET for differential diagnosis of low-grade gliomas. Neurology 1998;50(5):1316–22.

95. Tripathi M, Sharma R, Varshney R, et al. Comparison of F-18 FDG and C-11 methionine PET/CT for the evaluation of recurrent primary brain tumors. Clin Nucl Med 2012;37(2):158–63.

96. Li W, Ma L, Wang X, et al. 11)C-choline PET/CT tumor recurrence detection and survival prediction in post-treatment patients with high-grade gliomas. Tumour Biol 2014;35(12):12353–60.

97. Khangembam BC, Singhal A, Kumar R, et al. Tc-99m glucoheptonate single photon emission computed tomography-computed tomography for detection of recurrent glioma: a prospective comparison with N-13 ammonia positron emission tomography-computed tomography. Indian J Nucl Med 2019;34(2):107–17.

98. Geisler S, Stegmayr C, Niemitz N, et al. Treatment-related uptake of O-(2-(18)F-Fluoroethyl)-l-Tyrosine and l-[Methyl-(3)H]-methionine after tumor resection in rat glioma models. J Nucl Med 2019; 60(10):1373–9.

99. Zhu A, Lee D, Shim H. Metabolic positron emission tomography imaging in cancer detection and therapy response. Semin Oncol 2011;38(1): 55–69.

100. Stern PH, Wallace CD, Hoffman RM. Altered methionine metabolism occurs in all members of a set of diverse human tumor cell lines. J Cell Physiol 1984; 119(1):29–34.

101. Di Chiro G, DeLaPaz RL, Brooks RA, et al. Glucose utilization of cerebral gliomas measured by [18F] fluorodeoxyglucose and positron emission tomography. Neurology 1982;32(12):1323–9.

102. Alavi JB, Alavi A, Chawluk J, et al. Positron emission tomography in patients with glioma. A predictor of prognosis. Cancer 1988;62(6):1074–8.

103. Herholz K, Pietrzyk U, Voges J, et al. Correlation of glucose consumption and tumor cell density in astrocytomas. A stereotactic PET study. J Neurosurg 1993;79(6):853–8.

104. Patronas NJ, Di Chiro G, Kufta C, et al. Prediction of survival in glioma patients by means of positron emission tomography. J Neurosurg 1985;62(6): 816–22.

105. Barker FG 2nd, Chang SM, Valk PE, et al. 18-Fluorodeoxyglucose uptake and survival of patients with suspected recurrent malignant glioma. Cancer 1997;79(1):115–26.

106. Schwarzenberg J, Czernin J, Cloughesy TF, et al. Treatment response evaluation using 18F-FDOPA PET in patients with recurrent malignant glioma on bevacizumab therapy. Clin Cancer Res 2014; 20(13):3550–9.

107. Mohammed W, Xunning H, Haibin S, et al. Clinical applications of susceptibility-weighted imaging in detecting and grading intracranial gliomas: a review. Cancer Imaging 2013;13(2):186–95.

108. Kracht LW, Miletic H, Busch S, et al. Delineation of brain tumor extent with [11C]L-methionine positron emission tomography: local comparison with stereotactic histopathology. Clin Cancer Res 2004; 10(21):7163–70.

109. Galldiks N, Stoffels G, Filss C, et al. The use of dynamic O-(2-18F-fluoroethyl)-l-tyrosine PET in the diagnosis of patients with progressive and recurrent glioma. Neuro Oncol 2015;17(9):1293–300.

110. Rapp M, Heinzel A, Galldiks N, et al. Diagnostic performance of 18F-FET PET in newly diagnosed cerebral lesions suggestive of glioma. J Nucl Med 2013;54(2):229–35.

111. Bund C, Heimburger C, Imperiale A, et al. FDOPA PET-CT of nonenhancing brain tumors. Clin Nucl Med 2017;42(4):250–7.

112. Khangembam BC, Karunanithi S, Sharma P, et al. Perfusion-metabolism coupling in recurrent gliomas: a prospective validation study with 13N-

ammonia and 18F-fluorodeoxyglucose PET/CT. Neuroradiology 2014;56(10):893–902.

113. Khangembam BC, Sharma P, Karunanithi S, et al. 13N-Ammonia PET/CT for detection of recurrent glioma: a prospective comparison with contrast-enhanced MRI. Nucl Med Commun 2013;34(11):1046–54.

114. Albert NL, Winkelmann I, Suchorska B, et al. Early static (18)F-FET-PET scans have a higher accuracy for glioma grading than the standard 20-40 min scans. Eur J Nucl Med Mol Imaging 2016;43(6):1105–14.

115. Lohmann P, Herzog H, Rota Kops E, et al. Dual-time-point O-(2-[(18)F]fluoroethyl)-L-tyrosine PET for grading of cerebral gliomas. Eur Radiol 2015;25(10):3017–24.

116. Tian M, Zhang H, Higuchi T, et al. Oncological diagnosis using (11)C-choline-positron emission tomography in comparison with 2-deoxy-2-[(18)F]fluoro-D-glucose-positron emission tomography. Mol Imaging Biol 2004;6(3):172–9.

117. Tian M, Zhang H, Oriuchi N, et al. Comparison of 11C-choline PET and FDG PET for the differential diagnosis of malignant tumors. Eur J Nucl Med Mol Imaging 2004;31(8):1064–72.

118. Takenaka S, Shinoda J, Asano Y, et al. Metabolic assessment of monofocal acute inflammatory demyelination using MR spectroscopy and (11)C-methionine-, (11)C-choline-, and (18)F-fluorodeoxyglucose-PET. Brain Tumor Pathol 2011;28(3):229–38.

119. Galldiks N, Ullrich R, Schroeter M, et al. Volumetry of [(11)C]-methionine PET uptake and MRI contrast enhancement in patients with recurrent glioblastoma multiforme. Eur J Nucl Med Mol Imaging 2010;37(1):84–92.

120. Terakawa Y, Tsuyuguchi N, Iwai Y, et al. Diagnostic accuracy of 11C-methionine PET for differentiation of recurrent brain tumors from radiation necrosis after radiotherapy. J Nucl Med 2008;49(5):694–9.

121. Herrmann K, Czernin J, Cloughesy T, et al. Comparison of visual and semiquantitative analysis of 18F-FDOPA-PET/CT for recurrence detection in glioblastoma patients. Neuro Oncol 2014;16(4):603–9.

122. Galldiks N, Stoffels G, Ruge MI, et al. Role of O-(2-18F-fluoroethyl)-L-tyrosine PET as a diagnostic tool for detection of malignant progression in patients with low-grade glioma. J Nucl Med 2013;54(12):2046–54.

123. Galldiks N, Dunkl V, Stoffels G, et al. Diagnosis of pseudoprogression in patients with glioblastoma using O-(2-[18F]fluoroethyl)-L-tyrosine PET. Eur J Nucl Med Mol Imaging 2015;42(5):685–95.

124. Kebir S, Fimmers R, Galldiks N, et al. Late pseudo-progression in glioblastoma: diagnostic value of dynamic O-(2-[18F]fluoroethyl)-L-Tyrosine PET. Clin Cancer Res 2016;22(9):2190–6.

125. Nioche C, Soret M, Gontier E, et al. Evaluation of quantitative criteria for glioma grading with static and dynamic 18F-FDopa PET/CT. Clin Nucl Med 2013;38(2):81–7.

126. Galldiks N, Kracht LW, Burghaus L, et al. Use of 11C-methionine PET to monitor the effects of temozolomide chemotherapy in malignant gliomas. Eur J Nucl Med Mol Imaging 2006;33(5):516–24.

127. Hutterer M, Nowosielski M, Putzer D, et al. O-(2-18F-fluoroethyl)-L-tyrosine PET predicts failure of antiangiogenic treatment in patients with recurrent high-grade glioma. J Nucl Med 2011;52(6):856–64.

128. Galldiks N, Rapp M, Stoffels G, et al. Response assessment of bevacizumab in patients with recurrent malignant glioma using [18F]Fluoroethyl-L-tyrosine PET in comparison to MRI. Eur J Nucl Med Mol Imaging 2013;40(1):22–33.

129. Galldiks N, Langen KJ, Holy R, et al. Assessment of treatment response in patients with glioblastoma using O-(2-18F-fluoroethyl)-L-tyrosine PET in comparison to MRI. J Nucl Med 2012;53(7):1048–57.

130. Moreau A, Febvey O, Mognetti T, et al. Contribution of different positron emission tomography tracers in glioma management: focus on glioblastoma. Front Oncol 2019;9:1134.

131. Ito K, Matsuda H, Kubota K. Imaging spectrum and pitfalls of (11)C-methionine positron emission tomography in a series of patients with intracranial lesions. Korean J Radiol 2016;17(3):424–34.

132. Floeth FW, Pauleit D, Sabel M, et al. 18F-FET PET differentiation of ring-enhancing brain lesions. J Nucl Med 2006;47(5):776–82.

133. Hutterer M, Nowosielski M, Putzer D, et al. Response to "reply to [18F]-fluoro-ethyl-L-tyrosine PET: a valuable diagnostic tool in neuro-oncology, but not all that glitters is glioma" by Hutterer et al. Neuro Oncol 2013;15(7):814–5.

134. Harat M, Małkowski B, Makarewicz R. Pre-irradiation tumour volumes defined by MRI and dual time-point FET-PET for the prediction of glioblastoma multiforme recurrence: a prospective study. Radiother Oncol 2016;120(2):241–7.

135. Sala Q, Metellus P, Taieb D, et al. 18F-DOPA, a clinically available PET tracer to study brain inflammation? Clin Nucl Med 2014;39(4):e283–5.

136. Ohtani T, Kurihara H, Ishiuchi S, et al. Brain tumour imaging with carbon-11 choline: comparison with FDG PET and gadolinium-enhanced MR imaging. Eur J Nucl Med 2001;28(11):1664–70.

137. Albano D, Tomasini D, Bonù M, et al. 18)F-Fluciclovine ((18)F-FACBC) PET/CT or PET/MRI in gliomas/glioblastomas. Ann Nucl Med 2020;34(2):81–6.

138. Bogsrud TV, Londalen A, Brandal P, et al. 18F-fluciclovine PET/CT in suspected residual or recurrent high-grade glioma. Clin Nucl Med 2019;44(8):605–11.

# Fibroblast Activation Protein Inhibitor Theranostics

Shobhana Raju, MBBS, MD[a], Jaya Shukla, MSc, PhD[b],
Rakesh Kumar, MBBS, DRM, DNB, MNAMS, PhD[c],*

## KEYWORDS

- Fibroblast activation protein inhibitor • Fibroblast activation protein • PET

## KEY POINTS

- Tumor microenvironment consisting of stromal cells can be targeted with FAPI, an inhibitor of fibroblast activation protein(FAP).
- Based on the UAMC1110 scaffold molecule, two molecules with specific binding to human and murine FAP were developed, namely FAPI-01 and FAPI-02.
- The limitations in the FAPI-02 led to development of new molecules with improved specificity and stability such as [68]Ga-DOTA.SA
- FAPI and [68]Ga-DATA[5m].SA.FAPI.
- These novel molecules were used for imaging studies of non-oncological and oncological conditions like head and neck carcinomas, brain tumors, hepatic tumors, gastrointestinal malignancies, etc. with the theranostic counterpart of the molecules showing promising results in clinical studies.
- Whether FAPI will replace fluoro-2-deoxy-D-glucose in the next decade is a million-dollar question that needs to be considered.

## INTRODUCTION

PET has emerged as an advanced diagnostic imaging tool that allows the identification of the physiologic and biochemical alterations in various pathologic lesions. 2-[Fluorine-18] fluoro-2-deoxy-D-glucose ([18]F-FDG) was developed as a PET tracer later in the 1970s by labeling FDG with [18]F and was administered in human volunteers by Abass Alavi at the University of Pennsylvania in 1976.[1] Since then, [18]F-FDG has been the workhorse of PET and hybrid PET/computed tomographic (CT) imaging. [18]F-FDG, being a glucose analogue, is transported into tumor cells by glucose transporters and phosphorylated by hexokinase to FDG-6-phosphate. This metabolic trapping of [18]F-FDG constitutes the basis for in vivo distribution of radiotracer and metabolic mapping of whole-body disease dissemination. The oncologic indications of [18]F-FDG are diagnosis, staging, and restaging of non–small cell lung cancer, Hodgkin and non-Hodgkin lymphoma, colorectal cancer, breast cancer, esophageal cancer, colorectal cancer, and so forth.[2] The nononcologic indications are pyrexia of unknown origin, infections, especially bone infections like spondylodiscitis and diabetic foot, inflammations like sarcoidosis, rheumatoid arthritis, vasculitis, and pericarditis, and in neurology for neurocognitive disorders.[3] Other more specific tracers that came to the forefront in specific malignancies include [68]Ga-SSA (somatostatin analogue) for

Disclosure
The authors have nothing to disclose.
[a] Department of Nuclear Medicine, AIIMS, New Delhi 110029, India; [b] Department of Nuclear Medicine and PET, PGIMER, Chandigarh 160012, India; [c] Diagnostic Nuclear Medicine Division, Department of Nuclear Medicine, AIIMS, New Delhi 110029, India
* Corresponding author.
E-mail address: rkphulia@hotmail.com

PET Clin 17 (2022) 453–464
https://doi.org/10.1016/j.cpet.2022.03.005

neuroendocrine tumors and prostate-specific membrane antigen ($^{68}$Ga-PSMA) -based tracers for prostate cancer.[4,5] Other tracers like amino-acid analogues ($^{18}$F-FET, $^{18}$F-FLT) have also been evaluated in brain tumors owing to high physiologic activity of $^{18}$F-FDG in the brain.[6]

Even with the advent of these specific tracers in dedifferentiated tumors, the role of $^{18}$F-FDG PET/CT has not deteriorated, especially in poorly differentiated carcinomas. The clinical utility of $^{18}$F-FDG PET/CT can be limited by the physiologic distribution of the radiotracer in the brain, liver, renal system, digestive system, and head and neck mucosa. Mucin-producing low-grade carcinomas, such as ovarian, pancreatic, and sarcomas, exhibit low glycolytic activity and low $^{18}$F-FDG avidity. In this era of precision medicine and molecular targeted therapy, $^{18}$F-FDG falls short owing to the lack of a therapeutic pair.[7] Recently, a small molecule fibroblast activation protein inhibitor (FAPI) has been studied in various carcinomas with potential for targeted therapy. In this article, the biological basis of FAPI as theranostic agent, development and evolution of tracer, and role in various oncologic and non-oncologic conditions are evaluated. An insight into the recent query in the nuclear medicine community of whether FAPI will replace FDG is also considered.

## UNDERSTANDING THE TUMOR MICROENVIRONMENT

Tumors can be considered an assembly of not only tumor cells but also stroma. The stroma represents approximately 90% of tumor mass especially in tumors with a pronounced desmoplastic reaction, such as breast, pancreatic, and colon carcinoma. Fibroblasts are an important constituent of stroma, which are heterogeneous in origin. In tumors, a subgroup of fibroblasts, known as cancer-associated fibroblasts (CAFs), are associated with growth, migration, and progression of tumor and extracellular matrix production. CAFs are involved in the remodeling of the extracellular matrix by collagenolysis, which promotes tumor invasion and is involved in epithelial to mesenchymal transition. The CAFs are also involved in immunosuppression, angiogenesis, and metabolic cooperation with tumor cells. They differ from the normal fibroblast in terms of markers expressed, the most significant being fibroblast activation protein (FAP).[8] FAP is a membrane-bound glycoprotein of the dipeptidyl peptidase 4 (DPP4) family. DPP4 and FAP are membrane-bound enzymes, with DPP4 showing only exopeptidase activity and FAP showing both dipeptidyl peptidase and endopeptidase activity.[9] Because CAFs are more stable than cancer cells and less susceptible to

therapy resistance, these are suitable targets for anti-tumor therapy.

## MOLECULES TARGETING FIBROBLAST ACTIVATION

As FAP is broadly expressed in the tumor microenvironment and less susceptible to develop therapy resistance, these are explored for antitumor therapy. There have been approaches to target FAP, such as immunoconjugates, chimeric antigen receptor T cells, immunotherapy, peptide drug complexes, and FAP inhibitors and antibodies.[8] Several preclinical studies with FAP inhibitor molecules showed promising results. Oral DNA vaccine targeting FAP suppressed primary tumor cell growth and metastasis of multidrug-resistant murine colon and breast carcinoma through T-cell–mediated killing of tumor-associated fibroblasts.[10] In xenograft models, treatment with antibody-maytansinoid conjugate, namely mAB-FAP5-DM1, leads to complete regression of tumor growth.[11] These preclinical results were applied clinically in patients with metastatic colorectal carcinoma in an open-labeled multicentric study. Seventeen patients were given 8 weekly infusions of sibrotuzumab and evaluated. No complete or partial response was noted; rather, ongoing tumor progression was noted in all patients except 2 patients with stable disease.[12] Enzyme inhibitors targeting the NH2-Xaa-Pro motif, such as Val-boro-Pro (PT-100, talabostat), were developed with promising results in preclinical studies. These preclinical results failed to translate into clinical results owing to lack of receptor selectivity, which hindered further development of the molecule.[8,13]

Even though therapies targeting FAP were less successful, radionuclide-based imaging agents were simultaneously under development. Iodine-labeled FAP inhibitor MIP-1232 was used for the detection of atherosclerotic plaques with limited success.[14] $^{131}$I labeled anti-FAP antibody sibrotuzumab was used in the treatment of metastasized FAP-positive carcinomas. $^{131}$I-sibrotuzumab showed slow blood pool clearance with considerable tracer accumulation in lesions larger than 1.5 cm. The disadvantages of these initial tracers were poor energy resolution, limited sensitivity for detection of small lesions, and variations in number of FAP-positive cells in tumors.[15] Also, these FAP inhibitors lacked nanomolar affinity and selectivity toward propyl oligo-peptidase (PREP) and dipeptidyl-peptidases (DPPs). This led to the search for FAP-specific inhibitors that could bind with higher affinity and specificity.

A variety of structurally related small molecule inhibitors were developed, which were chemically 2-pyrrolidine derivatives.[16] One of the most promising molecules with low nanomolar affinity and high selectivity for DPPs and PREP was UAMC1110, quinoline-based FAP-specific inhibitor (4-quinoli-noyl)glycyl-2-cyano-4,4-difluoro-pyrrolidine. The high FAP selectivity of UAMC1110 is particularly attractive for tumor targeting, while considering the near-ubiquitous expression of the DPPs and PREP in humans. In addition, this molecule possessed a satisfactory pharmacokinetic profile.[16,17]

## EVOLUTION OF FIBROBLAST ACTIVATION PROTEIN INHIBITOR RADIOTRACERS

Based on the UAMC1110 scaffold molecule, 2 molecules with specific binding to human and murine FAP were developed, namely FAPI-01 and FAPI-02, by the Heidelberg group.[18] These molecules lacked nonspecific binding to closely related proteins, such as DPP4/CD26. FAPI-01 labeled with [125]I showed rapid internalization into cells but suboptimal performance owing to time-dependent enzymatic deiodination. [125]I-labeled FAPI-01 thus had low intracellular radioactivity after longer incubation periods ($3.25\% \pm 0.29\%$ after 24 hours). FAPI-02 was developed as a DOTA-linked compound and had better pharmacokinetic and biochemical properties. This molecule showed 10 times higher retention with slower elimination. The DOTA moiety of FAPI-02 allowed for easy incorporation of both diagnostic and therapeutic radionuclides.[19]

The initial diagnostic studies were done with [68]Ga-FAPI-02 after intravenous injection of 222 to 312 MBq and imaging at 10 minutes, 1 hour, and 3 hours. A robust accumulation of the tracer was noted in the primary tumor, lymph nodes, and skeletal metastasis, with a maximum standardized uptake value ($SUV_{max}$) of 13.3. There was a rapid clearance of radiotracer from the bloodstream, minimal uptake in normal tissues, and rapid renal clearance, providing high contrast images. In contrast to [18]F-FDG, there was minimal physiologic uptake in the brain and liver. The theranostics counterpart of FAPI-02 was developed with [177]Lu. [177]Lu-FAPI-02 showed rapid internalization into FAP-expressing cells, giving higher uptake rates and retention of 12% of the initial accumulated activity at 24 hours.[19] A further improvement of the FAPI-02 molecule was tried to optimize uptake and tumor retention, and 15 different compounds were developed. The most promising of these was FAPI-04, with a 3-fold reduction of the 50% effective concentration value compared with FAPI-02. There was a difference in affinity for the related enzymes FAP and DPP4/CD26. The FAP/DPP4 binding ratios for FAPI-02 and FAPI-04 were 45 and 750, respectively.[18] Diagnostic imaging with [68]Ga-FAPI-04 was performed in 2 patients with metastatic breast cancer yielding high contrast images with robust tracer accumulation in metastatic lesions. The therapeutic analogue with [90]Y-FAPI-04 yielded significant pain reduction in a treated patient.[18]

The 2 promising FAPI tracers, FAPI-02 and FAPI-04, were studied in terms of biodistribution and dosimetry in the featured article of August 2018 in the *Journal of Nuclear Medicine*.[20] This article also did an intraindividual comparison of [18]F-FDG and [68]Ga-FAPI in 6 different tumors. Even though both the agents performed equally with respect to tumor-to-background at 1 hour, the tumor uptake decline from 1 hour to 3 hours after injection was higher for FAPI-02 (mean decline of 75% for FAPI-02 vs 25% for FAPI-04). There was no statistically significant difference between the 2 tracers in the average $SUV_{max}$ values (8.37 for [68]Ga-FAPI-02 and 10.07 for [68]Ga-FAPI-04). Both the tracers correspond to an equivalent dose of 3 to 4 mSv at a dose of 200 MBq, similar to [18]F-FDG. The quantitative tumor uptake of [68]Ga-FAPI and [18]F-FDG was comparable in different cancers, such as pancreatic, esophageal, lung, head and neck, and colorectal carcinomas (average $SUV_{max}$ of 7.41 for [18]F-FDG and 7.37 for [68]Ga-FAPI-02; not statistically significant). The average background $SUV_{max}$ of [68]Ga-FAPI-02 was significantly lower compared with [18]F-FDG in the brain (0.32 vs 11.01), liver (1.69 vs 2.77), and oral/pharyngeal mucosa (2.57 vs 4.88). This improved the contrast ratios for liver metastases of pancreatic and colorectal cancer and delineation of the esophageal cancer.[20]

The favorable initial results of the [68]Ga-FAPI studies led to the search for delineation of the clinical utility of the tracer. In this search, the same Heidelberg group used the tracer on an experimental basis in patients facing an unmet diagnostic challenge. This included most patients in whom the conventional modalities did not solve the diagnostic challenge or in whom tumor delineation for the planning of radiotherapy was inaccurate. Eighty patients with 28 different histologically proven tumor types were evaluated. [68]Ga-FAPI-04 PET/CT was acquired 1 hour postinjection of 122 to 312 MBq of the tracer. The tumor uptake was quantified by $SUV_{max}$ and $SUV_{mean}$ with 60% isocontour. The tumors evaluated were categorized into highest (>12), intermediate (6–12), and lowest $SUV_{max}$ tumors (**Table 1**).

Several FAPI molecules were developed by structural variations mainly within the linker chain with low nanomolar affinities and longer tumor retention times. The relevance of those is FAPI-21 and FAPI-46 (50% inhibitory concentration [IC50] = 6.7 nM for FAPI-21 and IC50 = 13.5 nM for FAPI-46).[21] Moon and colleagues[22] developed FAPI molecules with squaramide coupled

**Table 1**
Classification of various tumors based on the maximum standardized uptake value values of $^{68}$Ga-FAPI-04 PET/computed tomography

| Highest SUV$_{max}$ (>12) | Intermediate SUV$_{max}$ (6–12) | Lowest SUV$_{max}$ (<6) |
|---|---|---|
| Sarcoma | Hepatocellular Ca | Pheochromocytoma |
| Esophageal Ca | Colorectal Ca | Renal cell Ca |
| Breast Ca | Head and neck Ca | Adenoid cystic Ca |
| Cholangiocarcinoma | Ovarian Ca | Gastric Ca |
| Lung Ca | Pancreatic Ca | Dedifferentiated thyroid Ca |
|  | Prostate Ca |  |

bifunctional DOTA and DATA$^{5m}$ chelators. The novel radiopharmaceuticals $^{68}$Ga-DOTA.SA.FAPI and 68Ga-DATA$^{5m}$.SA.FAPI had high radiochemical yields (>97%) and high molecular stability over 2 hours with high inhibitory efficiency to FAP and PREP. The advantages of squaramide compounds were high target-to-background ratio, longer biological half-life, improved pharmacokinetic properties, and potential for theranostics.

In the prospective study by Ballal and colleagues,[23] biodistribution, pharmacokinetics, and dosimetry of $^{68}$Ga-DOTA.SA.FAPI (in 3 patients) were evaluated with a head-to-head comparison of the tracer with $^{18}$F-FDG in 44 patients with 14 different cancers. Physiologic uptake was observed in liver, kidney, pancreas, and heart. In target lesions, uptake was noted in 10 minutes, with no additional lesion detection at delayed time point images. The highest absorbed dose was received by the pancreas (5.46E-02 mSv/MBq). In comparison with $^{18}$F-FDG, complete concordance was noted in the detection of primary, skeletal, and hepatic metastasis and second primary. Discordant imaging findings were noted in lymph nodal, lung, and brain metastatic lesions. A comparable SUL$_{peak}$ was noted in all regions of metastasis except brain metastasis, with significantly comparable SUL$_{peak}$ for brain metastasis with $^{68}$Ga-DOTA.SA.FAPI. Based on these imaging results, therapies targeting FAP with $^{177}$Lu-DOTA.SA.FAPI was tried in a patient with end-stage breast cancer by the same group. It was assumed that $^{177}$Lu-DOTA.SA.FAPi, guided by $^{68}$Ga-DOTA.SA.FAPI PET/CT, can be a novel therapeutic option, especially in patients refractory to conventional therapies, and can be a new milestone in this era of precision medicine.

## DIAGNOSTIC STUDIES
### Nononcologic

Fibroblast activation protein has been found activated in cardiac wound healing and remodeling in small-animal models. Based on these studies, retrospectively analyzing the cardiac findings in oncologic patients with cardiac pathology was initiated. Siebermair and colleagues[24] evaluated myocardial $^{68}$Ga-FAPI uptake in oncologic patients and demonstrated a significant correlation by univariate analysis between coronary artery disease (CAD), left ventricular ejection fraction, and age and SUV$_{mean}$ myocardial uptake. This paved the potential to access if fibroblast accumulation can be used for early detection, risk stratification, and progression of CAD, for which further studies are warranted. Heckmann and colleagues[25] observed that high left ventricular $^{68}$Ga-FAPI signals were significantly related to cardiovascular risk factors, such as overweight (odds ratio [OR] 2.6; $P = 0.023$) and type II diabetes mellitus (OR, 2.9; $P = .041$), chemotherapy received (platinum-based), and history of radiation exposure. Immune checkpoint inhibitor-associated myocarditis could be assessed at an early stage by $^{68}$Ga-FAPI PET/CT and correlated with electrocardiographic abnormalities, wall motion abnormalities on echocardiography, and lymphocytic infiltration of myocardium in biopsies.[26]

Preclinical studies with radiolabeled anti-FAP antibodies showed evidence of FAP expression in inflamed joints, which correlated with the severity of inflammation in experimental murine rheumatoid arthritis. On the basis of these, several studies evaluated the role in uncoupling inflammation from fibrotic disease in Immunoglobulin G4 (IgG4)-related disease, which is a fibroinflammatory disease. Schmidkonz and colleagues[27] demonstrated that a combination of $^{18}$F-FDG and $^{68}$Ga-FAPI PET/CT can provide a noninvasive tracking of IgG4-related disease evolution from inflammatory to fibrotic nature, which can change the management from anti-inflammatory to antifibrotic agents. Another study by Luo and colleagues[28] observed that $^{68}$Ga-FAPI PET/CT had a higher detection rate than $^{18}$F-FDG in involved organs, like pancreas, bile duct, lacrimal, and salivary gland in IgG4-related disease. However, IgG4-related lymphadenopathy was not FAPI avid. Systemic sclerosis–associated interstitial lung disease activity and disease progression were found to be related to the $^{68}$Ga-FAPI PET/CT uptake.[29]

## Oncologic

The initial work in $^{68}$Ga-FAPI PET/CT has mainly concentrated in biodistribution and kinetics study of the tracer, staging, and radiotherapy planning in the carcinomas of head and neck and abdominal malignancies. Initial kinetic studies of the tracer to study the optimal uptake time of the tracer compared the early ($\sim$ 10 minutes) and late ($\sim$ 60 minutes) FAPI imaging in various cancers. On per-patient level, it was found that there was no statistically significant difference in the $SUV_{max}$ of the hottest tumor lesion, and the significant early to late decrease in $SUV_{mean}$ was noted favoring early PET imaging in clinical research. The preliminary oncologic studies concentrated on the carcinomas in which unmet needs of $^{18}$F-FDG PET/CT prevailed, such as brain, liver, head, and neck, owing to high physiologic uptake.

### Head and neck carcinomas

The state-of-the-art $^{18}$F-FDG in head and neck carcinomas (HNCs) is less specific owing to false-positive results and fails to precisely assess local tumor spread in relation to the complex peritumoral structures. In the study conducted by Syed and colleagues[30] in 14 HNCs, all FAPI-based gross tumor volumes (GTVs) were significantly different from CT GTVs, with FAPI $\times$ 3 being the ideal threshold for precise tumor detection, allowing radiation therapy planning. The intratumoral uptake was also correlated with the grade of malignancy, invasion, and therapy resistance of the tumor. In another study by Serfling and colleagues,[31] 8 patients with malignant Waldeyer ring tumor $^{18}$F-FDG was compared with $^{68}$Ga-FAPI for primary and lymph nodal metastasis detection. The primary tumor detection was comparable with mean tumor-to-background ratio for $^{68}$Ga-FAPI (10.90) being markedly higher than $^{18}$F-FDG (4.11), but cervical lymph nodal metastasis detection was higher with $^{18}$F-FDG. A head-to-head comparison of $^{68}$Ga-FAPI-04 and $^{18}$F-FDG PET/MR in nasopharyngeal carcinoma noticed better delineation of the skull base and intracranial invasion by $^{68}$Ga-FAPI-04. By detection of additional small distant metastasis, $^{68}$Ga-FAPI-04 changed overall staging in 6/15 patients. Similar to the previous study, this group also noted the limitation of $^{68}$Ga-FAPI-04 in detecting lymph nodal metastasis.[32]

### Brain tumors

Targeting FAP in glioma was initially studied in glioblastoma cell lines U87MG and used for clinical imaging in 18 glioma patients, both isocitrate dehydrogenase (IDH) mutant gliomas and IDH-wild-type gliomas. $^{68}$Ga-FAPI-04 showed higher tumor accumulation in IDH wild-type glioblastomas and grade III/IV IDH mutant gliomas, allowing distinction between low-grade and high-grade gliomas.[33] Based on the findings of the previous study, the question of whether local tumor uptake can be related to local differences in perfusion and cell density was raised. Therefore, another study correlating FAP-specific signaling with relative cerebral blood volume (rCBV) and apparent diffusion coefficient was used to further characterize the FAPI uptake in gliomas. A moderate positive correlation between FAP-specific signals and rCBV was noted in T2-weighted/fluid-attenuated inversion recovery lesionsequence and no correlation with cell density, indicating that FAPI imaging is not a surrogate marker of perfusion or cell density.[34] Target volume delineation was evaluated with $^{68}$Ga-FAPI in 13 glioblastoma patients and compared with MR imaging, giving better GTV volumes containing tumor not covered by MR imaging–GTVs.

### Hepatic tumors

Kinetic modeling of the hepatic lesions was first evaluated in hepatic lesions to differentiate hepatocellular carcinoma (HCC) from non-HCC lesions. An image-derived input function based on the arterial and venous reversible compartmental model showed a significant difference in kinetic parameters between healthy liver regions, non-HCC lesions, and HCC lesions ($P<.01$).[35] In an initial pilot study for evaluation of the suspected hepatic nodules, fibroblast imaging uptake values were correlated by immunohistochemistry to FAP expression. $^{68}$Ga-FAPI-04 showed high sensitivity (75% of the primary HCC lesions) in detecting hepatic malignancies, with concordantly elevated FAP expression. A comparison of the 68Ga-FAPI-04 with $^{18}$F-FDG PET/CT was done by the same investigators, which revealed the superior potential of 68Ga-FAPI-04 in the detection of primary hepatic malignancies. In 17 patients with primary hepatic tumors,[16] HCC in 14 patients and 4 intrahepatic cholangiocarcinomas (IHCC) in 3 patients, $^{68}$Ga-FAPI-04 showed uptake in all the patients, whereas only 7 patients had FDG-avid disease.[36,37] A post hoc retrospective analysis of 34 patients (HCC = 20, IHCC = 12, and benign nodule = 2) revealed a sensitivity of contrast-enhanced CT (CECT), MR imaging, $^{68}$Ga-FAPI-04, and $^{18}$F-FDG PET/CT for detection of primary hepatic tumors to be 96%, 100%, 96%, and 65%, respectively. For malignant lesions, the detection rates of $^{68}$Ga-FAPI-04 were significantly higher than $^{18}$F-FDG PET/CT (87.4% vs 65%, $P<.001$).[38] **Figs. 1** and **2** represent cases of HCC and Ca gallbladder, respectively.

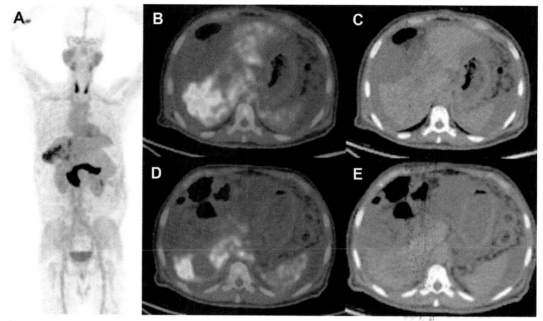

**Fig. 1.** Patient 1 (HCC): A 61-year-old man c/o HCC, decompensated NASH cirrhosis. CT abdomen showed liver cirrhosis with hepatic SOL with ascites. (*A*) $^{68}$Ga-FAPI PET/CT was performed for disease evaluation. WB PET/CT images were acquired 60 minutes after intravenous injection of 111 MBq (3 mCi) of $^{68}$Ga-FAPI. Intense FAPI avidity is noted in the periphery of hypodense necrotic lesion in segment VI of the liver (SUV$_{max}$: 12.9) (*B–E*) Physiological tracer uptake is noted in B/L salivary glands, liver (SUC$_{max}$: 6.4), thyroid, muscles, pancreas, and excretion via kidneys and urinary bladder.

## Gastrointestinal tumors

The major drawbacks of $^{18}$F-FDG PET/CT in gastrointestinal (GI) cancers, such as variable sensitivity in the detection of primary and lymph nodal, hepatic, and peritoneal metastasis, demanded a validated PET tracer in GI malignancies.[39] The first clinical experience of $^{68}$Ga-FAPI PET/CT in lower GI tract malignancies was reported by the Heidelberg group. The highest tumor uptake was noted in anal cancers and hepatic metastasis, and high target-to-background ratios were noted in most lesions. TNM staging was changed in 50% treatment-naïve patients, and new metastatic lesions were identified in 47% of the metastatic patients.[40] Comparison of $^{68}$Ga-FAPI-04 with $^{18}$F-FDG PET/CT in gastric, duodenal, and colorectal carcinomas revealed significantly higher uptake (gastric: 12.7 vs 3.7; $P = .003$; colorectal: 15.9 vs 7.9, $P = .03$; lymph node: 6.7 vs 2.4, $P<.001$; skeletal metastasis: 4.3 vs 2.2, $P<.001$, respectively). Higher sensitivity in lesion detection was noted not only of the primary lesion (100% [19/19] vs 53% [10/19]) but also of the lymph nodal (79% [22/28] vs 54% [15/28]), skeletal, and visceral metastasis (89% [31/35] vs 57% [20/35]).[39] Neoadjuvant radiotherapy planning of esophageal carcinomas demands better delineation of the GTV by CT, which demonstrates

the largest volume. $^{18}$F-FDG-based GTV could not differentiate between inflammation and malignancy, where $^{68}$Ga-FAPI based GTV delineation can be tried. The study by Zhao and colleagues[41] revealed that high target-to-background contrast allows for better tumor volume delineation, avoiding tumor geographic misses.

## Pancreatic tumors

In locally recurrent pancreatic carcinoma, the high interobserver variability in tumor delineation by radiation oncologists could be minimized by $^{68}$Ga-FAPI PET/CT-based automated GTVs. It was found to be superior to the current gold-standard CECT.[42] Another study assessing the impact of $^{68}$Ga-FAPI PET/CT imaging on therapeutic management of pancreatic adenocarcinoma showed that it could restage the disease when compared with CECT. An attempt to differentiate between pancreatitis and pancreatic adenocarcinoma based on different time point images was also made with differential uptake kinetics.[43] The role of $^{68}$Ga-FAPI PET/MR also has been evaluated in a recent case report by Shou and colleagues.[44]

Multiple studies have evaluated the role of $^{68}$Ga-FAPI PET/CT imaging in the staging and restaging of various carcinomas.[45–47] However, a few other studies tried to evaluate the role of

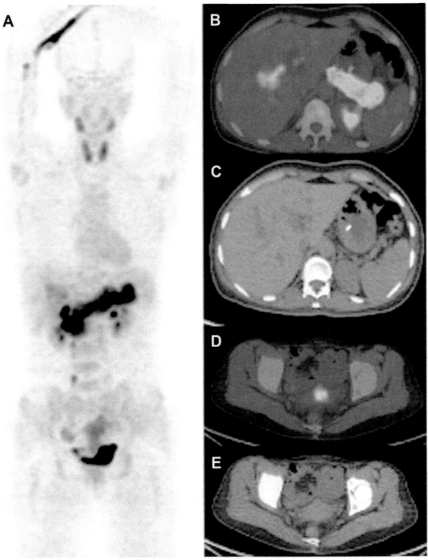

Fig. 2. Patient 2 (GB Ca): A 38-year-old woman c/o advanced GB Ca. CECT showed diffuse asymmetrical circumferential thickening in GB body and neck, complete obliteration of CBT lumen, loss of fat planes with D1, pylorus effacement of duodenal lumen, and ill-defined pancreatic head and adjacent liver decompensated NASH cirrhosis. (A) $^{68}$Ga-FAPI PET/CT was performed for disease evaluation. WB PET/CT images were acquired 60 minutes after intravenous injection of 111 MBq (3 mCi) of $^{68}$Ga-FAPI. (B and C) Faint FAPI uptake is noted in the GB (SUV$_{max}$: 7.7) neck along with ill-defined hypodense uptake in the liver parenchyma (SUC$_{max}$: 5.7) due to infiltration. (D and E) Physiological tracer uptake is noted in B/L salivary glands, liver, thyroid, muscles, pancreas, uterus (SUV$_{max}$: 11) and excretion via kidneys and urinary bladder.

$^{68}$Ga-FAPI PET/CT in patients with inconclusive $^{18}$F-FDG PET/CT findings, so that it can have a complementary role in characterizing lesions detected by conventional imaging, locating the primary site of carcinoma of unknown primary, staging and restaging, and recurrence detection. However, similar to $^{18}$F-FDG PET/CT, the tumors complicated with inflammation should be reported with caution.[48] The sensitivity, specificity, positive predictive value, negative predictive value, and accuracy of the 2 tracers were compared by the same group. In 12 different tumors, a favorable Target : Background contrast and high detection rate were noted for primary tumors compared with $^{18}$F-FDG PET/CT (98.2% vs82.1%; $P$ = .021). The sensitivity in the detection of lymph nodal, bone, and visceral metastasis was superior to $^{18}$F-FDG.[49]

Figs. 3–5 represent $^{68}$Ga-FAPI imaging in other carcinomas, such as breast carcinoma and ovary.

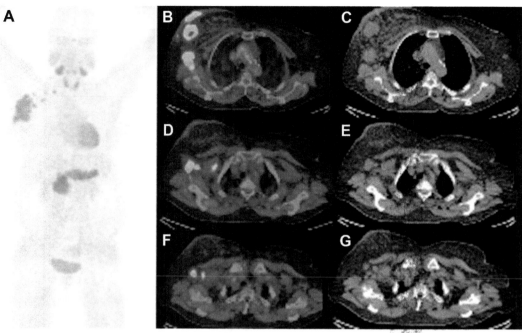

Fig. 3. Patient 3 (Breast Ca): A 65-year-old woman k/c/o right breast, IDC grade II; MMG: right breast (BIRADS 5), and left breast (BIRADS 2). WB PET/CT images were acquired 60 minutes after intravenous injection of 111 MBq (3 mCi) of (A) $^{68}$Ga-FAPI (A). Intense tracer avid soft tissue mass is noted in the upper quadrant of the right breast with central photopenia (SUV$_{max}$: 18.6) (B, C). FAPI-avid subcentrimetric satellite nodules, nodular cutaneous skin thickening (SUV$_{max}$: 18.6), and nipple areolar complex are noted in the right breast Tracer-avid subcentrimetric and enlarged level I to III axillary lymph nodes (SUC$_{max}$: 19.1) are noted (D–G).

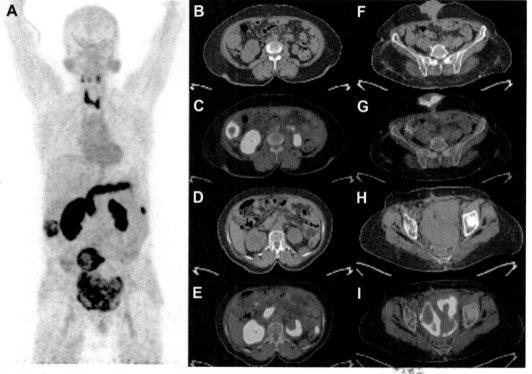

Fig. 4. Patient 4 (Ovary Ca): A 68-year-old woman diagnosed with ovary cancer underwent total abdominal hysterectomy (TAH) and bilateral salpingo-oophoroctomy (23/12/2019). Completed 12 cycles of chemotherapy (March 2020). $^{18}$F-FDG PET/CT revealed hypermetabolic B/L adrenal lesion with peritoneal deposits (02/09/2020). (A)$^{68}$Ga-FAPI was performed for disease evaluation. WB PET/CT images were acquired 60 minutes after intravenous injection of 148 MBq (4.0 mCi) of $^{68}$Ga-FAPI. Multiple serosal peritoneal deposits were noted (B–E). Soft tissue density lesion along the lower anterior abdominal wall (SUV$_{max}$: 14.2) was also noted (F, G). Avidity was noted in the pelvic region (SUV$_{max}$: 15.6) (H, I).

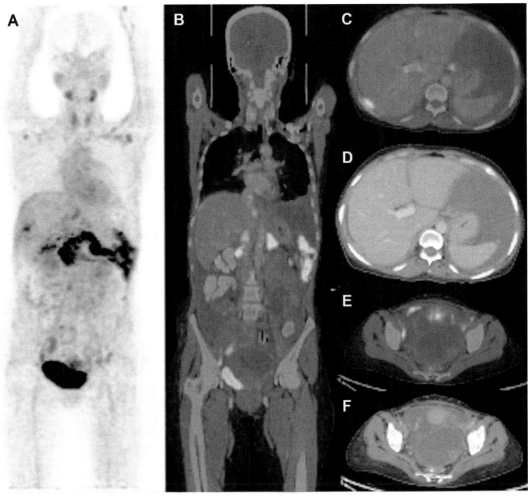

Fig. 5. Patient 5 (ovary Ca): A 37-year-old woman c/o abdominal pain and distension. Mammography showed necrotic lymph nodes in both axilla (right breast: BIRADS 3; left breast BIRADS 3). CECT abdomen showed abdominopelvic soft cystic mass lesion originating from B/L adnexa with extension consistent with ovarian Ca. Various soft tissue deposits were noted along small bowel, transverse mesocolon, and in omentum suggestive of peritoneal carcinomatosis. Inguinal, mesenteric, and retroperitoneal lymphadenopathy: likely metastatic. [68]GA-FAPI was performed for disease evaluation. WB PET/CT images (A, B) were acquired 30 minutes after intravenous injection of 125.8 MBq (3.4 mCi) of Ga-FAPI. Physiological tracer uptake was noted in the salivary glands, thyroid, liver, pancreas, and excretion via kidneys and bladder. FAPI-avid paraaortic, aortocaval, mesenteric, internal iliac, B/L external iliac, and right common iliac ($SUV_{max}$: 6.9) lymph nodes were noted. FAPI-avid soft tissue mass was noted in the right adnexa ($SUV_{max}$: 6.8) (E, F). Faint FAPI-avid peritoneal thickening ($SUV_{max}$: 3) was noted (C, D).

A recent systemic review and meta-analysis by Sollini and colleagues[50] evaluated 23 studies in various cancers and detected a pooled sensitivity of 0.99 (95% confidence interval [CI], 0.97–1.00) and a pooled specificity of 0.87 (95% CI, 0.62–1.00), both with negligible heterogeneity in patient-based analysis. The sensitivity and specificity had high heterogeneity on lesion-based analysis. Pooled sensitivities for the primary tumor and for distant metastasis were 1.00 (95% CI, 0.98–1.00) and 0.93 (95% CI, 0.88–0.97), respectively. Pooled sensitivity for lymph nodal metastasis showed high heterogeneity.

## THERAPEUTIC STUDIES

One of the initial molecules for therapeutic implication was obtained by labeling FAPI-02 with [177]Lu, which specifically binds to human and murine FAP-expressing cells. [177]Lu-FAPI-02 internalizes rapidly, showing more stable and higher uptake over time with minimal elimination in mice bearing HT-1080-FAP tumor. Tumor uptake was highest after 2 hours (4.7% ID/g).[19] In-human trial with therapeutic intent was first done with [90]Y-FAPI-04 in metastasized breast cancer with a dose of 2.9 GBq. The tracer accumulation was noted by bremsstrahlung imaging at 3 hours and 1 day post-injection, and a clinical response that manifested as a step down in the ladder of pain medication.[18] The novel alpha-targeted theranostic role of FAPI was evaluated in preclinical studies in xenograft mouse models with $^{64}$Cu and $^{225}$Ac-FAPI-04 with favorable results.[51] Another study compared the therapeutic effects of $^{177}$Lu-FAPI-46 and $^{225}$Ac-FAPI-46 in pancreatic cancer models. The therapeutic effects of $^{177}$Lu-FAPI-46 were found to be relatively slow but lasted longer than $^{225}$Ac-FAPI-46.[52] One of the promising studies in clinical patients was done in a case of Her2neu-positive breast carcinoma with progressive disease (new brain lesion) on the standard line of therapy. $^{68}$Ga-DOTA.SA.FAPI imaging showed a one-to-one matched lesion as compared with $^{18}$F-FDG, and brain metastasis was confirmed in MR imaging. $^{177}$Lu-DOTA.SA.-FAPI (3.2 GBq) was administered as slow intravenous infusion, and 24-hour posttherapeutic single-photon emission computerized tomography/CT images were acquired. Dosimetric studies in the same study revealed absorbed tumor doses of approximately 1.48E mGy/MBq and 3.46 mGy/MBq to the primary tumor and the brain metastasis, respectively.[53]

## FUTURE DIRECTIONS

With the advent of FAPI, it has emerged as a unique tracer over the past decades that has even brought a question of replacing $^{18}$F-FDG. "Whether FAPI will replace FDG in the next generation" is the question in the world of precision medicine of nuclear theranostics.[7] While considering this, a head-to-head comparison to prove the potential of $^{68}$Ga-FAPI to surmount[18] F-FDG is needed. The low background uptake and more sensitive detection of smaller lesions facilitating better tumor detection and delineation for radiotherapy planning bring an advantage to $^{68}$Ga-FAPI imaging. Another field where $^{68}$Ga-FAPI has an upper hand is in the detection of mucin-producing, low-grade cancers, including low-grade sarcoma, and some ovarian, pancreatic, breast cancer subtypes exhibiting low glycolytic phenotypes and low $^{18}$F-FDG uptake. The lack of a theranostic counterpart for $^{18}$F-FDG is another field where $^{68}$Ga-FAPI scores as a potential biomarker for response prediction to FAP-targeted therapeutics. Even with these advantages, to replace the age-old $^{18}$F-FDG, more prospective trials are needed that will bring to light the pros and cons of the tracer. The therapeutic potential and its efficacy need to be established by clinical trials of immense strength.[54] Thus, $^{68}$Ga-FAPI as an alternative of $^{18}$F-FDG in the near future seems too true to be realistic.

## SUMMARY

The evolution of the FAP inhibitor molecules over the past decade has brought into the forefront a novel theranostic agent that has the potential of matching the workhorse of PET/CT, the $^{18}$F-FDG. It is hoped that in the next decade it can act as a complementary tracer to $^{18}$F-FDG, in providing phenotypic and biomarker information and also in directing FAP-targeted therapies.

## CLINICS CARE POINTS

- From the diagnostic point $^{68}$Ga-FAPI can act as a complementary radiotracer with $^{18}$F-FDG.
- From therapeutic point there is an extensive realm to be explored and can be expected to be a revolution in the coming decades.

## REFERENCES

1. Ido T, Wan C-N, Casella V, et al. Labeled 2-deoxy-D-glucose analogs. 18F-labeled 2-deoxy-2-fluoro-D-glucose, 2-deoxy-2-fluoro-D-mannose and 14C-2-deoxy-2-fluoro-D-glucose. J Label Compd Radiopharm 1978;14(2):175–83.
2. Kostakoglu L, Agress H, Goldsmith SJ. Clinical role of FDG PET in evaluation of cancer patients. Radio-Graphics 2003;23(2):315–40.
3. Franz G, Schiappacasse G, Balcells A, et al. Rol del PET/CT con 18FDG en patología no neoplásica. Rev Chil Radiol 2017;23(3):116–29.
4. Kwekkeboom DJ, Kam BL, van Essen M, et al. Somatostatin receptor-based imaging and therapy of gastroenteropancreatic neuroendocrine tumors. Endocr Relat Cancer 2010;17(1):R53–73.
5. Fendler WP, Eiber M, Beheshti M, et al. 68Ga-PSMA PET/CT: joint EANM and SNMMI procedure guideline for prostate cancer imaging: version 1.0. Eur J Nucl Med Mol Imaging 2017;44(6):1014–24.
6. Juhász C, Dwivedi S, Kamson DO, et al. Comparison of amino acid positron emission tomographic radiotracers for molecular imaging of primary and metastatic brain tumors. Mol Imaging 2014;13(6). https://doi.org/10.2310/7290.2014.00015.
7. Calais J, Mona CE. Will FAPI PET/CT replace FDG PET/CT in the next decade? Point—an important diagnostic, phenotypic, and biomarker role. Am J Roentgenol 2021;216(2):305–6.
8. Lindner T, Loktev A, Giesel F, et al. Targeting of activated fibroblasts for imaging and therapy. EJNMMI Radiopharm Chem 2019;4(1):16.
9. Hamson EJ, Keane FM, Tholen S, et al. Understanding fibroblast activation protein (FAP): substrates,

activities, expression and targeting for cancer therapy. Prot Clin Appl 2014;8(5–6):454–63.

10. Loeffler M. Targeting tumor-associated fibroblasts improves cancer chemotherapy by increasing intratumoral drug uptake. J Clin Invest 2006;116(7):1955–62.

11. Ostermann E, Garin-Chesa P, Heider KH, et al. Effective immunoconjugate therapy in cancer models targeting a serine protease of tumor fibroblasts. Clin Cancer Res 2008;14(14):4584–92.

12. Hofheinz R-D, al-Batran S-E, Hartmann F, et al. Stromal antigen targeting by a humanised monoclonal antibody: an early phase II trial of sibrotuzumab in patients with metastatic colorectal cancer. Oncol Res Treat 2003;26(1):44–8.

13. Eager RM, Cunningham CC, Senzer N, et al. Phase II trial of talabostat and docetaxel in advanced non-small cell lung cancer. Clin Oncol 2009;21(6):464–72.

14. Meletta R, Müller Herde A, Chiotellis A, et al. Evaluation of the radiolabeled boronic acid-based FAP inhibitor MIP-1232 for atherosclerotic plaque imaging. Molecules 2015;20(2):2081–99.

15. Scott AM, Wiseman G, Welt S, et al. A phase I dose-escalation study of sibrotuzumab in patients with advanced or metastatic fibroblast activation protein-positive cancer. Clin Cancer Res 2003;9(5):1639–47.

16. Jansen K, Heirbaut L, Cheng JD, et al. Selective inhibitors of fibroblast activation protein (FAP) with a (4-quinolinoyl)-glycyl-2-cyanopyrrolidine scaffold. ACS Med Chem Lett 2013;4(5):491–6.

17. Jansen K, Heirbaut L, Verkerk R, et al. Extended structure–activity relationship and pharmacokinetic investigation of (4-quinolinoyl)glycyl-2-cyanopyrrolidine inhibitors of fibroblast activation protein (FAP). J Med Chem 2014;57(7):3053–74.

18. Lindner T, Loktev A, Altmann A, et al. Development of quinoline-based theranostic ligands for the targeting of fibroblast activation protein. J Nucl Med 2018;59(9):1415–22.

19. Loktev A, Lindner T, Mier W, et al. A tumor-imaging method targeting cancer-associated fibroblasts. J Nucl Med 2018;59(9):1423–9.

20. Giesel FL, Kratochwil C, Lindner T, et al. [68]Ga-FAPI PET/CT: biodistribution and preliminary dosimetry estimate of 2 DOTA-containing FAP-targeting agents in patients with various cancers. J Nucl Med 2019;60(3):386–92.

21. Loktev A, Lindner T, Burger E-M, et al. Development of fibroblast activation protein–targeted radiotracers with improved tumor retention. J Nucl Med 2019;60(10):1421–9.

22. Moon, EJNMMI Radiopharm Chem, 2020, https://doi.org/10.2310/7290.2014.00015. Submitted for publication.

23. Ballal S, Yadav MP, Moon ES, et al. Biodistribution, pharmacokinetics, dosimetry of [68Ga]Ga-DOTA.SA.FAPi,

and the head-to-head comparison with [18F]F-FDG PET/CT in patients with various cancers. Eur J Nucl Med Mol Imaging 2021;48(6):1915–31.

24. Siebermair J, Köhler MI, Kupusovic J, et al. Cardiac fibroblast activation detected by Ga-68 FAPI PET imaging as a potential novel biomarker of cardiac injury/remodeling. J Nucl Cardiol 2021;28(3):812–21.

25. Heckmann MB, Reinhardt F, Finke D, et al. Relationship between cardiac fibroblast activation protein activity by positron emission tomography and cardiovascular disease. Circ Cardiovasc Imaging 2020;13(9).

26. Finke D, Heckmann MB, Herpel E, et al. Early detection of checkpoint inhibitor-associated myocarditis using 68Ga-FAPI PET/CT. Front Cardiovasc Med 2021;8:614997.

27. Schmidkonz C, Rauber S, Atzinger A, et al. Disentangling inflammatory from fibrotic disease activity by fibroblast activation protein imaging. Ann Rheum Dis 2020;79(11):1485–91.

28. Luo Y, Pan Q, Yang H, et al. Fibroblast activation protein–targeted PET/CT with [68]Ga-FAPI for imaging IgG4-related disease: comparison to [18]F-FDG PET/CT. J Nucl Med 2021;62(2):266–71.

29. Bergmann C, Distler JHW, Treutlein C, et al. 68Ga-FAPI-04 PET-CT for molecular assessment of fibroblast activation and risk evaluation in systemic sclerosis-associated interstitial lung disease: a single-centre, pilot study. Lancet Rheumatol 2021;3(3):e185–94.

30. Syed M, Flechsig P, Liermann J, et al. Fibroblast activation protein inhibitor (FAPI) PET for diagnostics and advanced targeted radiotherapy in head and neck cancers. Eur J Nucl Med Mol Imaging 2020;47(12):2836–45.

31. Serfling S, Zhi Y, Schirbel A, et al. Improved cancer detection in Waldeyer's tonsillar ring by 68Ga-FAPI PET/CT imaging. Eur J Nucl Med Mol Imaging 2021;48(4):1178–87.

32. Qin C, Liu F, Huang J, et al. A head-to-head comparison of 68Ga-DOTA-FAPI-04 and 18F-FDG PET/MR in patients with nasopharyngeal carcinoma: a prospective study. Eur J Nucl Med Mol Imaging 2021. https://doi.org/10.1007/s00259-021-05255-w.

33. Röhrich M, Loktev A, Wefers AK, et al. IDH-wildtype glioblastomas and grade III/IV IDH-mutant gliomas show elevated tracer uptake in fibroblast activation protein–specific PET/CT. Eur J Nucl Med Mol Imaging 2019;46(12):2569–80.

34. Röhrich M, Floca R, Loi L, et al. FAP-specific PET signaling shows a moderately positive correlation with relative CBV and no correlation with ADC in 13 IDH wildtype glioblastomas. Eur J Radiol 2020;127:109021.

35. Geist BK, Xing H, Wang J, et al. A methodological investigation of healthy tissue, hepatocellular

carcinoma, and other lesions with dynamic 68Ga-FAPI-04 PET/CT imaging. EJNMMI Phys 2021;8(1):8.

36. Shi X, Xing H, Yang X, et al. Fibroblast imaging of hepatic carcinoma with 68Ga-FAPI-04 PET/CT: a pilot study in patients with suspected hepatic nodules. Eur J Nucl Med Mol Imaging 2021;48(1):196–203.

37. Shi X, Xing H, Yang X, et al. Comparison of PET imaging of activated fibroblasts and 18F-FDG for diagnosis of primary hepatic tumours: a prospective pilot study. Eur J Nucl Med Mol Imaging 2021;48(5):1593–603.

38. Guo W, Pang Y, Yao L, et al. Imaging fibroblast activation protein in liver cancer: a single-center post hoc retrospective analysis to compare [68Ga]GaFAPI-04 PET/CT versus MRI and [18F]-FDG PET/CT. Eur J Nucl Med Mol Imaging 2021;48(5):1604–17.

39. Pang Y, Zhao L, Luo Z, et al. Comparison of 68Ga-FAPI and 18F-FDG uptake in gastric, duodenal, and colorectal cancers. Radiology 2021;298(2):393–402.

40. Koerber SA, Staudinger F, Kratochwil C, et al. The role of 68Ga-FAPI PET/CT for patients with malignancies of the lower gastrointestinal tract: first clinical experience. J Nucl Med 2020;61(9):1331–6.

41. Zhao L, Chen S, Chen S, et al. 68Ga-fibroblast activation protein inhibitor PET/CT on gross tumour volume delineation for radiotherapy planning of oesophageal cancer. Radiother Oncol 2021;158:55–61.

42. Liermann J, Syed M, Ben-Josef E, et al. Impact of FAPI-PET/CT on target volume definition in radiation therapy of locally recurrent pancreatic cancer. Cancers 2021;13(4):796.

43. Röhrich M, Naumann P, Giesel FL, et al. Impact of 68Ga-FAPI PET/CT imaging on the therapeutic management of primary and recurrent pancreatic ductal adenocarcinomas. J Nucl Med 2021;62(6):779–86.

44. Shou Y, Xue Q, Yuan J, et al. 68Ga-FAPI-04 PET/MR is helpful in differential diagnosis of pancreatitis from pancreatic malignancy compared to 18F-FDG PET/CT: a case report. Eur J Hybrid Imaging 2021;5(1):12.

45. Kratochwil C, Flechsig P, Lindner T, et al. 68Ga-FAPI PET/CT: tracer uptake in 28 different kinds of cancer. J Nucl Med 2019;60(6):801–5.

46. Dendl K, Koerber SA, Finck R, et al. 68Ga-FAPI-PET/CT in patients with various gynecological malignancies. Eur J Nucl Med Mol Imaging 2021. https://doi.org/10.1007/s00259-021-05378-0.

47. Hathi DK, Jones EF. 68Ga FAPI PET/CT: tracer uptake in 28 different kinds of cancer. Radiol Imaging Cancer 2019;1(1):e194003.

48. Chen H, Zhao L, Ruan D, et al. Usefulness of [68Ga]Ga-DOTA-FAPI-04 PET/CT in patients presenting with inconclusive [18F]FDG PET/CT findings. Eur J Nucl Med Mol Imaging 2021;48(1):73–86.

49. Chen H, Pang Y, Wu J, et al. Comparison of [68Ga]Ga-DOTA-FAPI-04 and [18F] FDG PET/CT for the diagnosis of primary and metastatic lesions in patients with various types of cancer. Eur J Nucl Med Mol Imaging 2020;47(8):1820–32.

50. Sollini M, Kirienko M, Gelardi F, et al. State-of-the-art of FAPI-PET imaging: a systematic review and meta-analysis. Eur J Nucl Med Mol Imaging 2021. https://doi.org/10.1007/s00259-021-05475-0.

51. Watabe T, Liu Y, Kaneda-Nakashima K, et al. Theranostics targeting fibroblast activation protein in the tumor stroma: 64Cu- and 225Ac-labeled FAPI-04 in pancreatic cancer xenograft mouse models. J Nucl Med 2020;61(4):563–9.

52. Liu Y, Watabe T, Kaneda-Nakashima K, et al. Fibroblast activation protein targeted therapy using [177Lu]FAPI-46 compared with [225Ac]FAPI-46 in a pancreatic cancer model. Review 2021. https://doi.org/10.21203/rs.3.rs-602564/v1.

53. Ballal S, Yadav MP, Kramer V, et al. A theranostic approach of [68Ga]Ga-DOTA.SA.FAPi PET/CT-guided [177Lu]Lu-DOTA.SA.FAPi radionuclide therapy in an end-stage breast cancer patient: new frontier in targeted radionuclide therapy. Eur J Nucl Med Mol Imaging 2021;48(3):942–4.

54. Moradi F, Iagaru A. Will FAPI PET/CT replace FDG PET/CT in the next decade? Counterpoint—no, not so fast. Am J Roentgenology 2021;216(2):307–8.

# PET-CTBased Quantitative Parameters for Assessment of Treatment Response and Disease Activity in Cancer and Noncancerous Disorders

Rahul V. Parghane, MBBS, MD[a,b], Sandip Basu, MBBS, DRM, DNB, MNAMS[a,b],*

## KEYWORDS

• SUVmax • SUVmean • MTV • TLG • TMTV • [18]F-FDG PET/CT • Quantitative techniques
• Global assessment of disease activity

## KEY POINTS

- In clinical practice, qualitative or visual assessment of FDG uptake on PET/CT images is the most common approach for the evaluation of disease burden. SUVmax is the most commonly used semiquantitative tool for measuring FDG uptake.
- MTV and TLG are being investigated as novel quantitative parameters on [18]F-FDG PET-CT scan. MTV is defined as the volume of lesion with active FDG uptake, and TLG is determined by multiplying SUVmean of the lesion by MTV for a single lesion.
- For measurement of global disease activity, TLG of all lesions are summed up as total metabolic tumor volume (TMTV).
- Segmentation process involves target volume delineation from the surrounding tissue by using SUV or voxel grayscale value. Thresholding and adaptive thresholding methods are commonly used algorithms for the evaluation of global disease activity.
- Nowadays, commercial software are available for providing easy, less time consuming, highly reproducible, and more accurate measurement of global disease activity on PET-CT imaging in evaluation of malignant as well as benign disorders with heterogeneous and/or widespread lesions.

## INTRODUCTION

PET is a noninvasive imaging tool that provides tomographic images of radioactive tracer distribution in tissues through detection of annihilation photons that are emitted when positron-emitting radionuclides are introduced into the body and release positrons. [18]F, the most commonly used radioisotope of fluorine in PET imaging, is labeled with various molecules that are found in living cells and commonly labeled with fluorodeoxyglucose (FDG). FDG is a glucose analogue that is incorporated into the first step of the normal glycolytic pathway in living cells via cell membrane glucose transporters (GLUT).[1,2] [18]F-FDG PET and computed tomography (CT) are established imaging modalities in medical field. In the last decade, hybrid PET-CT study has been extensively validated in routine clinical settings, in which PET and CT data are acquired in a single imaging device. This hybrid PET-CT study provided both molecular/functional and morphologic information of lesion in a single imaging machine. Measurement

[a] Radiation Medicine Centre (BARC), Tata Memorial Hospital Annexe, Parel, Mumbai, India; [b] Homi Bhabha National Institute, Mumbai, India
* Corresponding author. Radiation Medicine Centre, Bhabha Atomic Research Centre, Tata Memorial Hospital, Annexe Building, Jerbai Wadia Road, Parel, Mumbai 400 012, India.
E-mail address: drsanb@yahoo.com

PET Clin 17 (2022) 465–478
https://doi.org/10.1016/j.cpet.2022.03.006
1556-8598/22/© 2022 Elsevier Inc. All rights reserved.

of in vivo distribution and quantification of $^{18}$F-FDG uptake is one major aspect of hybrid PET-CT imaging in the evaluation of malignant and benign disorders. Assessment of $^{18}$F-FDG uptake in hybrid PET-CT imaging can be divided into (1) qualitative/visual and (2) quantitative analysis.

## Qualitative/Visual Analysis of Fluorodeoxyglucose Uptake

In tissues, FDG uptake is proportional to the amount of glucose utilization, and this is related to overexpression of GLUT, increased hexokinase activity, and glucose-6-phosphatase level in cells. Physiologic accumulation of FDG activity is seen in the brain, heart, mediastinal blood pool, liver, kidneys, and urinary tract at 60 minutes after injection of $^{18}$F-FDG. In pathologic condition, depending on GLUT, hexokinase activity, and glucose-6-phosphatase level in cells, there is "metabolic contrast" between surrounding background activity/physiologic FDG uptake and FDG uptake in target lesions on PET images. This "metabolic contrast" is used as a tool for quality/visual analysis of FDG uptake in various pathologic conditions. The qualitative/visual FDG PET-CT assessment is best performed on 3-dimensional maximum intensity projection or coronal images, which facilitates comparison with the standard references of liver and mediastinal pool. The Deauville 5-point scoring system (D5PS) is such an example of analysis of FDG uptake, in which comparisons between FDG uptake in target lesions with mediastinal blood pool and liver FDG uptake are used as standard references.[3] In clinical oncology practice, D5PS is routinely used for the response assessment of Hodgkin and FDG-avid non-Hodgkin lymphomas during midtreatment and end-of-treatment evaluation. A similar 5-point scale and Hopkins 5-point score is used as visual analysis of $^{18}$F-FDG PET-CT in patients with locally advanced cervix carcinoma and head and neck squamous cell carcinoma, respectively, for response evaluation and survival prediction.[4,5] In view of being a simple method for evaluation of the target lesions as global disease in body, qualitative/visual analysis of $^{18}$F-FDG PET-CT is the most commonly used tool in routine clinical practice. The accuracy of this analysis depends on the interpreter's experience and his or her knowledge about normal physiologic FDG distribution in the body. The accuracy also depends on knowledge about common artifacts in $^{18}$F-FDG PET-CT imaging, inflammatory/infective nature of disease, histopathology of tumor, various treatment modalities, and posttreatment changes in target lesions. Despite simplicity of visual assessment, this method suffers several limitations, which include problem for defining and use of a threshold for FDG concentration evaluation in target lesion, issue of poor both interobserver and intraobserver reliability, nonavailability of analysis scales for most malignancies, and futile analysis in pathologic conditions that are not substantially FDG avid. Hence, objective quantitative analysis is essential for disease burden evaluation in various benign and malignant disorders.

## Quantitative Analysis of Fluorodeoxyglucose Uptake

Quantitative analysis of FDG uptake on PET scan ranges from simple detection and determination of FDG concentrations in units of kBq/mL or µCi/mL to more sophisticated mathematical algorithms that show rate of FDG transportation or exchange among different tissue spaces. This complexity of quantitative analysis of FDG uptake depends on the objective of the PET study and clinical/research requirement in various conditions. Quantitative analysis of FDG uptake in PET imaging may be classified into 2 major types, namely, absolute measurements of FDG uptake using kinetic modeling analysis and semiquantitative analysis using standardized uptake value (SUV) and its variants. In PET-CT study, 2 major types of data acquisition are available that allow quantification analysis, namely, dynamic and static imaging. Dynamic PET-CT study captures FDG metabolic information in a real-time fashion enabling one to derive valuable physiologic quantitative parameters. Static PET-CT study is normally acquired after a time gap of $^{18}$F-FDG injection so that an adequate clearance of FDG from plasma and accumulation of FDG into the tissue have occurred to detect target lesions and improve target-to-nontarget ratio.[6]

### Kinetic modeling analysis
In PET imaging, FDG tracer kinetic depends on the region or voxel of interest. Dynamic acquisition of PET imaging is required to calculate absolute quantification of data based on compartmental or noncompartmental methods such as nonlinear regression, Patlak graphical analysis and derived methods, and simplified quantitative methods. The advantages of tracer kinetic quantitative analysis include low dependency on imaging time, measurement of absolute rate of FDG metabolism, and giving insights about various components of glucose metabolism such as transport and phosphorylation. In the clinical scenario, use of kinetic modeling for quantitative analysis of FDG uptake is precluded because of the complex and time-consuming study procedure with requirement for

arterial blood sampling or dynamic imaging of a blood-pool structure to obtain a precise input function. In dynamic acquisition of PET imaging, field of view is limited to a single bed position. Hence, this is another factor that prevents the use of tracer kinetic modeling analysis in various clinical conditions (benign and malignant disorders) with multiple sites of involvement and heterogeneous lesions throughout the body. However, whole-body dynamic PET imaging is possible, but is technically advanced with nonavailability and nonfeasibility at the moment in most commercial PET imaging. Therefore, global disease burden cannot be assessed by using dynamic PET imaging on a single image acquisition.[7–10]

### Semiquantitative analysis

In PET imaging, SUV is the most commonly used quantitative index. Calculation of SUV is very simple and is available in all commercial PET scanners. Hence, SUV analysis is widely acceptable in clinical practices. SUV is a quantity derived from a region of interest (ROI) or voxel taken at a certain single region where FDG metabolic concentration is of considerable clinical value on PET imaging. Normalized injected activity is administered dose of $^{18}$F-FDG normalized to the patient body weight (BW), body surface area (BSA), or lean body mass, and decay corrected to PET acquisition start time. SUV is determined by the following formula:

$$SUV = \frac{\text{Tissue Activity (voxel or volume of interest)}}{\text{Normalized injected activity (BW, LBW or BSA)}}$$

SUV indices have several variants based on the complexity of computation and analytical methods used.[11] SUVmean, SUVmax, and SUVpeak are commonly used SUV metrices in clinical practices. SUVmean is calculated by using the aforementioned formula in which numerator is taken as mean FDG activity within the region or volume of interest (VOI). SUVmax is maximal activity in a pixel within ROI in selected lesion. SUVpeak is average SUV within a small, fixed-size ROI centered on a high-activity part of lesion. There are certain limitations of SUV-based quantitative analysis, such as SUVmean depends on ROI drawn by operator and its value underestimates in small lesions due to partial volume effect, whereas SUVmax is affected by noise and has increased positive bias as noise increases.[12,13] SUVmax does not represent true value in heterogeneous mass lesions. SUVpeak with Lean Body weight, that is, SUL, is recommended in PET Response Criteria in Solid Tumor (PERCIST) as an index for tumor response evaluation.[14] SUVpeak has several technical definitions related to ROI shape, size, and dimensions. The shape of ROI for SUVpeak calculation may be square or cuboidal of side length 7 to 15 mm.[15] Size of ROI is an influential factor in SUVpeak calculation. Hence, ROI in SUVpeak calculation should be optimally chosen based on a well-defined specific criterion for accurate lesion assessment in patients. Brendle and colleagues[16] demonstrated SUVpeak as most robust and more stable variant of SUV in various reconstruction methods, especially in small-sized lesions, when compared with SUVmean and SUVmax. Measurements of SUV are considered as "surrogate" biomarker and reference gold standard for treatment response strategy in malignant disorders.[17] In SUV-based quantitative analysis in most patients, the number of lesions all over the body is not assessed and also metabolic volume or global metabolic activity all over the body is not quantified. Therefore, these factors lead to a relative sampling and assessment error in quantitative analysis particularly in patients with widespread disease. Hence, there is a growing interest in the assessment of patients based on quantitative analysis, which evaluates global disease activity.

### Global Assessment of Disease Activity

PET-CT scanners provide an accessible and reliable score for evaluating global disease activity (GDA) throughout the body and demonstrate extent of disease within minutes, which consists of metabolic tumor volume (MTV) and total lesion glycolysis (TLG). MTV is defined as the volume of lesion with active FDG uptake and TLG is calculated by multiplying SUVmean of the lesion by MTV for a single lesion. To calculate global disease activity, the values of TLG of all lesions are summed up for determination of total metabolic tumor volume (TMTV).[18–20]

Measurement of global metabolic activity by using PET scan was first introduced by Alavi and colleagues[21] in evaluation of the brain in patients of Alzheimer disease and age-matched controls. The investigators used MR imaging of the brain for determination of segmented brain volumes. These segmented brain volumes were multiplied with mean cerebral glycolytic activity. Final results in their study showed that partial volume-corrected metabolic rates per unit weight of the brain were not significantly different in the 2 groups; however, global brain metabolism was significantly lower in patients with Alzheimer disease.[21] Similar approach of structural segmentation by using PET-CT imaging was proposed by the same investigators for the evaluation of global normal organ function and global disease activity in various other conditions such as oncology and nononcology. In this approach by using hybrid PET-CT imaging, structural (volumetric) and metabolic data were combined and summarized into a whole-body metabolic assessment instead of evaluation of these parameters independently and on per-lesion basis. At present, automated or semiautomated software are available in most commercial PET-CT scanners for computing both tissue segmentation and measurement of global disease metabolism. These software are easier and faster and provide a highly reproducible and accurate assessment of global disease activity than manually performed tissue segmentation.

Basically, in PET-CT imaging target volumes are delineated from the surrounding tissue by using SUV or voxel grayscale value, and this process is called segmentation. This segmentation has 2 related tasks: (1) recognition and (2) delineation. Recognition is the detection of target in PET-CT image without precise specification of the region occupied by the target. Delineation is the process of separating target's precise spatial extent and composition including gradation. This delineation can be broadly classified as boundary-based, region-based, and hybrid approaches. In boundary-based approach, target is described in the form of a boundary surface that separates the target from background. In region-based approach, targets are described in the form of the region occupied by target, whereas in hybrid approach, combined information of boundaries and regions-based approaches is used for processing delineation of target.

In PET-CT imaging, there are several methods for creating a segmented target volume, and commonly used ones include the following. (1) Manual delineation approach—manually drawing a boundary around metabolically active lesion is a common method used in clinical practice. This approach is challenged by lack of clear edges between lesions and normal tissues in noisy PET images and also prone to errors. This approach is operator dependent and suffers from intravariability and intervariability for evaluation of multiple lesions throughout body. (2) Thresholding—in this method, a percentage of mean or maximum voxel value is set as a threshold and voxels are either included (above threshold) or excluded (below threshold) from segmented volume based on their intensity. (3) Adaptive thresholding—in this method, SUVmean plus a constant is used with an initial guess of percentage. The threshold value and SUVmean is updated by regression until convergence is reached. (4) Region growing—a single or a set of voxels is chosen as a starting point, and this connected region is grown based on a voxel threshold value until no more voxels can be added to the region. (5) Gradient-based methods—change in voxel values are used to characterize target contours and enable edge detection. (6) Classifiers—in this method, predetermined features, for example, voxel intensities, region textures, and voxel gradients, of different tissues are used for determining a set of class. The regions of image are labeled with their respective class based on a pattern recognition algorithm by using predetermined features.[22] The details of medical image segmentation algorithms are available and written elsewhere.[23–26]

## Assessment of Treatment Response and Disease Activity

An international standard RECIST 1.1 criterion with the help of anatomic imaging is used commonly in the assessment of treatment responses for solid tumors. Anatomic imaging by using RECIST criteria for treatment response assessment has several intrinsic limitations such as moderate reproducibility for size measurement, late occurrence of anatomic response compared with early metabolic changes, and not useful with nonmeasurable anatomic lesions (skeletal lesions, lymphangitis, and effusions) and in treatment with cytostatic therapies. The metabolic activity measured in PET-CT studies is used for assessment of treatment response in oncological and nononcological disorders. Changes of SUVmax and SUVpeak are commonly used quantitative parameters for evaluating treatment response and predicting prognosis in oncological disorders with help of the European Organization for Research and Treatment of Cancer and PERCIST criteria, respectively. MTV, TLG, and TMTV are less commonly used PET/CT-based quantitative parameters in routine clinical practice. Recently, these parameters have been suggested as promising indices for treatment response evaluation in various oncological disorders as shown in **Fig. 1**.

PET-CT-Based Quantitative Techniques for Assessment of Treatment Response and Global Disease Activity

In hybrid PET-CT, global disease activity is evaluated by using quantitative parameters such as MTV, TLG, and TMTV. From clinical point of view, global disease activity assessment is important in malignant disorder at initial staging, during treatment response monitoring and predicting

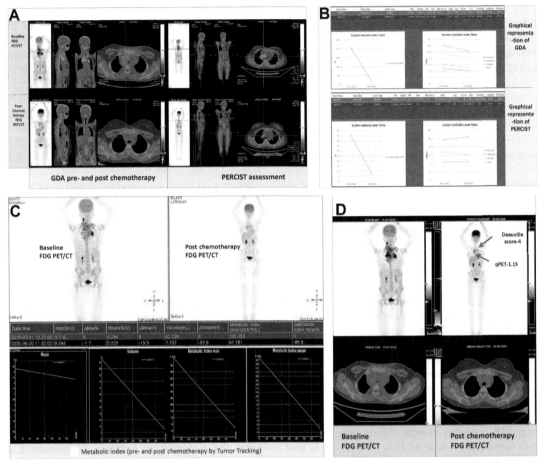

Fig. 1. A 16-year-old female patient, diagnosed case of Hodgkin lymphoma, had undergone chemotherapy. The response to chemotherapy was evaluated in terms of quantitative and qualitative analysis of FDG uptake on PET-CT images by using commercially available software. The GDA was measured by using Segami Oasis software at thresholding of SUVmax40% as shown in left panel (*A*) and upper panel (*B*) with significant reduction of TMTV value from 1227.6 to 96.3 after chemotherapy. PERCIST criteria for mediastinal lymph nodes showed (*right panel* in *A* and *lower panel* in *B*) slight increase in SUVmax from 9.72 to 10.38 with significant reduction of TLG value from 306.7 to 39.3 after chemotherapy. The metabolic index max and metabolic index mean (by tumor tracking software, EBW, Philips) demonstrated (*C*) similar result as shown by Segami Oasis software. Qualitative analysis showed (*D*) Deauville score of 4 and qPET value of 1.15 indicating that quantitative analysis (MTV, TLG, and TMTV) may prove better parameter than qualitative analysis and SUVmax alone in response evaluation of patients with lymphoma.

survival. Similarly, this approach can be used in benign systemic disorders such as in patients with atherosclerosis, tuberculosis, inflammatory bowel disease, and so on.

## Malignant disorders

Assessment of global disease activity is an important aspect in the evaluation of malignant disorders in which widespread disease involvement and heterogeneous lesions exist and also demonstrate variable degree of FDG uptake in several lesions throughout the body such as in hematolymphoid malignancy, skeleton system involvement, head and neck malignancy, lung malignancy, gynecologic malignancy, and neuroendocrine tumors (NETs). Measurement of global disease activity by using $^{18}$F-FDG PET-CT provides an efficient means for the disease quantification in a reproducible and objective manner on a single imaging modality as shown in **Fig. 2**. This measurement has great potential for objective treatment response evaluation after therapeutic intervention and as a prognostic tool in various oncological conditions as shown in **Fig. 3**.[27–32]

In one of the earliest studies, Francis and colleagues[33] determined global disease activity by using [18]F-FDG PET-CT in 23 patients of mesothelioma. The investigators used a semiautomated 3D volume-based region-growing algorithm to calculate volume-based parameters in patients with mesothelioma after 1 cycle of chemotherapy. The investigators found a statistically significant relationship between a decrease in volume-based parameter and improved patient survival. Nowak and colleagues[34] used the same method to measure global disease activity (volume-based parameters) in 89 patients with mesothelioma. The investigators proposed volume-based parameters as the new prognostic model in the evaluation of patients with mesothelioma. Lee and colleagues[35] studied volume-viewer software on a commercial workstation (Advantage Workstation 4.4, General Electric, New York, USA) in 13 patients with mesothelioma. This software provided an automated tumor volume delineation by using an isocontour threshold method, and they found MTV and TLG as independent predictive factors for tumor progression in patients with mesothelioma. Veit-Haibach et al[36] and Schaefer and colleagues[37] used similar methods for calculation of volume-based parameters on [18]F-FDG PET in patients with mesothelioma. Both investigators used a commercially available workstation (Advanced Workstation, General Electrics); they determined volume-based parameters by drawing a rectangular VOI over the corresponding hemithorax in all 3 planes with minimal SUV of 2.5 levels and found that these parameters were predictor of overall survival in patients with mesothelioma treated with chemotherapy. Marin-Oyaga and colleagues[38] evaluated a quantitative global disease assessment method in 19 patients with mesothelioma. The investigators used an adaptive contrast-oriented thresholding algorithm for determination of global disease by using region of interest visualization, evaluation, and image registration (ROVER) software (ABX, Radeberg, Germany). In this algorithm, disease burden was calculated by taking both volumetric and metabolic characteristics of the disease. The investigators calculated MTV, TLG, and SUVmean by using ROVER software and also determined global tumor glycolysis (GTG) by summing up all TLG. It was found that an adaptive contrast-oriented thresholding algorithm in [18]F-FDG PET imaging provided an efficient means for quantification of extensive disease throughout in a highly reproducible and accurate manner. The investigators concluded that this approach has great potential in monitoring treatment response.

Similarly, several studies are available in the literature for evaluation of tumor burden in various malignant disorders by using MTV and TLG values for prediction of overall survival, progression-free survival, and treatment response. In most of the studies, MTV was determined by either using a fixed background SUV cutoff, all voxels containing SUV values above this threshold constituting MTV, for example, MTV 2.5, 3, or 4 times or 2SD above that of the normal liver activity, and so on, or using SUVmax values of individual tumor site involved region growing up to a prefixed percentage of SUVmax, for example, MTV 40%, 50%, and so on as shown in **Fig. 4**. Van de Wiele and colleagues[39] reviewed the literature data of tumor burden evaluation by using MTV and TLG values in patients suffering from squamous cell carcinoma of the head and neck, lung carcinoma, esophageal carcinoma, and gynecologic malignancies. The investigators found that the range of fixed SUV thresholds values of SUV 2.0 to 3.0 (MTV 2/3) and percentage cutoff values of SUVmax 40% to 50% (MTV 40%/50%) for MTV calculation showed significant findings in many reported studies. The investigators also found that commercially available gradient-based segmentation method was used in a limited number of studies, in which MTV was calculated from gradient between high SUV in tumor cells and lower SUV in adjacent normal tissue. This method provided similar information to that obtained using threshold techniques. The investigators concluded that MTV and TLG values in [18]F-FDG PET imaging have the potential to become prognostic biomarkers, to improve clinical cancer staging, and to help in assessment of treatment response in various malignant disorders.

Husby and colleagues[40] investigated specific quantitative parameters on [18]F-FDG PET imaging in 129 consecutive patients with endometrial carcinoma. The investigators used a commercially available software (Segami Oasis, version 1.9.4.2; Segami Corp, Columbia, USA.) for measurements of MTV and TLG, in which voxels with an SUV of more than 2.5 were included in VOI for MTV calculation. It was found that MTV and TLG were significantly related to deep myometrial invasion, presence of lymph node metastases, and high histologic grade and that these parameters were an independent predictor of deep myometrial invasion, lymph node metastases, and histologic risk in patients with endometrial carcinoma. The investigators concluded that measurements of specific quantitative parameters (by using commercially available Segami Oasis software) were a clinically valuable tool in the preoperative evaluation of lymph node metastases. They also concluded that these parameters increased diagnostic accuracy of [18]F-FDG PET imaging and aided preoperative

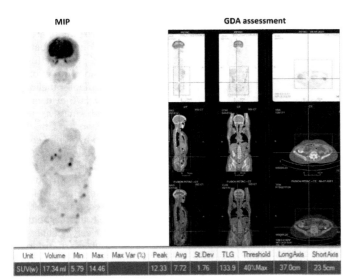

Fig. 2. A 54-year-old female patient, diagnosed case of ovarian cancer, had undergone total abdominal hysterectomy and bilateral salpingo-oophorectomy and omentectomy and adjuvant chemotherapy. In the follow-up period, the patient became symptomatic and developed metastatic disease. Postsurgery and postchemotherapy, [18]F-FDG PET-CT images demonstrated multiple foci FDG-avid lesions in abdominopelvic regions as shown in Maximum Intensity Projection (MIP) image. GDA was evaluated by using commercial automated software (Segami Oasis, version 1.9.4.2; Segami Corp.) at thresholding of SUVmax40%, which provided various quantitative parameters of GDA on single click even in widespread metastatic disease in patients with cancer.

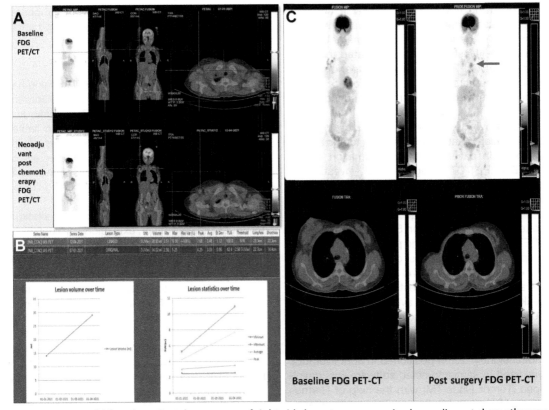

Fig. 3. A 40-year-old female patient, known case of right-side breast cancer, received neoadjuvant chemotherapy. Response to neoadjuvant chemotherapy was evaluated by using [18]F-FDG PET-CT images (A). No new lesion with stable disease was noticed on qualitative analysis. Quantitative analysis (GDA, by Segami Oasis software) showed (B) significant increase in TMTV value from 42.4 to 100.8 after neoadjuvant chemotherapy. Subsequently, the patient underwent right-side modified radical mastectomy. Within 6 months of breast surgery, the patient developed metastatic skeletal lesions as shown by arrow (C) suggesting that quantitative analysis has potential for predicting disease prognosis in patients with cancer.

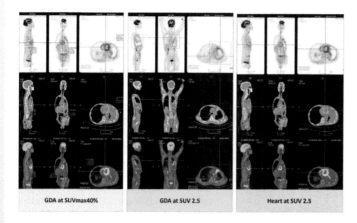

GDA at SUVmax40%          GDA at SUV 2.5          Heart at SUV 2.5

Fig. 4. A 47-year-old male patient, known case of chronic obstructive pulmonary disease and history of smoking. The patient presented with left-sided pleural effusion and was evaluated for cancerous etiology and diagnosed as a case of mesothelioma. $^{18}$F-FDG PET-CT showed FDG-avid entire pleural thickening with massive non-FDG-avid pleural effusion on the left side. GDA was evaluated by using Segami Oasis software at thresholding of SUV-max40% and at thresholding of SUVmax 2.5. In the presence of high physiologic myocardial FDG uptake, mesothelioma lesion was not delineated at thresholding of SUVmax40%, whereas at thresholding of SUV 2.5 there was clearly delineated mesothelioma in the entire left hemithorax suggesting that evaluation of GDA requires judicious use of different thresholding methods for delineation of lesions in various clinical conditions, depending on FDG uptake in lesions and background activity in the vicinity of lesions.

identification of high-risk patients in endometrial carcinoma. Fasmer and colleagues[41] measured MTV (SUV of more than 2.5 for volume delineation) by using commercially available software (Segami Oasis) and MR imaging markers in 215 consecutive patients with endometrial carcinoma. The investigators demonstrated that MTV from $^{18}$F-FDG PET-CT imaging outperforms MR imaging markers for the prediction of lymph node metastases in patients with endometrial carcinoma.[41]

Hasenclever and colleagues[42] developed a novel semiautomated quantification tool to assess response in patients with lymphoma on interim $^{18}$F-FDG PET-CT imaging. The investigators calculated SUVpeak of residual tumors and average FDG uptake of liver with standardized VOI and demonstrated quotient of SUVpeak of hottest tumor lesion over SUVmean of liver as *qPET value* in 898 pediatric patients with Hodgkin lymphoma after 2 cycles of OEPA (vincristine, etoposide, prednisone, and doxorubicin) chemotherapy regimen. The investigators defined SUV-peak of tumor lesions as average over maximum SUV voxel and 3 hottest adjacent ones. For calculation of average liver uptake, a cuboid VOI with a volume of 30 mL (edge length proportion: length:width:height = 2:2:1) positioned in right liver lobe was used. A semiautomated software was developed (Tumor FinderTM) with the help of Hermes Medical Solutions AB, Sweden, which allows positioning of 2 VOIs with simple clicks in respective regions and displayed them for visual control and calculation of predefined parameters. The investigators demonstrated that Deauville categories 3, 4, and 5 correspond to qPET values of 0.95, 1.3, and 2.0, respectively, in their study shown in

Fig. 1. They concluded that, qPET values by using semiautomated quantification approach provided easy-to-use method for interim $^{18}$F-FDG PET response evaluation in patients with lymphoma extending ordinal Deauville scoring to a continuous scale.[42]

### Benign disorders
In clinical practice, $^{18}$F-FDG PET-CT imaging had a limited role for evaluation of benign disorders; this is because of nonspecific FDG uptake in a number of benign conditions resulting in limited accuracy and specificity of this imaging modality. Introduction of novel quantitative parameters on $^{18}$F-FDG PET/CT imaging improves and adds values in the evaluation of number of benign disorders shown in Fig. 5.

Bural and colleagues[43] developed a technique for quantification and extension evaluation in atherosclerosis (benign disorder involving large-sized and medium-sized arteries) by using combined SUV and volumetric data in large-sized arteries (aorta). In their study, 18 patients underwent $^{18}$F-FDG PET imaging for calculation of mean SUV in aorta and contrast-enhanced CT of chest and abdomen regions for measurement of arterial wall volume. The investigators determined atherosclerotic burden in aorta by multiplying SUV with wall volume in each age group of patients and found that atherosclerotic burden values increased with age of patients. They concluded that use of combined metabolic and morphologic data by using $^{18}$F-FDG PET imaging and contrast-enhanced CT, respectively, provides atherosclerotic burden, which can be used as an indicator for an extension of atherosclerotic process in body and leading to optimal screening,

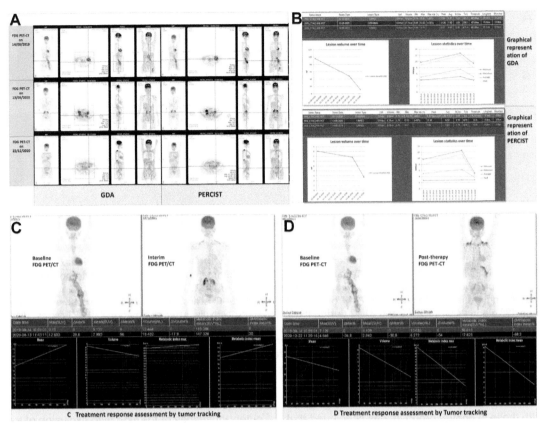

**Fig. 5.** A 45-year-old female, diagnosed case of Koch abdomen, was evaluated for response to antituberculosis drugs during and after treatment on ${}^{18}$F-FDG PET-CT images by using commercial software (Segami Oasis software [*A, B*] and tumor tracking software of EBW [*C, D*]). FDG-avid abdominal paraspinal lesions seen during initial course of antituberculosis drug treatment showed near-complete metabolic response after treatment on visual analysis of ${}^{18}$F-FDG PET-CT images (*A, C*). TMTV value decreased from 475.4 to 358.1, whereas SUVmax increased from 9.75 to 12.63 during treatment (*B*). Posttreatment, TMTV value was further reduced to 53.2 and SUVmax reduced to 9.35. Similar results were demonstrated for metabolic index mean and metabolic index max on tumor tracking software of EBW (*C, D*). PET-CT-based quantitative parameters were found to perform better than qualitative or SUV-alone parameters even in benign disorders for treatment response evaluation.

diagnosis, and management of these patients with atherosclerosis.

Rose and colleagues[44] quantitatively evaluated blood vessel inflammation in patients with psoriasis and rheumatoid arthritis, and also in healthy subjects by using ${}^{18}$F-FDG PET-CT imaging. The investigators used semiautomated image analysis software (Extended Brilliance Workstation (EBW); Philips Healthcare, Bothell, WA, USA) on a dedicated PET-CT scanner, in which circular 2-dimensional ROI was manually drawn around external aortic contour of serial transverse sections extending from aortic root to iliac bifurcation. They calculated mean metabolic volumetric product (MVPmean) for each aortic subsegment as SUV-mean per slice × ROI area (in mm²) × slice thickness (in mm), in each slice. It was found that values of MVPmean in patients with psoriasis and rheumatoid arthritis were increased when

compared with healthy subjects. The investigators concluded that quantitative analysis of ${}^{18}$F-FDG PET-CT imaging is an operator-independent and highly reproducible technique and that this analysis may greatly improved assessment of vascular inflammatory condition in various benign disorders.

Bural and colleagues[45] studied hepatic SUVs and hepatic metabolic volumetric products (HMVP) values in patients with diffuse hepatic steatosis and normal liver control subjects. Mean and maximum hepatic SUVs were determined on FDG-PET scan and hepatic volumes on MR imaging for both subject groups. HMVP in each subject was subsequently measured by multiplication of hepatic volume by mean hepatic SUV. The investigators found that values of HMVPs, mean hepatic SUVs, and maximum hepatic SUVs were greater in subjects with diffuse hepatic steatosis compared

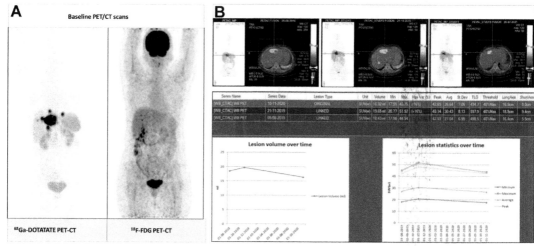

**Fig. 6.** A 53-year-old female, known patient of small bowel NET with liver metastasis (Ki-67 index = 4%–5%, WHO grade II). Baseline [68]Ga-DOTATATE and [18]F-FDG PET-CT MIP images showed (*A*) SSTR-avid and non-FDG-avid multiple liver lesions, respectively. Patient received 4 cycles of PRRT. The response to treatment was evaluated during and after completion of PRRT on [68]Ga-DOTATATE PET-CT scans. TMTV and SUVmax values increased from 498.5 and 44.94 to 597.9 and 51.92 during PRRT cycles, respectively. After completion of PRRT cycles, TMTV and SUVmax values decreased to 434.7 and 43.79, respectively (*B*). During and after PRRT cycles Krenning score = 4 liver lesions were seen suggestive of stable disease on visual analysis, whereas quantitative parameters were reduced after completion of PRRT cycles indicating favorable response PRRT. Similar to [18]F-FDG analysis on PET-CT scan, quantitative analysis of non-FDG tracers could be potentially useful for response evaluation in various oncological disorders.

with those in control group. It was concluded that active inflammatory process in patients with diffuse hepatic steatosis resulted in the increase in hepatic metabolic activity in these patients on FDG-PET scan.

Malherbe and colleagues[46] developed a technique for quantification of lesions in patients with pulmonary tuberculosis on PET and CT imaging. The investigators calculated metabolic lesion volume (MLV), SUVmean, and total glycolytic activity (TGA = MLV × SUVmean) by using different approaches, namely, optimal adaptive thresholds for semiautomated segmentation approach and manual segmentation approach on PET imaging. It was found that semiautomated thresholding approach saved time in delineations of multiple lesions and seemed highly sensitive as compared with manual approach. The investigators concluded that the semiautomatic approach allowed quantification of multiple pulmonary lesions with widespread distribution, variable FDG uptake, size, and morphology and that this approach reduces interreader variability, especially after interventions in patients with tuberculosis.

Abdulla and colleagues[47] quantified global lung inflammation in patients with lung cancer following radiation therapy by using FDG PET-CT imaging. The investigators drew ROIs manually around outer boundaries of the lung with exclusion of trachea and main stem bronchi from the ROIs; they used commercial software (EBW analysis software) for calculation of sectional lung volume (sLV) for each lung (determined from each slice by multiplying the lung area by slice thickness) and sectional lung glycolysis (sLG = sLV × lung sectional SUVmean). The lung volume (LV) and global lung glycolysis (GLG) were measured by adding all sLVs and by adding all sLGs from the lung, respectively. The result of their study demonstrated that lung parenchyma SUVmean and parenchymal GLG were significantly increased following radiation therapy in lung that received direct radiation therapy without significant change in lung SUVmean or GLG in contralateral lung. The investigators concluded that global lung parenchymal glycolysis and parenchymal SUVmean can be used as biomarkers to quantify lung inflammation following thoracic radiation therapy on [18]F-FDG PET-CT scan.

Saboury and colleagues[48] developed a new quantitative approach in the evaluation of disease activity in patients with Crohn disease (CD) by using [18]F-FDG PET-CT imaging. CD endoscopy index of severity, CD activity index (CDAI), and fecal calprotectin for determination of severity in CD were used. These parameters were compared with PET-CT-based quantitative parameters. The

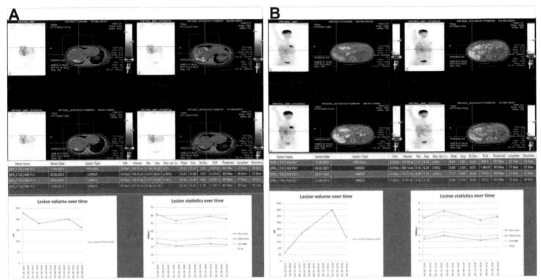

Fig. 7. A 47-year-old female patient with metastatic NET (Ki-67 index = 4%, WHO grade II), demonstrated large, multiple heterogeneous liver lesions on both $^{68}$Ga-DOTATATE and $^{18}$F-FDG PET-CT images. The patient received combined treatment of PRRT and chemotherapy. Response to this combined chemo-PRRT regimen was evaluated on both $^{68}$Ga-DOTATATE and $^{18}$F-FDG PET-CT scans (A, B). TMTV and SUVmax values of $^{68}$Ga-DOTATATE were reduced from 7159.7 and 61.35 to 4687.6 and 54.80, whereas the TMTV and SUVmax values of $^{18}$F-FDG increased from 253.2 and 6.70 to 699.5 and 6.75 after combined treatment, respectively. The findings were consistent with the visual assessment of the studies. This illustration emphasizes the role and requirement of dual-tracer PET-CT-based evaluation and quantitative analysis in response evaluation of patients with NET with heterogeneous lesions.

metabolically active volume (MAV), SUVmean, and SUVmax were determined on PET-CT scan. The investigators used automatically determined background correction, partial volume correction (PVC), and an adaptive contrast-oriented thresholding algorithm (ROVER software, ABX, Radberg, Germany) for calculation of volumetric-based FDG PET-CT parameters. Various VOIs were placed on segments of bowel such as terminal ileum, ascending colon and cecum, transverse colon, descending and sigmoid colon, and rectum with significant FDG uptake in lesions (SUVmax $\geq$3) for calculation of segmental parameters. The investigators first calculated lesional MAV, uncorrected TLG (TLG = MAV $\times$ SUVmean), and PVC-TLG (PVC-TLG = MAV $\times$ PVC-SUVmean) in the segment. Then segmental MAV, TLG, and PVC-TLG were calculated by adding measures of all VOIs in each segment. Finally, they calculated global CD activity score (GCDAS) as sum of PVC-TLG over all significant FDG-avid regions (SUVmax $\geq$ 3) in each subject and GLG as sum of TLG of the same lesions. Significant correlation of CDAI and fecal calprotectin level with global PET/CT parameters was found. Out of global parameters, GCDAS showed most robust correlations with CDAI and fecal calprotectin. The investigators concluded that use of this quantitative volumetric-based approach on FDG PET-CT imaging provided regional and global bowel disease activity in CD, which correlated with clinical and pathologic disease activity. $^{18}$F-FDG PET-CT imaging with these quantitative parameters is helpful in detecting and localizing lesion and also determining degree of bowel inflammation in patients with CD; this is particularly important for clinical management of patients with inflammatory bowel disease at the time of diagnosis and following treatment evaluation.

## PET-Computed Tomography-Based Quantitative Analysis with Nonfluorodeoxyglucose Radiopharmaceuticals

At present, $^{18}$F-FDG is the commonly used PET-based radiopharmaceutical in oncology as well as nononcological disorders. The main limitation of FDG is that it is a nonspecific radiopharmaceutical and several malignancies, for example, well-differentiated NET, prostate cancer, hepatocellular carcinoma, and renal cell carcinoma, cannot be adequately assessed by $^{18}$F-FDG (**Fig. 6**). Hence several newer radiopharmaceuticals have been developed that can provide more specific information in various oncological and nononco-logical disorders.

The discovery of overexpression of somato-statin receptors in NET led to the development of radiolabeled somatostatin analogues. PET-based [68]Ga-DOTA peptides are found to be excellent ra-diopharmaceuticals for localizing and staging of NET. Another advantage of PET-based assess-ment is analysis by the multitracer PET imaging ([68]Ga-DOTA-peptides and FDG) that provides useful information regarding tumor biology, thera-peutic workup, and for treatment response evalu-ation and correlation with clinical and pathologic findings for an accurate assessment (Fig. 7).[49–51]

Sharma and colleagues[52] evaluated quantitative [68]Ga-DOTATATE-based PET-CT parameters for response assessment and predication of clinical outcome after [177]Lu-DOTATATE therapy. The in-vestigators measured single-lesion SUVmax, tumor-to-spleen and tumor-to-liver SUV ratios, and SUVmax-av using up to 5 target lesions in multiple organ sites on [68]Ga-DOTATATE scan at baseline and follow-up and also determined PER-CIST. It was concluded that single lesion SUVmax and SUVmax-av were predicted response to [177]Lu-DOTATATE therapy.

Ortega and colleagues[53] determined quantita-tive parameters on [68]Ga-DOTATATE PET/CT for predicting response to therapy. The investigators calculated and divided tumor metrices into lesion-based measures (mean $SUV_{max}$ and ratio of the mean lesion $SUV_{max}$ to the $SUV_{max}$ in the liver or the $SUV_{max}$ in the spleen) and segmented [68]Ga-DOTATATE tumor volumes (DTTVs), $SUV_{max}$, and $SUV_{mean}$ obtained with the liver and spleen as thresholds. The investigators found that higher mean $SUV_{max}$ and ratio of the mean lesion $SUV_{max}$ to the $SUV_{max}$ in the liver were pre-dictive of therapeutic response. Higher $SUV_{max}$ and $SUV_{mean}$ obtained with the liver as a threshold and lower kurtosis for DTTV parameters were pre-dictors of a favorable response.

## SUMMARY

[18]F-FDG PET-CT is a routinely used imaging mo-dality for diagnosis, staging, recurrence detection, and response evaluation in many malignant disor-ders and also used in the evaluation of disease process and treatment response in several benign disorders. Hybrid PET-CT imaging provides both quality and quantitative parameters. SUVmax is a commonly used PET-CT parameter in clinical practice as well as in research. However, SUVmax is not a valid expression of global disease activity because it measures 1 index lesion and this is particularly true in the evaluation of heterogeneous

lesions and widespread disease throughout body. Therefore, quantitative parameters measuring whole-body metabolic burden or/and TLG is an important requisite for evaluation of these types of multiple lesions in malignant and benign disorders. Commercial software with various algo-rithms are available for assessment of metabolic-volumetric product on [18]F-FDG PET/CT imaging and can also be used on non-FDG radiopharma-ceuticals such as [68]Ga-DOTATATE. Available liter-ature on assessment of treatment response by using quantitative analysis and global disease ac-tivity is limited to measurement of MTV and TGL primarily in malignant and in a few benign systemic disorders. Literature data demonstrated that these parameters are potentially valuable tool of prog-nostic biomarkers for survival outcome, clinical staging, and response assessment to therapies. Most of the literature mentioned the requirement of validation of these global quantitative parame-ters in larger cohort along with comparison with biomarkers, prognosis, and clinical outcomes. Hence, standardization and validation of these so-phisticated software are required before routine clinical use.

## CLINICS CARE POINTS

- SUVmax is not a foolproof measure of global disease activity because it measures 1 index lesion and this is particularly true in the eval-uation of heterogeneous lesions and wide-spread disease throughout body.

- Commercial software with various algorithms are available for assessment of metabolic-volumetric product on [18]F-FDG PET/CT.

- Available literature on assessment of treat-ment response by using quantitative analysis and global disease activity with MTV and TLG demonstrated that these parameters are potentially valuable tool for response assess-ment to therapies clinical staging, and sur-vival outcome.

## DISCLOSURE

The authors have nothing to disclose.

## REFERENCES

1. Vander Heiden MG, Cantley LC, Thompson CB. Un-derstanding the Warburg effect: the metabolic re-quirements of cell proliferation. Science 2009;324: 1029–33.

2. Pauwels EK, Ribeiro MJ, Stoot JH, et al. FDG accumulation and tumor biology. Nucl Med Biol 1998;25: 317–22.

3. Gallamini A, Fiore F, Sorasio R, et al. Interim positron emission tomography scan in Hodgkin lymphoma: definitions, interpretation rules, and clinical validation. Leuk Lymphoma 2009;50:1761–4.

4. Scarsbrook A, Vaidyanathan S, Chowdhury F, et al. Efficacy of qualitative response assessment interpretation criteria at 18F-FDG PET-CT for predicting outcome in locally advanced cervical carcinoma treated with chemoradiotherapy. Eur J Nucl Med Mol Imaging 2017;44:581–8.

5. Marcus C, Ciarallo A, Tahari AK, et al. Head and neck PET/CT: therapy response interpretation criteria (Hopkins criteria)—interreader reliability accuracy, and survival outcomes. J Nucl Med 2014; 55:1411–6.

6. von Schulthess GK, Steinert HC, Hany TF. Integrated PET/CT: current applications and future directions. Radiology 2006;238:405–22.

7. Klein R, Beanlands RS, deKemp RA. Quantification of myocardial blood flow and flow reserve: technical aspects. J Nucl Cardiol 2010;17:555–70.

8. Dimitrakopoulou-Strauss A, Pan L, Strauss LG. Parametric imaging: a promising approach for the evaluation of dynamic PET-18F-FDG studies – the DKFZ experience. Hell J Nucl Med 2010;13:18–22.

9. Muzi M, O'Sullivan F, Mankoff DA, et al. Quantitative assessment of dynamic PET imaging data in cancer imaging. Magn Reson Imaging 2012;30:1203–15.

10. Jones T, Rabiner EA. The development, past achievements, and future directions of brain PET. J Cereb Blood Flow Metab 2012;32:1426–54.

11. Carlier T, Bailly C. State-of-the-art and recent advances in quantification for therapeutic follow-up in oncology using PET. Front Med (Lausanne) 2015;2:18.

12. Lodge MA, Chaudhry MA, Wahl RL. Noise considerations for PET quantification using maximum and peak standardized uptake value. J Nucl Med 2012;53:1041–7.

13. Boellaard R, Krak NC, Hoekstra OS, et al. Effects of noise, image resolution, and ROI definition on the accuracy of standard uptake values: a simulation study. J Nucl Med 2004;45:1519–27.

14. Wahl RL, Jacene H, Kasamon Y, et al. From RECIST to PERCIST: evolving considerations for PET response criteria in solid tumors. J Nucl Med 2009; 50(Suppl 1):122S–50S.

15. Vanderhoek M, Perlman SB, Jeraj R. Impact of the definition of peak standardized uptake value on quantification of treatment response. J Nucl Med 2012;53:4–11.

16. Brendle C, Kupferschlager J, Nikolaou K, et al. Is the standard uptake value (SUV) appropriate for quantification in clinical PET imaging? – variability induced by different SUV measurements and varying reconstruction methods. Eur J Radiol 2014;84:158–62.

17. Weber WA. Assessing tumor response to therapy. J Nucl Med 2009;50(Suppl 1). 1S–0.

18. Manohar K, Mittal BR, Bhattacharya A, et al. Prognostic value of quantitative parameters derived on initial staging 18F-fluorodeoxyglucose positron emission tomography/computed tomography in patients with high-grade non-Hodgkin's lymphoma. Nucl Med Commun 2012;33:974–81.

19. Chung HH, Kwon HW, Kang KW, et al. Prognostic value of preoperative metabolic tumor volume and total lesion glycolysis in patients with epithelial ovarian cancer. Ann Surg Oncol 2011;19:1966–72.

20. Liao S, Penney BC, Wroblewski K, et al. Prognostic value of metabolic tumor burden on 18F-FDG PET in nonsurgical patients with non-small cell lung cancer. Eur J Nucl Med Mol Imaging 2012;39:27–38.

21. Alavi A, Newberg AB, Souder E, et al. Quantitative analysis of PET and MRI data in normal aging and Alzheimer's disease: atrophy weighted total brain metabolism and absolute whole brain metabolism as reliable discriminators. J Nucl Med 1993;34:1681–7.

22. Visser EP, Boerman OC, Oyen WJ. SUV: from silly useless value to smart uptake value. J Nucl Med 2010;51:173–5.

23. Alavi A, Reivich M, Greenberg J, et al. Mapping of functional activity in brain with 18F-fluoro-deoxyglucose. Semin Nucl Med 1981;11:24–31.

24. Zaidi H, Ruest T, Schoenahl F, et al. Comparative evaluation of statistical brain MR image segmentation algorithms and their impact on partial volume effect correction in PET. Neuroimage 2006;32: 1591–607.

25. Soret M, Bacharach SL, Buvat I. Partial-volume effect in PET tumor imaging. J Nucl Med 2007;48: 932–45.

26. Zaidi H, Alavi A. Current trends in PET and combined (PET/CT and PET/MR) systems design. PET Clin 2007;2:109–23.

27. Parghane RV, Basu S. PET/Computed tomography in treatment response assessment in cancer: an Overview with Emphasis on the evolving role in response evaluation to Immunotherapy and radiation therapy. PET Clin 2020;15:101–23.

28. Basu S, Zaidi H, Houseni M, et al. Novel quantitative techniques for assessing regional and global function and structure based on modern imaging modalities: implications for normal variation, aging and diseased states. Semin Nucl Med 2007;37(3):223–39.

29. Ziai P, Hayeri MR, Salei A, et al. Role of optimal quantification of FDG PET imaging in the clinical practice of Radiology. Radiographics 2016;36:481–96.

30. Basu S, Zaidi H, Salavati A, et al. FDG PET/CT methodology for evaluation of treatment response in lymphoma: from "graded visual analysis" and "semiquantitative SUVmax" to global disease burden assessment. Eur J Nucl Med Mol Imaging 2014;41: 2158–60.

31. Taghvaei R, Zadeh MZ, Werner TJ, et al. Critical role of PET/CT-based novel quantitative techniques for assessing global disease activity in multiple myeloma and other hematological malignancies: why it is time to abandon reliance on examining focal lesions. Eur Radiol 2021;31:149–51.

32. Basu S, Kumar R, Ranade R. Assessment of treatment response using PET. PET Clin 2015;10:9–26.

33. Francis RJ, Byrne MJ, van der Schaaf AA, et al. Early prediction of response to chemotherapy and survival in malignant pleural mesothelioma using a novel semiautomated 3-dimensional volume-based analysis of serial 18F-FDG PET scans. J Nucl Med 2007;48:1449–58.

34. Nowak AK, Francis RJ, Phillips MJ, et al. A novel prognostic model for malignant mesothelioma incorporating quantitative FDG-PET imaging with clinical parameters. Clin Cancer Res 2010;16:2409–17.

35. Lee HY, Hyun SH, Lee KS, et al. Volume-based parameter of 18F-FDG PET/CT in malignant pleural mesothelioma: prediction of therapeutic response and prognostic implications. Ann Surg Oncol 2010; 17:2787–94.

36. Veit-Haibach P, Schaefer NG, Steinert HC, et al. Combined FDGPET/CT in response evaluation of malignant pleural mesothelioma. Lung Cancer 2010;67:311–7.

37. Schaefer NG, Veit-Haibach P, Soyka JD, et al. Continued pemetrexed and platin-based chemotherapy in patients with malignant pleural mesothelioma (MPM): value of 18F-FDG-PET/CT. Eur J Radiol 2012;81:19–25.

38. Marin-Oyaga VA, Salavati A, Houshmand S, et al. Feasibility and performance of an adaptive contrast-oriented FDG PET/CT quantification technique for global disease assessment of malignant pleural mesothelioma and a brief review of the literature. Hell J Nucl Med 2015;18:11–8.

39. Van de Wiele C, Kruse V, Smeets P, et al. Predictive and prognostic value of metabolic tumour volume and total lesion glycolysis in solid tumours. Eur J Nucl Med Mol Imaging 2013;40:290–301.

40. Husby JA, Reitan BC, Biermann M, et al. Metabolic tumor volume on 18F-FDG PET/CT improves preoperative identification of high-risk endometrial carcinoma patients. J Nucl Med 2015;56:1191–8.

41. Fasmer KE, Gulati A, Dybvik JA, et al. Preoperative 18F-FDG PET/CT tumor markers outperform MRI-based markers for the prediction of lymph node metastases in primary endometrial cancer. Eur Radiol 2020;30:2443–53.

42. Hasenclever D, Kurch L, Mauz-Körholz C, et al. qPET-a quantitative extension of the Deauville scale to assess response in interim FDG-PET scans in lymphoma. Eur J Nucl Med Mol Imaging 2014;41:1301–8.

43. Bural GG, Torigian DA, Chamroonrat W, et al. Quantitative assessment of the atherosclerotic burden of the aorta by combined FDG-PET and CT image analysis: a new concept. Nucl Med Biol 2006;33:1037–43.

44. Rose S, Sheth NH, Baker JF, et al. A comparison of vascular inflammation in psoriasis, rheumatoid arthritis, and healthy subjects by FDG-PET/CT: a pilot study. Am J Cardiovasc Dis 2013;3:273–8.

45. Bural GG, Torigian DA, Burke A, et al. Quantitative assessment of the hepatic metabolic volume product in patients with diffuse hepatic steatosis and normal controls through use of FDG-PET and MR imaging: a novel concept. Mol Imaging Biol 2010;12:233–9.

46. Malherbe ST, Dupont P, Kant I, et al. A semi-automatic technique to quantify complex tuberculous lung lesions on 18F-fluorodeoxyglucose positron emission tomography/computerised tomography images. EJNMMI Res 2018;8:55.

47. Abdulla S, Salavati A, Saboury B, et al. Quantitative assessment of global lung inflammation following radiation therapy using FDG PET/CT: a pilot study. Eur J Nucl Med Mol Imaging 2014;41:350–6.

48. Saboury B, Salavati A, Brothers A, et al. FDG PET/CT in Crohn's disease: correlation of quantitative FDG PET/CT parameters with clinical and endoscopic surrogate markers of disease activity. Eur J Nucl Med Mol Imaging 2014;41:605–14.

49. Basu S, Sirohi B, Shrikhande SV. Dual tracer imaging approach in assessing tumor biology and heterogeneity in neuroendocrine tumors: its correlation with tumor proliferation index and possible multifaceted implications for personalized clinical management decisions, with focus on PRRT. Eur J Nucl Med Mol Imaging 2014;41(8):1492–6.

50. Basu S, Ranade R, Thapa P. Correlation and discordance of tumour proliferation index and molecular imaging characteristics and their implications for treatment decisions and outcome pertaining to peptide receptor radionuclide therapy in patients with advanced neuroendocrine tumour: developing a personalized model. Nucl Med Commun 2015; 36(8):766–74.

51. Basu S, Ranade R, Ostwal V, et al. PET-based molecular imaging in Designing personalized management strategy in Gastroenteropancreatic neuroendocrine tumors. PET Clin 2016;11(3):233–41.

52. Sharma R, Wang WM, Yusuf S, et al. 68Ga-DOTATATE PET/CT parameters predict response to peptide receptor radionuclide therapy in neuroendocrine tumours. Radiother Oncol 2019; 141:108–15.

53. Ortega C, Wong RKS, Schaefferkoetter J, et al. Quantitative 68Ga-DOTATATE PET/CT parameters for the prediction of therapy response in patients with progressive metastatic neuroendocrine tumors treated with 177Lu-DOTATATE. J Nucl Med 2021;62:1406–14.

# Positron Emission Tomography-Based Assessment of Cognitive Impairment and Dementias, Critical Role of Fluorodeoxyglucose in such Settings

Andrew B. Newberg, MD[a,b,*], Roger Coble, BA[a,c], Mohsen Khosravi, MD[a], Abass Alavi, MD[d]

## KEYWORDS

• Alzheimer disease • Cognitive impairment • Dementia • Parkinson disease • FDG

## KEY POINTS

• Fluorodeoxyglucose positron emission tomography (FDG PET) imaging is highly useful in diagnosing Alzheimer disease.
• FDG PET imaging can also help distinguish other neurologic and psychological conditions from each other including fronto-temporal dementia and depression.
• FDG PET provides different clinical information compared with current tracers for amyloid and tau deposition.
• PET imaging of various neurotransmitter systems can complement FDG PET imaging in the evaluation of dementias.
• PET imaging is a useful tool for assessing therapeutic interventions in patients with dementia.

## INTRODUCTION

Positron emission tomography (PET) has provided substantial contributions to understanding the neurophysiological basis of neurodegenerative diseases. Used for more than 40 years, [18]F-fluorodeoxyglucose (FDG) is the most frequently used tracer in the measurement of cerebral glucose metabolism. FDG has not only been used as the predominant PET tracer in evaluating neurodegenerative diseases in research contexts but is also prominently used in clinical applications. FDG has served to be so useful because it both permits specific brain regions to be individually evaluated, as well as the demonstration of disease-specific patterns of abnormal cerebral metabolism. The use of neurotransmitter tracers in PET imaging has helped in further elucidating the pathophysiologic mechanisms of neurodegenerative diseases, even though they have primarily

The authors have nothing to disclose.
[a] Marcus Institute of Integrative Health, Thomas Jefferson University, 789 East Lancaster Avenue, Suite 110, Villanova, PA 19085, USA; [b] Department of Radiology, Thomas Jefferson University, Philadelphia, PA, USA; [c] University of California Berkeley, Berkeley, CA, USA; [d] Department of Radiology, University of Pennsylvania, Philadelphia, PA, USA
* Corresponding author. Marcus Institute of Integrative Health, Thomas Jefferson University, 789 East Lancaster Avenue, Suite 110, Villanova, PA 19085.
E-mail address: Andrew.newberg@jefferson.edu

PET Clin 17 (2022) 479–494
https://doi.org/10.1016/j.cpet.2022.03.009

been used in research studies. Overall, PET has provided an enormous amount of data and information regarding the nature, diagnosis, and treatment of neurodegenerative diseases. Specifically, Alzheimer disease (AD) has been most extensively evaluated using PET imaging. AD was a predominant target in early PET imaging studies due to its dual status as both the most common neurodegenerative disease and the most common cause of dementia. PET imaging studies continue to focus on exploring AD as a primary disease of interest while also demonstrating that PET is useful in the evaluation of other neurodegenerative diseases such as Parkinson disease, frontotemporal dementia, and dementia with Lewy bodies (DLB)—both in terms of studying these disorders individually, as well as comparing them to each other. Although the existing body of literature focuses on using PET in the evaluation of cerebral glucose metabolism, several studies exist that demonstrate the use of PET in exploring the various neurotransmitter systems at play in such disorders, as well as pathophysiological mechanisms of disease. Key neurotransmitter systems implicated in neurodegenerative disease that have been evaluated with PET include dopamine, serotonin, gamma amino butyric acid, acetylcholine, and others. Pathophysiological processes that have been evaluated include the accumulation of abnormal tau and amyloid proteins as well as various inflammatory markers. For example, PET using FDG as the primary radiopharmaceutical (FDG PET) provides a map of the brain's function based on metabolic activity, whereas a PET scan specific to amyloid (amyloid PET) illustrates where in the brain the amyloid tracer binds—showing amyloid deposition (Figs. 1 and 2). A nuclear medicine physician can then qualitatively or quantitatively review these results in the context of the patient's diagnosis and treatment plan.

However, many PET scans are read without substantial consideration of the patient's condition or potential diagnosis. This brings to light the importance of an informed reader in determining the clinical significance of the implementation of PET imaging of neurodegenerative diseases in a clinical setting. This is a critical point, as the clinician reading the PET scan must contextualize the PET finings within the primary question at hand—that is, differentiating a patient's diagnosis of AD from frontotemporal dementia (FTD), or distinguishing depression from AD. Furthermore, it is helpful to know the patient's symptoms and cognitive findings as several studies considered below demonstrate how metabolic abnormalities in specific brain regions correlate with cognitive impairment. A more specific reading can be provided

when knowledge of the patient and the key clinical question is known. This article will review the variety of applications of PET in the study and evaluation of neurodegenerative diseases.

## ALZHEIMER DISEASE

The foundation of the criteria for the diagnosis of AD originates from the 1984 Working Group of the National Institute of Neurological and Communicative Disorders and Stroke and the Alzheimer Disease and Related Disorders Association.[1] The clinical criteria for diagnosing AD include evidence of progressive cognitive deficits in middle-aged or elderly patients with no identifiable underlying cause. Potential underlying causes of impaired cognition that should always be considered include thyroid disease; B12, folate, or other vitamin deficiencies; renal or liver dysfunction; medication effects; depression; or infectious and inflammatory diseases. Most neurologists specializing in neurodegenerative disorders can make an accurate diagnosis in patients with severe symptoms or after following the patient clinically for 6 to 12 months. However, it is often difficult to differentiate between the various dementing disorders when patients are in the early phases of the disease and presenting with mild symptoms.[2,3]

Due to this ambiguity of diagnosis in patients with mild disease, the definition of AD was revised in 2011 by the National Institute on Aging and the Alzheimer's Association. The current clinical guidelines present AD as a continuum of pathologies. In other words, these guidelines conceptualize AD as a spectrum from mild disease states, such as asymptomatic neurologic changes, to those of greater severity, such as full-onset dementia, as a way of mapping out criteria for the symptomatic predementia phase of AD—otherwise referred to as mild cognitive impairment (MCI).[4,5] MCI is a heterogenous nosologic clinical concept referring to elderly people with mild cognitive deficits but not severe enough to deserve the diagnosis of dementia. Several attempts have been made in recent years to classify the boundaries between MCI and Alzheimer dementia. For example, the European Consortium on AD MCI group clearly identifies 3 individual stages of the MCI diagnosis. However, even with these new MCI criteria, they suggest that additional tests, such as neuroimaging, are needed to determine the underlying cause to distinguish it from AD.[6] Furthermore, the combination of PET neuroimaging data and classic clinical evaluation have been proposed to yield more accurate predictions of progression from MCI to AD than clinical diagnosis alone, thus demonstrating the

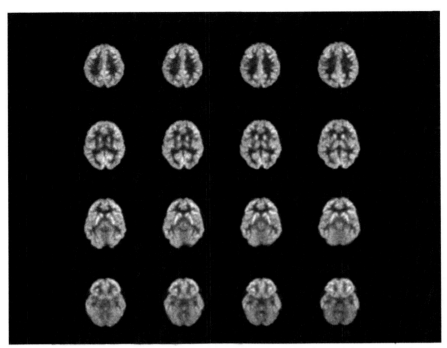

**Fig. 1.** Transaxial images of an FDG PET scan from a healthy individual with no neurologic or psychiatric disorder. The scan demonstrates uniform cerebral glucose metabolism throughout the cortical and subcortical structures.

importance of using neuroimaging techniques as a supplement to standard clinical evaluation.[7]

Most PET studies of AD have used FDG and found substantially reduced cerebral glucose metabolism (sometimes referred to as the cerebral metabolic rate of glucose or CMRGlu) in the whole brain, and particularly in the bilateral temporo-parietal regions.[8–15] This temporo-parietal hypometabolism (**Fig. 3**) has often been referred to as the "typical" pattern of AD and is thought to be more pronounced in patients aged less than 65 years or as patients develop more severe symptoms.

A large number of foundational studies show that this pattern of temporo-parietal hypometabolism has a sensitivity of approximately 85% to 90%, a specificity of approximately 60% to 70%, and a negative predictive value ranging from 77% to 95% in screening for AD.[16] However, because this pattern can be observed in patients with other conditions including Parkinson disease, DLB, bilateral parietal stroke, bilateral parietal

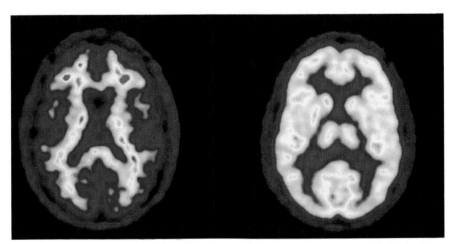

**Fig. 2.** FDG-PET scan (*right*) and florbetaben (amyloid) scan (*left*) of a healthy control subject showing uniform cerebral glucose metabolism throughout the cortex and no evidence of amyloid accumulation. Note the nonspecific tracer binding of florbetaben in the white matter regions.

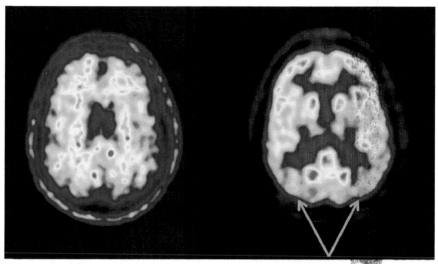

Fig. 3. FDG-PET scan (*right*) and florbetaben (amyloid) scan (*left*) of a patient with AD showing decreased cerebral glucose metabolism in the temporo-parietal regions (*arrows*) and substantial amyloid accumulation throughout the cortex.

subdural hematomas, and bilateral parietal radiation therapy ports, it is not considered to be pathognomonic for AD.[17] Furthermore, recent findings suggest that other patterns of hypometabolism, such as that within the entorhinal cortex, may be more specific to AD and thus provide more accurate diagnostic biomarkers of AD.[18] This highlights the importance of the proactive reevaluation of PET findings attributed to the differential diagnosis of underlying dementia pathologic condition due to the fast evolving body of PET literature in evaluating neurodegenerative diseases.

Although the current body of literature surrounding FDG PET suggests that regional glucose hypometabolism, specifically that of the temporoparietal region, is a prominent biological indicator of disease status in patients with AD, the inferior parietal lobe, frontal lobe, lateral temporal region, posterior cingulate, and precuneus have also been observed to show reduced CMRGlu values in patients with AD.[19] Hunt and colleagues found that patients with aging-associated cognitive decline (AACD) had significantly reduced glucose metabolism in the right precuneus, posterior cingulate, right angular gyrus, and bilateral middle temporal cortices compared with controls in an exploration of the differences in metabolic activity between patients with AACD, AD, and healthy controls. Although present in AACD patients, these metabolic deficits were more prominent in patients with AD, who also presented with hypometabolism in the frontal cortices. The key finding, however, was that AACD patients who subsequently converted to AD had greater hypometabolism involving the frontal and temporal cortices, right cingulate gyrus, right thalamus, and bilateral precuneus compared with those patients who did not progress to AD.[20]

The pattern of hypometabolism on FDG PET scans in patients with AD has also been demonstrated to be persistent and progressive in longitudinal studies. For example, Jagust and colleagues[21] demonstrated that over time the parietal cortex experienced significantly more severe hypometabolism than did the frontal and occipital cortices in an early longitudinal cohort of 6 patients with AD. This was expanded on by Smith and colleagues'[22] finding that hypometabolism in the temporal and parietal association areas within the same subjects increase in severity as they progresses into later stages of AD, yet show lesser degrees of deficit in subcortical gray matter structures. Furthermore, Alexander and colleagues[23] reported that patients with AD showed significant declines in glucose metabolism in the parietal, temporal, and frontal lobes, as well as the posterior cingulate cortex, at 1 year follow-up. Studies have also reported that patients with familial AD—both those associated with amyloid precursor protein mutation and chromosome 14 linkage—display similar temporo-parietal hypometabolism.[24]

It is important to note potential caveats to these findings. One prominent consideration is that it is possible for there to an absence of significant changes in glucose metabolism in patients with early mild AD—even if there are changes in glucose metabolism in these patients, they are generally minor decreases in the parietal lobes, leading such information to further complicate the implications of the above findings.[25] Additionally, other disorders, such as depression, may mimic the clinical findings of AD. However, there generally remains some distinction between depression and AD in FDG PET scans, as depression typically shows a more global cortical hypometabolism that particularly affects the frontal lobes (Fig. 4). This can, however, complicate the ability to adequately detect which patients will progress clinically. However, as more high-resolution PET scanners are used in clinical practice, it is conceivable that early AD can be better detected using FDG.

Considering both the aforementioned strengths and limitations of FDG PET imaging in assessing and diagnosing the AD process, the European Association of Nuclear Medicine and the European Academy of Neurology in their Delphi Consensus supported the clinical use of FDG PET over other PET-based biomarkers due to its potential of identifying underlying AD pathologic condition early in the disease process.[26]

One important interpretive issue with PET scans is that their spatial resolution makes it difficult to adequately separate metabolically active brain tissue from adjunct metabolically inactive ventricular and sulcal CSF spaces. Therefore, it has been suggested that the correction for brain atrophy is necessary for accurate PET-based measures of glucose metabolism.[27] MRI scans are currently used to correct for the CMRGlu values obtained by FDG PET because their volumetric determinations are significantly more accurate than CT scans at determining brain atrophy. Volumetric correction is of more significant urgency in PET scans of patients with AD because there tends to be greater atrophy when compared with controls, and thus a greater need to ensure that the hypometabolism is a result of the disease, and not solely related to a lack of brain tissue. However, there remains a debate on the necessity of correcting for atrophy in CMRGlu values of patients with AD. In an early study, before atrophy correction, patients with AD showed significant decreases in mean whole brain CMRGlu compared with controls, but there were no differences between the groups after correction.[28] However, Ibanez and colleagues[19] found that global CMRGlu was significantly lower in patients with AD compared with controls both before and after atrophy correction, thus reflecting a true metabolic reduction in AD.

In addition to volumetric correction, more quantitative approaches for evaluating FDG PET data might improve the overall ability to determine the course and severity of AD.[29] The region-specific quantitative analysis of cerebral metabolism continues to improve as techniques progress and is especially apparent in brain regions substantially affected by AD pathologic condition, such as the hippocampus. An interesting quantitative FDG PET study showed that resting CMRGlu significantly correlated with performance on a story recall test. However, there existed a significant difference between 2 subgroups of 20 patients, which differed in AD severity as classified by Mini-Mental State Examination. Of the 2 groups, the less severe subgroup showed correlation of task performance with the hippocampal cortex regions, posterior cingulate gyrus, and retrosplenial cortex, in addition to other limbic structures, whereas the subgroup with more severe impairment predominately displayed a correlation with the left temporal neocortex, which is implicated in semantic memory.[30] The authors argued that when episodic memory is mildly impaired, the limbic functions are still sufficient to support the remaining cognitive processes, but with more severe memory deficits, there is an inability to adequately compensate during task performance.

Although PET is still used to measure cerebral metabolic activity, there has been a recent focus on using PET to identify novel therapeutic targets and to monitor AD treatment outcomes. Because the identification of more therapeutic targets eventually leads to the development of efficacious interventions, PET imaging will play a more significant role in the effective evaluation and management of patients in the early stages of AD.[31–33]

Recent advances in neuroimaging of AD have been grounded in elucidating the specific pathophysiological processes underlying AD. One of the most prominent findings is the accumulation of amyloid proteins as plaques in the brain, which is now recognized as a central component of the pathologic diagnosis of AD.[8] Although the development of amyloid imaging has been important in developing a fuller understanding of AD pathologic condition, it has simultaneously become a topic of great controversy over the ethical consideration that there do not currently exist any treatment options in the case that an individual tests positive for AD. The value of amyloid imaging is in further question due to its inherent imaging characteristics. Ikonomovic and colleagues showed that in vivo [11]C-PiB binding may not be 100% sensitive for the presence of histologically detectable amyloid plaque. The short half-life of [11]C hindered the use of this tracer in a wider clinical setting, and thus, a second generation of [18]F-labeled radiotracers have been developed.[34] Currently, only

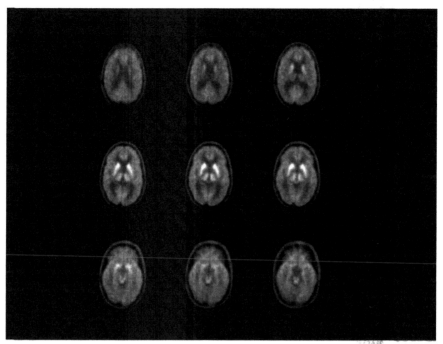

Fig. 4. Transaxial images of an FDG-PET scan from a patient with major depression showing a global cortical decrease in metabolism relative to the subcortical structures.

florbetapir, florbetaben, and flutemetamol have been approved for the clinical use by the Food and Drug Administration (FDA) and European regulatory authorities, and have done so under the respective names: Vizamyl@, Amyvid@, and Neuraceq@.[35–37] Although clinically approved, several studies have produced conflicting evidence when evaluating the ability of these particular tracers to diagnose AD through the accurate detection of amyloid burden in the brain (see **Fig. 3**; **Fig. 5**).[38,39]

When compared with autopsy, florbetapir PET was found to have a sensitivity of 96% and a specificity of 100% for the detection of Aβ plaques, whereas a similar study revealed a sensitivity of approximately 90% and specificity of 87% for flutametamol.[40,41] A PET imaging study aimed at evaluating the use of florbetapir in assessing the pathophysiology of AD in patients with early SCD and MCI observed that the first pathophysiological signs of Aβ plaques differing from healthy normal controls, as indicated by florbetapir retention, occurred in the anterior and posterior cingulate cortices, precuneus, and orbitofrontal cortex and later in the prefrontal cortex, inferior lateral temporal cortex, parietal cortex, and occipital cortex.[42] This suggests that such topological PET findings provide useful information in identifying early amyloid pathologic condition, and thus early signs of potential AD, that may not be demonstrated by neuropathological findings. The early detection of

amyloid deposition using PET imaging in SCD and MCI contributed to the construction of the early cutoff and definition of amyloid abnormality in the "gray zone" of florbetapir PET imaging. Yeo and colleagues[43] in their systematic review and meta-analysis on relevant studies published from January 1980 to March 2014 also demonstrated favorable sensitivity and specificity of amyloid imaging with novel fluorine tracers in diagnosis of AD, supporting their use as an adjunct in clinical practice. Again though, others have argued that there are significant technical and clinical problems with amyloid imaging such as the lack of therapeutic interventions, high positivity rates among healthy nondemented individuals, and the actual accuracy of binding of these tracers to amyloid versus other normal tissues.[44] A meta-analysis on diagnostic accuracy of [18]F amyloid PET tracers conducted by Moris and colleagues[45] indicated that all 3 [18]F-labeled tracers held similar diagnostic accuracy and generally high pooled sensitivity and specificity values, yet this performance was only useful in discriminating between patients with AD and healthy controls but not between patients with AD and MCI.

In analyzing quality-adjusted life years, costs, and incremental cost-effectiveness ratios, Hornberger and colleagues[46] concluded that [18]F-florbetapir PET imaging is a cost-effective supplemental diagnostic tool when paired with

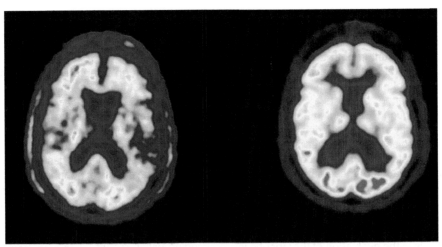

Fig. 5. FDG-PET scan (*right*) and florbetaben (amyloid) scan (*left*) of a patient with MCI showing normal cerebral glucose metabolism and substantial amyloid accumulation throughout the cortex. Such discrepant results require additional evaluation to determine which patients progress based on the specific findings of different types of PET scans.

standard AD diagnostic assessment. Conversely, due to overall poor sensitivity and specificity and high financial cost, Martinez and colleagues[47] recommended against the routine use of [18]F-florbetapir in clinical practice after evaluating the diagnostic test accuracy (DTA) of [18]F-florbetapir in predicting the progression from MCI to AD or any form of dementia. Furthermore, although the detection of Aβ plaques has been determined to be one of the characteristic pathologic findings of AD, one study of cognitively healthy elderly subjects (approximately 10%–15%) has also revealed significant Aβ burden in the brains of these individuals.[48] Additionally, longitudinal population-based estimates using [11C] PIB PET imaging suggest that the prevalence of testing positive for amyloid burden among elderly individuals aged 80 to 89 years is 41.3%.[49] These findings raise the critical point that the presence of Aβ plaques alone is not sufficient to produce cognitive impairment, especially when considering that amyloid PET studies have shown little association of brain amyloid load with clinical severity of dementia in patients with AD.[41,50] It is the combination of such findings and the lack of sufficient theoretic basis that fuel this dispute over the diagnostic value of amyloid PET in AD and other dementias.[51,52]

The accumulation of tau protein in the brain, manifesting as neurofibrillary tangles (NFTs), has been shown to be closely associated with neurodegeneration and cognitive impairment in a similar manner to Aβ plaques.[53] In vivo detection of tau protein deposits in the brain present helpful technique to diagnose tauopathies as well as to track and predict disease progression.[54] Recently,

several tau PET tracers including PBB3, T807, and THK-5117 have been developed and prospered in imaging neurofibrillary pathologic condition.[55] The first PET studies of [18F]T807 conducted in humans demonstrated significant tracer retention in the frequent areas of PHF-tau in the AD brain, which is thought to be associated with increased disease severity, when comparing severe cases of AD to both mild instances of AD and MCI.[56] Furthermore, very low levels of nonspecific binding of [18F]T807 in white matter have also been seen in these original studies, which is in contrast to most [18]F-labeled amyloid PET tracers. Similarly, [18F]THK-523, [18F]THK-5105, and [18F]THK-5117 have demonstrated high binding selectivity to tau over Aβ in the AD brain. In agreement with existing postmortem studies, these tracer retentions were also associated with dementia severity and brain atrophy.[57] However, patients with AD demonstrated significantly greater correlations between cortical atrophy and tau deposition in the entorhinal and middle temporal cortices, as measured by structural MRI and [18F]THK-5351 uptake respectively, when compared with healthy controls and MCI patients.[58] A specific correlation was found between atrophy of the hippocampus and [18F]THK-5351 uptake, yet was only observed in Aβ-positive subgroup and not in those with Aβ-negative PET readings.

In comparing the retention of [18]F-florbetaben and [18F]flortaucipir using PET imaging, Bullich and colleagues[42] observed a significant association between Aβ plaques and tau deposition. More specifically, the authors found that the amount of tau deposition was significantly elevated in individuals with existing amyloid pathologic condition. For example, this association was especially present in both the fusiform gyrus and lateral temporal cortex. Patients without significant Aβ pathologic condition, however, displayed very sparing amounts, if any, of tau deposition. Although PET imaging tracers for amyloid and tau may provide differing insights and both methodologies require further research, this study demonstrates the importance of acknowledging the association of these pathologic conditions underlying AD when conceptualizing the diagnostic utility of these biomarkers in assessing the disease process.

One of the most important potential roles for PET imaging is in the evaluation of therapeutic interventions for AD. During the last decade, there has been a spark in the push to develop pharmaceuticals and immunologically mediated therapies for the treatment of AD. Due to various methodological approaches that can be used in this space, PET imaging has the potential to serve many important roles in the development and evaluation of such AD treatments as this innovation continues. For example, PET imaging can be used before the administration of therapeutics as a way to determine what therapies and therapeutic targets have the most promise for a particular patient. Additionally, PET scans can also be performed longitudinally as an evaluative measure of a particular therapy to determine the pharmaceutical intervention's mechanism or effectiveness. One specific application of using PET imaging to evaluate the impact of a pharmacologic therapy was in the case of understanding the impact that donepezil has on acetylcholinesterase (AChE) activity.[59] Although it had been proposed that donepezil substantially inhibited cortical AChE activity, this study demonstrated an average of approximately 27% inhibition after donepezil administration, thus providing a specific metric. More recently, amyloid PET imaging was used in assessing the effects of cholinesterase inhibitors on amyloid burden and cognitive impairment. The authors observed there to be no significant association between the administration of cholinesterase inhibitors in amyloid-positive patients with AD and amyloid burden. There was also no significant association found between cholinesterase inhibitor administration and change in cognitive ability, even when using a multivariate linear regression analysis accounting for the potential effects of amyloid deposition.[60] Such findings reveal the value of PET in determining the underlying mechanisms of AD and thus in helping to guide the development of

future clinical trials to ensure appropriate use and dose of the pharmaceutical.

PET imaging was also used to evaluate the effect of 16 to 24 mg/d doses of glutamine, an AChE inhibitor, on cerebral blood flow and glucose metabolism. Glutamine seemed beneficial both by PET measures, because it had a positive outcome on brain perfusion and regional cerebral metabolism (CMRGlu), and cognitive assessments because it seemed to stabilize cognition during 12 months.[61] PET imaging has also been used in assessing the effects of nonpharmacological therapies in patients with AD. For example, a PET study demonstrated that acupuncture has beneficial effects in the treatment of dementia and AD.[62]

Some of the most significant applications of PET imaging within recent years have been its use to evaluate the effectiveness of vaccines eliciting immunologic responses against the amyloid protein as a therapeutic technique for patients with AD. For example, one study assessing the binding of lecozotan, a new potent 5-HT (1A) antagonist that could be useful for the treatment of AD, used $^{11}$C-labeled WAY 100635 PET to observe that lecozotan effectively binds to 5-HT (1A) receptors.[63] Specifically, after a single 5 mg dose of lecozotan in both elderly individuals and those with AD, this study found a maximum observed receptor occupancy of 50% to 60%.

Additionally, $^{18}$F-florbetapir PET was used to measure amyloid burden in a phase 2 randomized control trial of an investigational vaccine against AD, Vanutide Cridificar (ACC-001) with Quillaja saponaria (QS-21).[64] This study found neither of the 2 experimental groups given the vaccine, as compared with controls, to show any significant reduction in amyloid burden or clinical improvements. Notably, those administered either of the 2 vaccine doses actually presented with a more rapid loss of brain volume. This study calls into question the value of amyloid detection in the brain for developing appropriate therapies, as well as the use of amyloid burden as an indicator of clinical progression.

This has been further highlighted in the controversy created by the FDA's approval of aducanumab for clinical treatment against AD. Amyloid PET imaging played a key role in assessing the effect of aducanumab on amyloid burden in patients with AD in the experimental arms of the EMERGE and ENGAGE trials. Amyloid PET displayed what has been interpreted as a potential nonlinear effect on amyloid burden, and has been used as a justification for the observed dose–response relationship between aducanumab and cognitive improvement in patients with AD.[65] However, many experts disagree with the

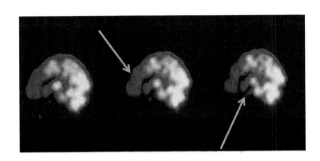

Fig. 6. Sagittal FDG-PET images of a patient with frontotemporal dementia showing markedly decreased metabolism in the frontal and temporal lobes (arrows).

standard of evidence for clinical benefit presented in these trials, highlighting the importance of the role of contextualizing PET imaging findings in this discourse and in future assessments of such AD therapeutics as aducanumab. More research will be necessary in understanding the best imaging techniques for the evaluation of AD progression, in addition to which therapeutic targets are most clinically successful in treating AD.

Overall, PET imaging has played an important role in both assessing and understanding all stages of the AD process. Building on this, PET techniques have and most likely will continue to play a key role in molecular imaging studies aimed at elucidating the pathophysiology of AD, the clinical management of the disease, and designing and assessing therapeutic interventions targeting AD pathologic condition.

## FRONTOTEMPORAL DEMENTIA

FTD is a clinical syndrome caused by the degeneration of the frontal lobes and anterior temporal lobes of the brain. The 3 clinical variants of FTD—behavioral variant frontotemporal dementia (bvFTD), nonfluent/agrammatic variant primary progressive aphasia (nfvPPA), and semantic variant primary progressive aphasia (svPPA)—all possess convergent and divergent behavioral symptoms that share many similarities with those of psychiatric disorders, thus making general FTD diagnosis and categorization into a specific FTD subtype very challenging.[66] Some clarity comes from there being 2 common classifications of FTD symptoms; those encompassing behavioral and affective alterations and those characterized by difficulties in language functioning.[67] Even though the current clinical understanding of FTD has allowed for clinicians to more readily distinguish the diagnosis of FTD from that of another neurodegenerative disease, the diagnosis of FTD remains to be challenging because its symptoms and findings continue to commonly overlap with other neurodegenerative diseases.

Because of these challenges in the clinical diagnosis of FTD, FDG PET scans have been used to identify affected brain regions and improve diagnostic accuracy of FTD. Such uses of FDG PET have shown that FTD generally presents as decreased cerebral metabolism and perfusion in the frontal lobes (Figs. 6 and 7) and anterior temporal lobes.[68] For example, when compared with controls, patients with FTD had significant decreases in cerebral metabolism in frontal cortical areas, caudate nuclei, and thalami, with marked concentration of this hypometabolism in the frontal cortex.[69] This hypometabolism was additionally seen to be more severe at approximately 18 months following the initial PET scan, an observation that occurred primarily in the orbitofrontal and subcortical frontal regions. According to the authors, these findings suggest that a region-specific reduction in cerebral glucose metabolism accompanies the progression of the clinical symptoms of FTD. A longitudinal study comparing metabolic and structural changes associated with the 3 FTD subtypes (bvFTD, svPPA, and nfvPPA), as measured by FDG PET and structural MRI respectively, additionally characterized metabolic patterns of the FTD disease process.[70] Among all 3 FTD syndromes, significant metabolic reductions were found in medial and inferolateral parietal regions, in addition to syndrome specific regions of hypometabolism, during a follow-up period of approximately 15 months when compared with healthy controls. The authors argue that this finding demonstrates that FDG PET patterns of hypometabolism in the medial and inferolateral parietal regions may not be a characteristic diagnostic marker of AD, as is a standard convention, and will complicate the differentiation of FTD and AD using FDG PET imaging. Furthermore, this study observed that the FDG PET and structural MRI are important tools in assessing the FTD disease process because structural MRI was seen to be more sensitive to capturing brain changes associated with early disease, whereas FDG PET was more adept for displaying brain changes in later disease

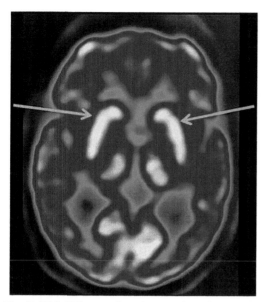

**Fig. 7.** FDG PET scan of patients with Parkinson disease showing increased metabolic activity in the basal ganglia (*arrows*).

progression. Volumetric changes from structural MRI were generally more significant and held less variability than metabolic changes from FDG PET; however, the findings illustrated by FDG PET displayed greater percent changes annually than those of structural MRI. These findings demonstrate the significance of FDG PET in elucidating the underlying brain changes associated with FTD, whereas highlighting the importance of including such neuroimaging techniques as a part of a broader battery of assessments.

Patients with FTD have overwhelmingly concentrated metabolic dysfunction in the frontal and anterior temporal lobes and associated subcortical structures, however, bring a new understanding to the overall FTD disease process. This study revealed that although prominent in the frontal and anterior temporal regions, the overall progression of FTD and associated metabolic deficits occur more globally than was previously conceived.[71] In an FDG PET study of cerebral metabolic activity in patients with sporadic bvFTD, Cerami and colleagues[72] found that individual differences in social cognition, as determined by variable performance on emotion regulation, attribution, and other such assessments, were associated with unique patterns of hypometabolism in limbic structures and prefrontal cortices.

Tau tangles have also been implicated as a pathologic contributor underlying various clinical presentations of FTD. Tsai and colleagues conducted an [18]F-flortaucipir PET study to further investigate the potential usefulness of tau PET

imaging in understanding the role of tau pathologic condition in FTD syndromes. The study observed varying degrees of [18]F-flortaucipir uptake in patients within each of 4 FTD syndrome groups and 3 FTD-associated mutation groups.[73] Overall, the authors found that [18]F-flortaucipir uptake was consistent with previously demonstrated patterns of tau pathologic condition in patients clinically characterized with corticobasal syndrome, bvFTD, nfvPPA, and carries of the MAPT gene. Additionally, they suggest that [18]F-flortaucipir may provide a longitudinal illustration of tau progression in these FTD syndromes and presents a potential methodology, when paired with amyloid PET imaging, to differentiate primary FTD syndromes from those caused by underlying AD pathologic condition. It is important, however, to note the variability of these findings and the need for larger scale studies of the utility of [18]F-flortaucipir PET in patients with FTD in comparison with postmortem pathologic assessment.

PET imaging has also been used to detect neuroinflammation in patients with FTD through the development of radiopharmaceuticals specifically targeting the translocator protein. For example, significant increases in mean [[11]C]-PK11195 binding in the left dorsolateral prefrontal cortex and the right hippocampus and parahippocampus of FTD patients, observed by Cagnin and colleagues,[74,75] demonstrate the importance of PET imaging in identifying specific regions of neuroinflammation associated with FTD, particularly the frontal and temporal regions. Although the aforementioned findings present a strong case for the significance of PET in assessing FTD, more studies of well-known PET radiopharmaceuticals for metabolism, as well as novel tracers that shed light into the underlying neurotransmitters and pathophysiology of FTD are necessary to establish a better understanding of this disease.

## DEMENTIA WITH LEWY BODIES

DLB is a neurodegenerative disease that is histopathologically characterized by having Lewy bodies and clinically characterized by cognitive impairment. PET studies of DLB have targeted the dopamine receptor system because it is known to be particularly affected. Additionally, an [11]C-altropane PET study found increased cognitive impairment to be associated with greater levels of regional DAT concentration in the anterior cingulate and decreased levels in the caudate in PD patients.[76]

In PET imaging, DLB is commonly characterized by the cingulate island sign (CIS), which refers to the preservation of the mid and posterior cingulate gyrus. Graff-Radford and colleagues[77] used FDG PET to explore this foundational relationship between the presence of the CIS and both clinical and postmortem neuropathological diagnoses of DLB using Braak NFT stage. This study quantified CIS metabolism using the FDG CIS ratio, which is the ratio of FDG uptake in the posterior cingulate to the sum of FDG uptake in the precuneus and cuneus. There was a significant association between FDG CIS ratio and Braak stage among patients at any point in the DLB disease process, thus supporting the utility of FDG CIS ratios gathered through PET imaging as a biomarker for DLB and clinical progression. However, it is important to note that the authors did not find a significant association between FDG CIS ratio and DLB subtypes (transitional vs diffuse), suggesting the need for a greater number of studies focusing on biomarkers to differentiate between each DLB types.

Due to the clinical difficulty of differentiating DLB from other dementia subtypes, PET shows promise in allowing for more accurate distinction and thus diagnosis of DLB. For example, an [11]C-PiB study aimed at elucidating the underlying role of Aβ-amyloid in DLB through investigating underlying AD and LBD pathologic condition demonstrated reduced [11]C-PiB uptake in patients with DLB compared with patients with AD.[78] Additionally, patients with DLB demonstrated greater [11]C-PiB uptake compared with patients with LBD-AD, and patients with AD showed increased [11]C-PiB uptake in the occipital cortices when compared with patients in the LBD-AD group. The authors also observed that PiB standardized uptake value ratios of global [11]C-PiB uptake in the cortex demonstrated the ability to differentiate the AD and DLB groups from one another with a sensitivity of 80%, specificity of 86%, and accuracy of 93%. These studies demonstrate the potential importance of PET imaging in both differentiating DLB from other similarly presenting neurodegenerative diseases, such as AD, and in better understanding the underlying pathologic condition of DLB and the ways in which it may overlap with pathologic condition previously attributed to different underlying causes of dementia.

Furthermore, FDG PET proved to be better equipped for distinguishing between DLB and AD when compared with [123]I-beta-CIT SPECT. Specifically, this study found that hypometabolism in the lateral occipital cortex had a sensitivity of 88%, which proved to hold the greatest sensitivity in diagnosing DLB. The region with the highest specificity, being 100%, was the CIS. Interestingly, [123]I-beta-CIT achieved 100% accuracy and greater effect size than did FDG PET most likely because the former preferentially measures the dopaminergic system, which is specifically impaired in DLB and not affected much in AD.[79]

In a related study, PET imaging with N-[[11]C]-methyl-4-piperidyl acetate to measure brain AChE activity was performed in 18 patients with PD, 21 patients with PDD/DLB, and 26 healthy controls.[80] AChE activity was significantly decreased in the cerebral cortex of PD patients and especially in the medial occipital cortex, but AChE activity was even lower in patients with PDD/DLB. However, no significant regional differences in AChE activity were able to differentiate between early PD and advanced PD groups or between the DLB and PDD groups. Thus, neurotransmitter imaging using PET as described above might be helpful in the research and clinical applications in patients with DLB, but more studies will be necessary.

## STUDIES COMPARING DIFFERENT DEMENTIAS

This final section will be dedicated to outlining applications of PET imaging that allow for the direct comparison of patients with differing neurodegenerative diseases. Studies of this nature hold the dual significance of providing techniques for more accurate differentiation and diagnosis of specific neurodegenerative disorders, in addition to building a framework to determine the most appropriate imaging methodologies to accomplish this task.

Foster and colleagues[81] indicated that FDG-PET is a powerful supplement to clinical diagnosis, and that FDG-PET + clinical diagnosis for both AD and FTD increased the diagnostic accuracy and confidence. These findings were especially significant in cases with ambiguous clinical diagnoses. Additionally, the ABIDE Project found that the use of PET [18]F-florbetaben amyloid imaging provided clinicians with important insight into the cause of MCI and SCD and increased the confidence in their diagnoses.[82] Specifically, the authors found that in a large sample of 507 patients, clinicians informed by amyloid PET imaging changed the clinical diagnosis in 25% of patients and demonstrated a 10% increase in confidence of diagnoses. PET findings also drove clinicians to alter the course of treatment in 24% of patients. These findings highlight the importance of amyloid PET imaging in disease diagnosis, informing disease management, and specifying appropriateness of treatments of AD and other related dementias.

Ishii and colleagues focused on using FDG PET to identify unique patterns of cerebral glucose metabolism specific to FTD that could be used to distinguish FTD from metabolic patterns in patients with AD and elderly controls. This study concluded that patients with FTD have standard cerebral glucose metabolism, as indicated by observed CMRGlu values, unilaterally in the left cerebellum and right sensorimotor area, and bilaterally in the occipital lobes. However, when compared with the AD group, patients with FTD displayed significantly lower CMRGlu values in the hippocampi, orbital gyri, anterior temporal lobes, anterior cingulate gyri, basal ganglia, thalami, middle and superior frontal gyri, and left inferior frontal gyrus.

In a study using FDG-PET imaging to characterize differential patterns of hypometabolism to distinguish AD from DLB, Ye and colleagues[83] found that both patients with AD and patients with DLB generally demonstrated hypometabolism in the bilateral lateral temporal, temporoparietal junction, posterior cingulate, and precuneus cortices when compared with healthy controls. Furthermore, this study observed significant hypometabolism bilaterally in the entorhinal cortices and hippocampi of patients with AD, but not in patients with DLB, proposing that this pattern of hypometabolism can be used to differentiate AD from DLB. Conversely, the authors found that patients with DLB, and not patients with AD, demonstrated bilateral hypermetabolism in the central cerebellum, posterior putamen, and somatomotor cortices, suggesting that this pattern of hypermetabolism may be used to distinguish DLB from AD.

An additional longitudinal study used FDG PET to examine the differentiation of patients with MCI who later progressed to prodromal DLB (MCI-prodromal DLB) from patients with MCI who proceeded to AD (MCI-AD).[84] Consistent with the current state of the literature, these authors found that preserved metabolism in the posterior cingulate and medial temporal lobe distinguished MCI-prodromal DLB from MCI-AD, as patients with MCI-AD presented with significant hypometabolism in these regions relative to patients with MCI-prodromal DLB.

Garibotto and colleagues[85] evaluated the use of FDG-PET and DaTScan SPECT in 27 patients with neurodegenerative dementia associated with parkinsonism to observe which imaging methodology most accurately distinguished patients into diagnostic groups consistent with standardized clinical diagnosis. The subjects were grouped according to diagnosis based on clinically established criteria, including probable Alzheimer disease (5 subjects), corticobasal degeneration (6 subjects), Lewy body dementia (8 subjects), FTD (4 subjects), and Parkinson disease with dementia (4 subjects). Individual analyses of each scan concluded that 85% of the patients were classified into the correct clinically established diagnostic group using FDG PET, whereas only 59% of participants were correctly classified using DaTScan. However, when FDG PET and DaTScan SPECT were combined, their integrated classifications were 100% consistent with the clinical diagnoses. The authors postulated, with the caveat that these results came from a small sample size, that the most effective approach for classifying individual patients with dementia and parkinsonism would be an automated analysis approach combining imaging data measuring FDG uptake and DAT binding.

Klein and colleagues used PET imaging with FGD, FDOPA, and N-($^{11}$C-methy;-4-piperidyl-acetate-(MP4A) in an investigation of the role that the cholinergic system may play in various physiologic aspects of dementia. The study used these PET scans in 8 patients with PDD, 6 patients with DLB, and 9 patients with PD without dementia, all of whom were compared with age-matched controls.[86] The authors concluded that patients with DLB and PD with dementia share the same dopaminergic and cholinergic deficit profile in the brain and suggested that such breakdown of the cholinergic system is a necessary contributing factor to the development of dementia, as well as some motor symptoms. Due to these observed similarities in the patterns of cholinergic and dopaminergic deficits, this study proposed that DLB and PD with dementia may not be 2 unique disorders but rather a continuum of Lewy Body diseases.

Although PET imaging demonstrates great potential to differentiate between distinct dementia classifications, many discrepancies still exist between clinical and PET-based diagnoses, thus presenting a need for more comprehensive studies of this application of PET. This is demonstrated by one study that compared clinical, PET $^{11}$C-dihydrotetrabenazine, and PET $^{11}$C-Pittsburgh compound-B classification of dementia types in 75 subjects with mild dementia. When using only a clinical evaluation to group these 75 participants, 36 individuals were classified as having AD, 25 as having FTD, and 14 as having DLB. Based on PET imaging alone (combined $^{11}$C-dihydrotetrabenazine and $^{11}$C-Pittsburgh compound-B findings), 47 subjects were classified as having AD, 15 as having DLB, and 13 as having FTD. This study reported only a moderate agreement between clinical consensus and neuroimaging classifications across all dementia subtypes, with discordant classifications in ~35% of subjects. It is important to note that the use of expert clinical consensus alone as the gold-standard of dementia classification, without comparing clinical and PET classifications to more accurate postmortem diagnosis, creates ambiguity in drawing conclusions from this study's results and should be considered when interpreting these findings.[87]

## SUMMARY

PET imaging has been a powerful tool for evaluating patients with neurodegenerative diseases. The variety of components of the disease process that PET can be used to image, from cerebral blood flow and glucose metabolism to changes in neurotransmitter systems to Aβ-amyloid and other disease related molecules, has allowed PET imaging to play a significant role in developing the current understanding these disease processes and their underlying pathophysiology within a research context. PET imaging has also served as a useful clinical tool showing a great potential for increasing the accuracy of evaluating, diagnosing, and assigning a prognosis of neurodegenerative diseases at various stages within the disease process and may additionally provide insight into therapeutic effectiveness on an individual level. Another future application of PET studies will be the ability to determine the patients who are most appropriate for medical or surgical interventions. Overall, PET imaging of patients affected by neurodegenerative diseases will continue to be a powerful tool in understanding and studying the disease course, underlying causes, and long-term implications both for research and clinical purposes.

## CLINICS CARE POINTS

1. It is important to have as much clinical information on a given patient when reading brain positron emission tomography (PET) scans to be able to provide the most useful imaging reports.

2. PET imaging is an important tool for helping clinicians with the diagnosis and management of patients with dementia.

3. Clinical reading of PET scans should follow established guidelines for consistency and accuracy.

4. Appropriate processing and analysis (including quantitative analysis) of scans is helpful for accurate diagnosis of PET scans.

## REFERENCES

1. McKhann G, Drachman D, Folstein M, et al. Clinical diagnosis of alzheimer's disease: report of the NINCDS-ADRDA work group under the auspices of department of health and human Services task force on alzheimer's disease. Neurol 1984;34:939–44.

2. Tierney MC, Gisher RH, Lewis AJ, et al. The NINCDS-ADRDA Workgroup criteria for the clinical diagnosis of probable Alzheimer's disease. A clinical pathological study of 57 cases. Neurol 1988; 38:359–64.

3. Joachim CL, Morris JH, Selkow DJ. Clinical diagnosed Alzheimer's disease. autopsy results in 150 cases. Ann Neurol 1988;24:50–6.

4. Alzheimer's Association. zheimer's disease facts and figures. Alzheimer's Dement 2017;13:325–73 [Internet].

5. Albert MS, DeKosky ST, Dickson D, et al. The diagnosis of mild cognitive impairment due to Alzheimer's disease: recommendations from the National Institute on Aging-Alzheimer's Association workgroups on diagnostic guidelines for Alzheimer's disease. Alzheimers Dement 2011;7(3):270–9.

6. Portet F, Ousset PJ, Visser PJ, et al. Mild cognitive impairment (MCI) in medical practice: a critical review of the concept and new diagnostic procedure. Report of the MCI Working Group of the European Consortium on Alzheimer's Disease. J Neurol Neurosurg Psychiatr 2006;77(6):714–8.

7. Blazhenets G, Ma Y, Sörensen A, et al. Predictive value of 18 F-florbetapir and 18 F-FDG PET for conversion from mild cognitive impairment to alzheimer dementia. J Nucl Med 2020;61(4):597–603.

8. Heiss WD, Kessler J, Szelies B, et al. Positron emission tomography in the differential diagnosis of organic dementias. J Neural Transm Suppl 1991; 33:13–9.

9. Jamieson DG, Chawluck JB, Alavi A, et al. The effect of disease severity on local cerebral glucose metabolism in Alzheimer's disease. J Cereb Blood Flow Metab 1987;7:S410.

10. Kumar A, Schapiro MB, Grady C, et al. High-resolution PET studies in Alzheimer's disease. Neuropsychopharmacology 1991;4:35–46.

11. Faulstich ME, Sullivan DC. Positron emission tomography in neuropsychiatry. Invest Radiol 1991;26: 184–94.

12. Bonte FJ, Hom J, Tinter R, et al. Single photon tomography in Alzheimer's disease and the dementias. Semin Nucl Med 1990;20:342–52.

13. Friedland RP, Grady CL, Shapiro MB, et al. Family history of dementia and regional cerebral glucose utilization (rCMRgle) in dementia of the Alzheimer type (AD) [Abstract]. Neurol 1989;39(Suppl 1):168.

14. Rapoport SI, Horowitz B, Grady CL, et al. Abnormal brain glucose metabolism in Alzheimer's disease as

measured by positron emission tomography. Adv Exp Med Biol 1991;291:231–48.

15. Croteau E, Castellano CA, Fortier M, et al. A cross-sectional comparison of brain glucose and ketone metabolism in cognitively healthy older adults, mild cognitive impairment and early Alzheimer's disease. Exp Gerontol 2018;107:18–26.

16. Arbizu J, Festari C, Altomare D, et al. Clinical utility of FDG-PET for the clinical diagnosis in MCI. Eur J Nucl Med Mol Imaging 2018;45:1497–508.

17. Mazziotta JC, Frackowiak RSJ, Phelps ME. The use of positron emission tomography in the clinical assessment of dementia. Semin Nucl Med 1992; 22:232–46.

18. Lee YH, Seun J, Yoo HS, et al. Effect of Alzheimer's disease and lewy body disease on metabolic chnages. J Alzheimer's Dis 2021;79(4):1471–87.

19. Ibáñez V, Pietrini P, Alexander GE, et al. Regional glucose metabolic abnormalities are not the result of atrophy in Alzheimer's disease. Neurology 1998; 50(6):1585–93.

20. Hunt A, Schönknecht P, Henze M, et al. Reduced cerebral glucose metabolism in patients at risk for Alzheimer's disease. Psych Res Neuroimag 2007; 155(2):147–54.

21. Jagust WJ, Friedland RP, Budinger TF, et al. Longitudinal studies of regional cerebral metabolism in Alzheimer's disease. Neurology 1988;38(6):909.

22. Smith GS, de Leon MJ, George AE, et al. Topography of cross-sectional and longitudinal glucose metabolic deficits in Alzheimer's disease: pathophysiologic implications. Arch Neurol 1992;49(11): 1142–50.

23. Alexander GE, Chen K, Pietrini P, et al. Longitudinal PET evaluation of cerebral metabolic decline in dementia: a potential outcome measure in Alzheimer's disease treatment studies. Am J Psychiatry 2002; 159(5):738–45.

24. Kennedy AM, Newman SK, Frackowiak RS, et al. Chromosome 14 linked familial Alzheimer's disease: a clinico-pathological study of a single pedigree. Brain 1995;118(1):185–205.

25. Newberg A, Cotter A, Udeshi M, et al. A metabolic imaging severity rating scale for the assessment of cognitive impairment. Clin Nucl Med 2003;28(7):565–70.

26. Nobili F, Arbizu J, Drezega A, et al. European Association of Nuclear Medicine and the European Academy of Neurology recommendations for the use of brain 18F-flourodeoxyglucose positron emission tomography in neurodegenerative cognitive impairment and dementia: delphi Consensus. Eur J Neurol 2018;25(10):1201–17.

27. Labbé C, Froment JC, Kennedy A, et al. Positron emission tomography metabolic data corrected for cortical atrophy using magnetic resonance imaging. Alzheimer Dis Assoc Disord 1996;10(3):141–70.

28. Alavi A, Newberg AB, Souder E, et al. Quantitative analysis of PET and MRI data in normal aging and Alzheimer's disease: atrophy weighted total brain metabolism and absolute whole brain metabolism as reliable discriminators. J Nucl Med 1993;34(10): 1681–7.

29. Landau SM, Harvey D, Madison CM, et al. Associations between cognitive, functional, and FDG-PET measures of decline in AD and MCI. Neurobiol Aging 2011;32(7):1207–18.

30. Desgranges B, Baron JC, Lalevée C, et al. The neural substrates of episodic memory impairment in Alzheimer's disease as revealed by FDG-PET: relationship to degree of deterioration. Brain 2002; 125(5):1116–24.

31. Nordberg A, Rinne JO, Kadir A, et al. The use of PET in Alzheimer disease. Nat Rev Neurol 2010;6(2):78.

32. Heiss WD, Kessler J, Slansky I, et al. Activation PET as an instrument to determine therapeutic efficacy in Alzheimer's disease. Ann N Y Acad Sci 1993;695(1): 327–31.

33. Mueller SG, Weiner MW, Thal LJ, et al. Ways toward an early diagnosis in Alzheimer's disease: the Alzheimer's disease neuroimaging initiative (ADNI). Alz Demen 2005;1(1):55–66.

34. Ikonomovic MD, Klunk WE, Abrahamson EE, et al. Post-mortem correlates of *in vivo* PiB-PET amyloid imaging in a typical case of Alzheimer's disease. Brain 2008;131(6):1630–45.

35. Dupont AC, Ribeiro MJ, Guilloteau D, et al. β-amyloid PET neuroimaging: a review of radiopharmaceutical development. Médecine Nucléaire 2017;41(1): 27–35.

36. Sabri O, Tiepolt S, Hesse S, et al. PET imaging of dementia. InDiseases of the brain, head & neck, spine 2012–2015. Milano: Springer; 2012. p. 244–50.

37. Bao W, Xie F, Zuo C, et al. PET neuroimaging of Alzheimer's disease: radiotracers and their utility in clinical research. Front Aging Neurosci 2021;13: 624330.

38. Wong DF, Rosenberg PB, Zhou Y, et al. In vivo imaging of amyloid deposition in Alzheimer disease using the radioligand 18F-AV-45 (flobetapir F 18). J Nucl Med 2010;51(6):913–20.

39. Clark CM, Schneider JA, Bedell BJ, et al. Use of florbetapir-PET for imaging β-amyloid pathology. J Amer Med Assoc 2011;305(3):275–83.

40. Salloway S, Gamez JE, Singh U, et al. Performance of [18F]flutemetamol amyloid imaging against the neuritic plaque component of CERAD and the current (2012) NIA-AA recommendations for the neuropathologic diagnosis of Alzheimer's disease. Alzheimers Dement (Amst) 2017;9:25–34.

41. Jack CR Jr, Lowe VJ, Weigand SD, et al. Serial PIB and MRI in normal, mild cognitive impairment and Alzheimer's disease: implications for sequence of

pathological events in Alzheimer's disease. Brain 2009;132:1355–65.

42. Bullich S, Roé-Vellvé N, Marquié M, et al. Early detection of amyloid load using 18F-florbetaben PET. Alzheimers Res Ther 2021;13:67.

43. Yeo JM, Waddell B, Khan Z, et al. A systematic review and meta-analysis of 18F-labeled amyloid imaging in Alzheimer's disease. Alz Demen 2015; 1(1):5–13.

44. Høilund-Carlsen PF, Barrio JR, Werner TJ, et al. Amyloid hypothesis: the emperor's new clothes? J Alzheimers Dis 2020;78(4):1363–6.

45. Morris E, Chalkidou A, Hammers A, et al. Diagnostic accuracy of 18 F amyloid PET tracers for the diagnosis of Alzheimer's disease: a systematic review and meta-analysis. Eur J Nucl Med Mol Imaging 2016;43(2):374–85.

46. Hornberger J, Michalopoulos S, Dai M, et al. Cost-effectiveness of florbetapir-PET in alzheimer's disease: a Spanish Societal perspective. J Ment Health Policy Econ 2015;18(2):63–73.

47. Martínez G, Vernooij RW, Fuentes Padilla P, et al. 18F PET with florbetapir for the early diagnosis of Alzheimer's disease dementia and other dementias in people with mild cognitive impairment (MCI). Cochrane Database Syst Rev 2017;11: CD012216.

48. Aizenstein HJ, Nebes RD, Saxton JA, et al. Frequent amyloid deposition without significant cognitive impairment among the elderly. Arch Neurol 2008; 65(11):1509–17.

49. Roberts RO, Aakre JA, Kremers WK, et al. Prevalence and outcomes of amyloid positivity among persons without dementia in a longitudinal, population-based setting. JAMA Neurol 2018;75(8): 970–9.

50. Rabinovici GD, Jagust WJ. Amyloid imaging in aging and demen- tia: testing the amyloid hypothesis in vivo. Behav Neurol 2009;21:117–28.

51. Moghbel MC, Saboury B, Basu S, et al. Amyloid-β imaging with PET in Alzheimer's disease: is it feasible with current radiotracers and technologies? Eur J Nucl Med Mol Imaging 2012;39(2):202–8.

52. Rice L, Bisdas S. The diagnostic value of FDG and amyloid PET in Alzheimer's disease—a systematic review. Eur J Radiol 2017;94:16–24.

53. Small GW, Kepe V, Ercoli LM, et al. PET of brain amyloid and tau in mild cognitive impairment. N Eng J Med 2006;355(25):2652–63.

54. Dani M, Brooks DJ, Edison P. Tau imaging in neurodegenerative diseases. Eur J Nucl Med Mol Imaging 2016;43(6):1139–50.

55. Okamura N, Harada R, Furumoto S, et al. Tau PET imaging in Alzheimer's disease. Curr Neurol Neurosci Rep 2014;14(11):500.

56. Chien DT, Bahri S, Szardenings AK, et al. Early clinical PET imaging results with the novel PHF-tau radioligand [F-18]-T807. J Alzheimers Dis 2013;34: 457–68.

57. Okamura N, Furumoto S, Fodero-Tavoletti MT, et al. Non-invasive assessment of Alzheimer's disease neurofibrillary pathology using 18F-THK5105 PET. Brain 2014;137:1762–71.

58. Park JE, Yun J, Kim SJ, et al. Intra-individual correlations between quantitative THK-5351 PET and MRI-derived cortical volume in Alzheimer's disease differ according to disease severity and amyloid positivity. PLoS One 2019;14(12):e0226265.

59. Kuhl DE, Minoshima S, Frey KA, et al. Limited donepezil inhibition of acetylcholinesterase measured with positron emission tomography in living Alzheimer cerebral cortex. Ann Neurol 2000;48(3): 391–5.

60. Pyun JM, Ryoo N, Park YH, et al. Change in cognitive function according to cholinesterase inhibitor use and amyloid PET positivity in patients with mild cognitive impairment. Alzheimers Res Ther 2021;13:10.

61. Keller C, Kadir A, Forsberg A, et al. Long-term effects of galantamine treatment on brain functional activities as measured by PET in Alzheimer's disease patients. J Alzheimers Dis 2011;24(1):109–23.

62. Xu JY, Wang FQ, Shan BC, et al. PET and fMRI to evaluate the results of acupuncture treatment of the cognition of alzheimer's disease. Chin Imaging J Int Trad West Med 2004;2:85–7.

63. Raje S, Patat AA, Parks V, et al. A positron emission tomography study to assess binding of lecozotan, a novel 5-hydroxytryptamine-1A silent antagonist, to brain 5-HT1A receptors in healthy young and elderly subjects, and in patients with Alzheimer's disease. Clin Pharmacol Ther 2008;83(1):86–96.

64. Ketter N, Liu E, Di J, et al. A randomized, double-blind, phase 2 study of the effects of the vaccine Vanutide cridificar with QS-21 adjuvant on immunogenicity, Safety and amyloid imaging in patients with mild to moderate alzheimer's disease. J Prev Alzheimers Dis 2016;3(4):192–201.

65. Knopman DS, Jones DT, Greicius MD. Failure to demonstrate efficacy of aducanumab: an analysis of the EMERGE and ENGAGE trials as reported by Biogen, December 2019. Alzheimers Dement 2021;17(4):696–701.

66. Bang J, Spina S, Miller BL. Frontotemporal dementia. Lancet 2015;386(10004):1672–82.

67. Forman MS, Farmer J, Johnson JK, et al. Frontotemporal dementia: clinicopathological correlations. Ann Neurol 2006;59(6):952–62.

68. Diehl J, Grimmer T, Drzezga A, et al. Cerebral metabolic patterns at early stages of frontotemporal dementia and semantic dementia, a PET study. Neurobiol Aging 2004;25:1051–6.

69. Grimmer T, Diehl J, Drzezga A, et al. Region-specific decline of cerebral glucose metabolism in patients with frontotemporal dementia: a prospective 18F-

FDG-PET study. Dement Geriatr Cogn Disord 2004; 18:32–6.

70. Bejanin A, Tammewar G, Marx G, et al. Longitudinal structural and metabolic changes in frontotemporal dementia. Neurology 2020;95(2):e140–54.

71. Ishii K, Sakamoto S, Sasaki M, et al. Cerebral glucose metabolism in patients with frontotemporal dementia. J Nucl Med 1998;39(11):1875–8.

72. Cerami C, Dodich A, Iannaccone S, et al. Right limbic FDG-PET hypometabolism correlates with emotion recognition and attribution in probable behavioral variant of frontotemporal dementia patients. PLoS One 2015;10(10):e0141672.

73. Tsai RM, Bejanin A, Lesmen-Segev O, et al. 18F-flortaucipir (AV-1451) tau PET in frontotemporal dementia syndromes. Alzheimers Res Ther 2019;11:13.

74. Cagnin A, Rossor M, Sampson EL, et al. In vivo detection of microglial activation in frontotemporal dementia. Ann Neurol 2004;56:894–7.

75. Lant SB, Robinson AC, Thompson JC, et al. Patterns of microglial cell activation in frontotemporal lobar degeneration. Neuropathol Appl Neurobiol 2014; 40(6):686–96.

76. Marquie M, Locascio JJ, Rentz DM, et al. Striatal and extrastriatal dopamine transporter levels relate to cognition in Lewy body diseases: an 11 C altropane positron emission tomography study. Alzheimers Res Ther 2014;6(5–8):52.

77. Graff-Radford J, Lesnick TG, Savica R, et al. 18F-fluorodeoxyglucose positron emission tomography in dementia with Lewy bodies. Brain Commun 2020; 2(1):fcaa040.

78. Kantarci K, Lowe VJ, Chen Q, et al. β-amyloid PET and neuropathology in dementia with Lewy bodies. Neurology 2020;94(3):e282–91.

79. Lim SM, Katsifis A, Villemagne VL, et al. The 18F-FDG PET cingulate island sign and comparison to 123I-beta-CIT SPECT for diagnosis of dementia with Lewy bodies. J Nucl Med 2009;50(10):1638–45.

80. Shimada H, Hirano S, Shinotoh H, et al. Mapping of brain acetylcholinesterase alterations in Lewy body disease by PET. Neurology 2009;73(4):273–8.

81. Foster NL, Heidebrink JL, Clark CM, et al. FDG-PET improves accuracy in distinguishing frontotemporal dementia and Alzheimer's disease. Brain 2007; 130(10):2616–35.

82. de Wilde A, van der Flier WM, Pelkmans, et al. Association of amyloid positron emission tomography with changes in diagnosis and patient treatment in an unselected memory clinic Cohort: the ABIDE project. JAMA Neurol 2018;75(9):1062–70.

83. Ye BS, Lee S, Yoo H, et al. Distinguishing between dementia with Lewy bodies and Alzheimer's disease using metabolic patterns. Neurobiol Aging 2020;87: 11–7.

84. Kantarci K, Boeve BF, Przybelski SA, et al. FDG PET metabolic signatures distinguishing prodromal DLB and prodromal AD. Neuroimage Clin 2021;31: 102754.

85. Garibotto V, Montandon ML, Viaud CT, et al. Regions of interest-based discriminant analysis of DaTSCAN SPECT and FDG-PET for the classification of dementia. Clin Nucl Med 2013;38(3):e112–7.

86. Klein JC, Eggers C, Kalbe E, et al. Neurotransmitter changes in dementia with Lewy bodies and Parkinson disease dementia in vivo. Neurology 2010; 74(11):885–92.

87. Burke JF, Albin RL, Koeppe RA, et al. Assessment of mild dementia with amyloid and dopamine terminal positron emission tomography. Brain 2011;134(Pt 6):1647–57.

# Nonmalignant Thoracic Disorders

## An Appraisal of Fluorodeoxyglucose and Non-fluorodeoxyglucose PET/Computed Tomography Applications

Vandana Kumar Dhingra, DNB[a], Dikhra Khan, MD[b],
Rakesh Kumar, MBBS, DRM, DNB, MNAMS, PhD[b],
Sandip Basu, MBBS, DRM, DNB, MNAMS[c,d,*]

KEYWORDS

• FDG-PET/CT • Nonmalignant thoracic disorders • Tuberculosis • Infection • Inflammation
• Sarcoidosis • Pyrexia of unknown origin • Interstitial lung disease

KEY POINTS

- Thorax consists of various vital and non-vital organs which require routine evaluation with various molecular imaging techniques. We focus on PET/CT based assessment of key non-malignant conditions of the thorax in this review.
- We also focus on the normal patterns and variants of various organs, understanding of which is of key significance in accurately differentiating disease from normal physiological uptake. We discuss various PET tracers like 18F-FDG, 11C- Acetate, 18F- Fluorothymidine (FLT) and 18F- DOPA PET-CT, used for molecular PET imaging in routine practice.
- The most challenging infections like fungal infections, tuberculosis, non-infective inflammatory conditions like sarcoidosis and fever of unknown origin commonly involve thorax, and they are also the common malignancy mimics; we discuss state of the art of PET/CT in these conditions.
- We discuss benign tumours like thymomas, interstitial lung disease and lung transplant assessment using PET/CT.
- It has been seen that the COVID-19 lungs appear to have peripheral ground-glass opacities and/or lung consolidations with increased 18F-FDG uptake and lymph node involvement as a regular feature, the present status of PET/CT in COVID-19 has been briefed.

## INTRODUCTION

Over the past two decades, more than 50,000 papers with keyword PET/computed tomography (CT) have been published. Most of these pertain to the role of PET/CT in malignant diseases or clinical oncology practice. The key words PET/CT and thorax resulted in nearly 1000 papers on the PubMed database. If only systematic reviews and meta-analysis are considered in the area of

The authors have nothing to disclose.
[a] Department of Nuclear Medicine, All India Institute of Medical Sciences, Rishikesh, Uttarakhand 249203, India; [b] Department of Nuclear Medicine, All India Institute of Medical Sciences, Sri Aurobindo Marg, Ansari Nagar, Ansari Nagar East, New Delhi, Delhi 110029, India; [c] Radiation Medicine Centre (B.A.R.C), Tata Memorial Hospital Annexe, Jerbai Wadia Road, Parel, Mumbai, Maharashtra 400012, India; [d] Homi Bhabha National Institute, 2nd floor, BARC Training School Complex, Anushaktinagar, Mumbai, Maharashtra 400094, India
* Corresponding author. Radiation Medicine Centre (B.A.R.C), Tata Memorial Hospital Annexe, Jerbai Wadia Road, Parel, Mumbai 400012, India
E-mail address: drsanb@yahoo.com

PET Clin 17 (2022) 495–515
https://doi.org/10.1016/j.cpet.2022.03.008
1556-8598/22/© 2022 Elsevier Inc. All rights reserved.

thorax, most of the literature is based on oncology, especially lung cancer with emphasis on staging of non–small cell lung cancer. Limited literature exists on PET/CT in nononcologic thoracic diseases including systemic reviews and meta-analyses. The first significant observation of the potential of PET/CT in nonmalignant disorders of the thorax was made in 2002 by Alavi and colleagues,[1] followed by its importance highlighted in another review by Basu and colleagues[2] of the same group. It was thus evident that PET/CT would play a significant role in evaluation of chest even for nonmalignant disorders in the future.

PET/CT evaluation of benign/nonmalignant conditions predominantly involves use of tracer [18]F-fluorodeoxyglucose (FDG). This was largely based on the premise that there is an increase in glucose metabolism in inflammation and infection similar to that in malignant conditions. With the advent of newer PET tracers and PET/MR imaging, the outlook of evaluation of various benign conditions has been changing. In this review, we highlight current developments and areas where PET/CT has a potential to impact the clinical management of nonmalignant thoracic conditions with special focus on non-FDG tracers.

## NORMAL PATTERNS AND COMMON PITFALLS ON PET/COMPUTED TOMOGRAPHY IMAGING OF THE THORAX
### [18]F-Fluorodeoxyglucose PET/Computed Tomography

Normally the vital organs and major structures of the thorax (lungs, heart, thymus, esophagus, bone marrow, and great vessels) show varying (low to moderate) levels of FDG uptake.[3] Such structures as muscles and brown fat may show variations in physiologic uptake depending on temperature and patient activity and metabolic milieu (**Fig. 1**). Focally increased FDG uptake could be observed in associated inflammation and granulation tissues related to various postintervention clinical situations, such as tracheostomy, sternotomy, biopsy with/without chest tubes, and central lines (**Figs. 2 and 3**). These are confounding factors to be noted while interpreting scans. Therapeutic situations, such as radiation (**Fig. 4**), talc pleurodesis, postchemotherapy (**Fig. 5**), and colony-stimulating factors (**Fig. 6**), are known to cause increase in uptake of FDG; however, these may be reported with caution and correlated with corresponding CT findings.

Radiation-induced pneumonitis sets in soon during radiation and reaches its peak between 6 and 12 weeks after radiation therapy. It may be seen in one of the following patterns: subpleural or patchy, diffuse, or peripheral surrounding an area of low or no uptake (primary tumor) (see **Fig. 4**). These could be observed separate from tumors. All patterns were seen nearly in the same frequency by Iravani and colleagues[4,5] in the setting of non–small cell lung cancer. New or progressive pleural effusion postradiation without evidence of tumor progression may also hint toward postradiation effects.

### Non-fluorodeoxyglucose PET Tracers: Normal Physiologic Distribution in the Thorax

#### [11]C-Acetate PET
Lung and mediastinal structures show faint uptake of [11]C-acetate with nearly absent uptake in the normal myocardium on routine protocol of 20 minutes postinjection. Lung uptake is considered to be abnormal whether diffuse (suggestive of parenchymal disease) or focal. A symmetric pattern of lymph node uptake usually represents reactive or inflammatory cause. Any lymphadenopathy related to tumor would be asymmetrical, so in addition to the intensity of uptake and size of lymph nodes the pattern of uptake in [11]C-acetate PET serves as an added advantage to differentiate benign (inflammatory) from malignant lymphadenopathy.[6]

#### [18]F-Fluorothymidine PET
The lung parenchyma shows minimal uptake of this tracer, hence any focal uptake needs evaluation. The heart region may show increased accumulation caused by blood pool and left ventricular myocardial (muscle) uptake. However, this has been overcome by observing that imaging at 45 minutes leads to significant clearance of the blood pool. In a method of kinetic filtering developed by Gray and colleagues,[7] differentiating the physiologic uptake of the healthy heart from breast tumor was possible. This is potentially useful for diagnosing and assessing response assessment of benign disorders.

#### [18]F-DOPA PET
Resembling natural L-DOPA biochemically and possessing similar biokinetics, this neutral amino acid enters the catecholamine metabolic pathway of endogenous L-DOPA in the brain and peripherally. In the thorax, mild uptake is seen physiologically in the myocardium, peripheral muscles, and esophagus; sometimes faint uptake is also noted in the mammary glands (**Fig. 7**). Any kind of uptake seen focally in the lungs is usually considered abnormal; the thorax is the only region where there are no potential confounding factors/pitfalls. With the radiopharmaceutical carbidopa, pretreatment has found to increase uptake in the lungs and

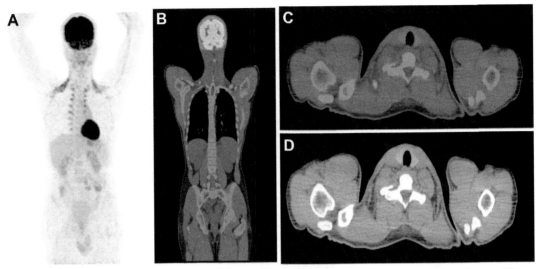

Fig. 1. A 22-year-old male patient came for FDG-PET/CT following treatment of Hodgkin lymphoma. Bilateral FDG uptake was noted at the supraclavicular region and also along the paravertebral region suggestive of brown adipose tissue uptake of FDG at these regions. Maximum intensity projection (MIP) (*A*), coronal (*B*), and axial sections (*C, D*) shows the same.

myocardium in the thorax and must be kept in mind while interpreting the scans after pretreatment with this drug (see **Fig. 7**).[8]

## PET/COMPUTED TOMOGRAPHY IN NON-MALIGNANT DISEASES OF THE THORAX
### Infections

#### Fungal infections
Patients with HIV infection, recipients of solid organ or hematologic stem cell transplants, oncologic patients, and patients with long-standing diabetes mellitus are most prone for systemic or invasive fungal infections. These infections pose a challenge for diagnosis, ascertaining extent of involvement especially at occult sites, and response assessment during and after treatment. Treatments often last for many months, and response seems challenging to monitor; however, PET/CT with FDG has shown promising results in this area.[9]

**Candidiasis** The most serious but rare form of candidiasis is the chronic disseminated form,

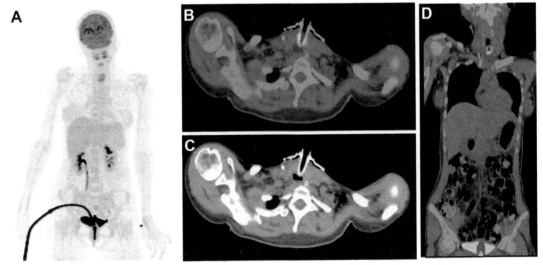

Fig. 2. A 26-year-old female patient diagnosed with autoimmune encephalitis with complaints of seizure underwent FDG-PET/CT. The MIP (*A*), transaxial PET (*B*), CT (*C*), and coronal (*D*) PET/CT images showed increased FDG activity along the vicinity of tracheostomy tube.

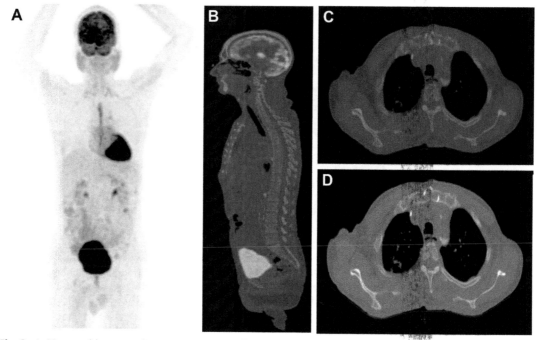

Fig. 3. A 47-year-old man underwent FDG-PET/CT for baseline lung lesion evaluation that revealed FDG uptake along the sternal region on MIP (*A*), fused sagittal (*B*), transaxial PET/CT (*C*), and CT transaxial (*D*) images. Retrospectively it was clarified that he underwent coronary artery bypass graft procedure 4 months back.

encountered in the immunocompromised patients. Currently, [18]F-FDG PET/CT has shown its major impact in two areas: for assessing the extent of involvement in systemic candidiasis including occult sites; and in assessing response to therapy, which is not clearly detected with anatomic/radiologic modalities. In *Candida*- induced lung abscess, normalization of uptake was noted by 8 to 10 weeks with FDG-PET/CT.[10] Soon, FDG-PET/CT may guide monitoring and therapy for systemic candidiasis.

Cryptococcosis *Cryptococcus neoformans* is a ubiquitous encapsulated yeast-like fungus. It is a rare infection transmitted through inhalation and involves lungs most exclusively in immunocompromised patients. It commonly appears as single nodule or masslike and bronchopneumonic pattern and is challenging to differentiate from malignancy with imaging alone.

Recently [68]Ga-Pentixafor was described to demonstrate uptake in cryptococcosis of lungs and this tracer may have potential to be used for

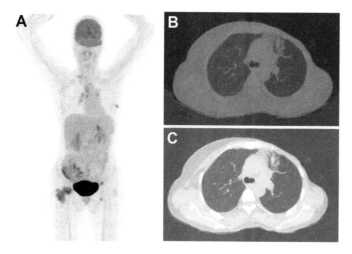

Fig. 4. A 41-year-old female patient with a known case of left carcinoma breast underwent surgery and received neoadjuvant chemotherapy and radiotherapy for metastatic disease. Post radiation therapy FDG-PET/CT showed multiple FDG-avid skeletal and soft tissue lesions in the chest region (residual disease) along with fibroreticular changes and air bronchogram and pleural-based patchy consolidation in left lung upper lobe suggestive of post-radiation pneumonitis on MIP (*A*), transaxial PET (*B*), and CT (*C*) images.

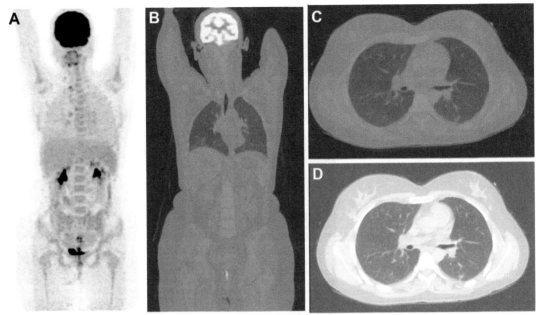

Fig. 5. A 31-year-old woman presented with a known case of Hodgkin lymphoma and who was treated with five cycles of ABVD chemotherapy regimen, underwent FDG-PET/CT as part of follow-up. The MIP and transaxial images of the lungs (A–C) show mild diffusely increased FDG uptake observed in bilateral lungs with no CT changes (D), a sign of early bleomycin toxicity.

this condition.[11] The postulated mechanism for this was the upregulated CXCR4 expression found in activated inflammatory cells in addition to the tumor cells.

**Histoplasmosis** Histoplasmosis, caused by *Histoplasma capsulatum*, causes cavitating pulmonary fungal lesions. Pulmonary findings include consolidation in the acute form of the disease and sharply defined nodules in the chronic form of the disease.[9] FDG-avid solitary pulmonary nodules posing a diagnostic dilemma may be imaged in dual time point. The trend of reduced FDG uptake after antifungal treatment may support the diagnosis of histoplasmosis.[12]

**Pulmonary aspergillosis** [18]F-FDG-PET/CT can help to differentiate between invasive (multiple hypermetabolic nodules with higher standardized *uptake* value [SUV]) and noninvasive (solitary isometabolic nodules with a halo pattern) aspergillosis.[9] As in oncology, detecting extrapulmonary lesions is of importance in aspergillosis. Among benign lesions of the lungs, fungal infections show the highest SUV of about 7.0.[13] [18]F-FDG-PET/CT has shown potential in monitoring antifungal therapy (especially for aspergillosis) through global total lesional glycolysis and metabolic volume, potentially useful parameters to predict metabolic response. Ankrah and colleagues[14]

showed that PET/CT led to change in management in 93%, prolongation of therapy in 64%, and change in plan for 28% of cases. A newer mAb-based PET tracer [64]Cu-DOTA-JF5 has been tried for imaging aspergillosis in the preclinical setting, and has shown clinical potential.[15] [68]Ga-labelled siderophores have also been used as potential probes for aspergillosis.[16]

**Coccidiomycosis** Coccidiomycosis is a fungal disease secondary to inhalation of the arthroconidia form of *Coccidioides immitis*. The commonly known three clinical stages are acute phase (manifests as infiltrates, consolidation, adenopathies, and pleural effusion), chronic phase (as nodular coccidioidomas, lung cavities, fibrosis, bronchiectasis, and scarring), and the disseminated phase (often harbor extrapulmonary lesions).[9,17] Most commonly confused with malignancy, nonresponse to antineoplastic therapy may be a clue.

**Mucormycosis and blastomycosis** Both these fungal infections involve lungs in systemic disease and the former is more common in persons with diabetes. Lung involvement may present with nonspecific symptoms, such as fever, cough, hemoptysis, chest pain, and dyspnea, with lesions showing increased FDG uptake. Pulmonary blastomycosis may appear as pulmonary nodules not differentiable from malignancy/metastasis.

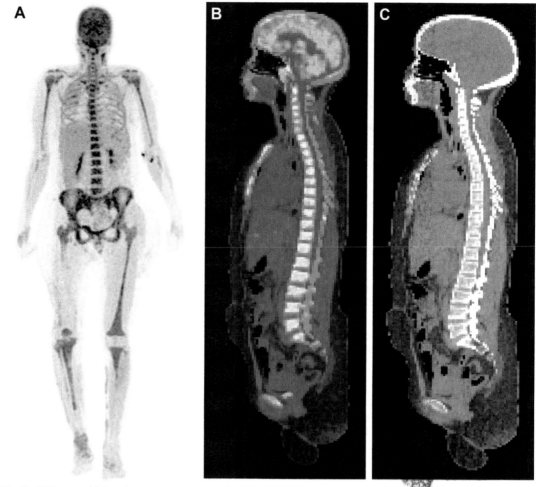

Fig. 6. A 23-year-old female patient, diagnosed with Ewing sarcoma in right thigh, underwent FDG-PET/CT post-surgery and postchemotherapy. She was also administered granulocyte colony–stimulating factor for bone marrow stimulation. The illustrated images show increased tracer uptake noted in marrow of long bones, pelvis, and vertebrae in the MIP (A) and sagittal PET (B) and CT (C) sectional slides of the patient.

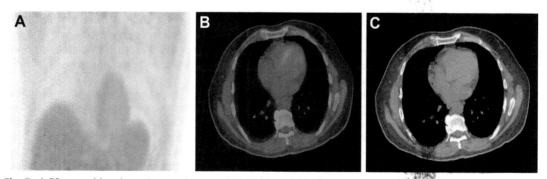

Fig. 7. A 50-year-old male patient underwent 18F-FDOPA PET/CT for assessment of cardiac uptake of 18F-FDOPA in patients with heart failure. The pre-treatment with carbidopa has shown mildly increased uptake in lungs and myocardium in the thorax as shown in MIP (A) and transaxial PET (B) and CT (C) section slices of thorax.

### Bacterial infections

**Syphilis** Predominant among the young, syphilis is a sexually transmitted systemic disease caused by the spirochete *Treponema pallidum*. Various stages of this disease (primary, secondary, tertiary, and latent), which occur when left untreated, mimic malignancies and are diagnosed on [18]F-FDG PET/CT scan, especially tertiary syphilis. Five types of patterns were observed (uptake at the site of inoculation or in the regional lymph nodes in primary syphilis). In secondary syphilis depending on organ involved increased uptake was seen in lung, bone, gastrointestinal involvement, or generalized lymphadenopathy. In tertiary syphilis variable pattern of increased glucose metabolic activity, hypometabolic lesions, or normal glucose uptake were seen. The mean pretreatment maximum SUV (SUVmax) was observed to be 6.99 ± 2.47 (range, 3.60–10.30).[18]

Pulmonary involvement of secondary syphilis is characterized by increased tracer uptake in nodules, except small nodules of subcentimetric size that do not show [18]F-FDG uptake. Hilar and mediastinal lymphadenopathy may be observed in the thorax in secondary syphilis with generalized lymphadenopathy. In these scenarios, the diagnosis may be clinched by the resolution of lesions after adequate penicillin therapy. Differential diagnosis includes other malignant conditions, such as primary lung tumor and metastasis, and other benign conditions, such as tuberculosis, fungal infection, and sarcoidosis. Tertiary syphilis presents as space-occupying lesions in visceral organs and hence often poses a diagnostic dilemma mimicking cancer.

Early or latent syphilis manifesting as aortitis is diagnosed on [18]F-FDG-PET/CT and holds prognostic significance because if left undiagnosed and untreated it may lead to aortic root dilatation and thus aortic insufficiency. A subtype of neurosyphilis may present as hypermetabolic enlarged lymph node in the symmetric bilateral cervical, axillary, hilar, tracheobronchial, portocaval, iliac, or inguinal regions, without abnormal FDG uptake in the brain.

In syphilitic aortitis, [18]F-FDG-PET showed marked radiotracer enhancement along the ascending aortic wall or in the thoracoabdominal aorta with involvement of the brachiocephalic and left carotid arteries. In syphilitic thoracic aneurysm, [18]F-FDG-PET shows increased metabolic activity, or no enhanced uptake. [18]F-FDG-PET may be useful in differentiating syphilitic aortic aneurysm from active vasculitis and is useful in assessing disease extent. It has been shown that follow-up [18]F-FDG PET scan after prescribed therapy with antibiotics resulted in resolution of abnormal uptakes, which corresponded to clinical improvement and serologic markers. Non-FDG tracers have not been highlighted in the management of syphilis.

### Tuberculosis

An important communicable disease in the developing world, tuberculosis has often posed a diagnostic and therapeutic enigma to attending physicians. In **Table 1**, the role of PET/CT (mainly FDG) is enumerated, as elaborated in the scientific literature.[19–21]

**Parenchymal disease with consolidation and associated lymphadenopathy** This is the commonest presentation of children with tuberculosis. Lymphadenopathy is the hallmark of primary tuberculosis in the pediatric age group but may be indistinguishable from lymphoma or sarcoidosis-associated lymphadenopathy. CT characteristic of a central hypodense lymphadenopathy, which is larger than 2 cm, indicates active disease. [18]F-FDG PET/CT helps to diagnose active pulmonary tuberculomas effectively because active tuberculomas have a high FDG uptake up to an SUV of 42 (**Fig. 8**). Postprimary tuberculosis seen in adolescents and young adults shows cavitary upper lobe involvement with absence of lymphadenopathy.

**Miliary tuberculosis** Although uncommon (<2%), this form is seen in immunocompromised children as diffusely increased FDG uptake in less than 2-mm-sized diffuse pulmonary and extrapulmonary miliary infiltrates (**Fig. 9**).[19] Miliary tuberculosis is a therapeutic challenge because of hepatotoxicity with common drugs. [18]F-FDG PET/CT for response assessment and early intervention for stoppage may be of potential in this subgroup.[22]

**Pleural effusion/involvement** Considered as an early complication of the primary infection and as extrapulmonary disease commonly in older individuals, pleural effusions are usually unilateral with ipsilateral lung involvement (see **Fig. 8**). With moderate to high FDG uptake, effusions may show diffuse variable degrees of uptake.[23]

**Extrapulmonary tuberculosis in thorax** Nearly half of skeletal tuberculosis involves spine (Pott disease); it typically begins at the anterior vertebral body near end plates and spondylitis with involvement of posterior elements. Sclerosis with bony destruction with increased FDG uptake involving posterior elements and soft tissue involvement is seen, with later complications, such as gibbous deformity (**Fig. 10**). A negative PET/CT study practically rules out active disease.[24]

**Table 1**
**The Potential roles of PET/CT in Tuberculosis**

| Time Point in Management | Utility Areas (Advantage of PET) |
| --- | --- |
| At initial diagnosis | Assessment of fever of unknown origin (whole-body imaging) |
| | Characterization/evaluation of lung nodule (metabolic activity) |
| | Characterization/evaluation of lymphadenopathy (pattern, metabolic uptake) |
| | Characterization/evaluation of asthenia, cachexia, and anorexia (whole-body imaging) |
| | Occult sites (high-resolution hybrid imaging PET/CT, PET/MR imaging) |
| | Guiding site selection for biopsy (PET/CT-guided biopsy) |
| For evaluation of disease extent | Detection of sites of tuberculosis lesions including extrapulmonary and occult sites (whole-body imaging) |
| | Assessment of disease activity (corresponding to the metabolic activity and degree of uptake) |
| | Differentiation between active and latent disease (anatomic vs metabolic abnormality) |
| | Assessment of disease extent (whole-body imaging) |
| Treatment response related | Interim assessment for change of ineffective therapy (semiquantitative methods) |
| | Early stoppage or limiting use of toxic therapies |
| | End of treatment response assessment: residual disease requiring further therapy |
| | In challenging situations, such as spinal tuberculosis and genital tuberculosis |
| | Recurrent disease assessment |
| | Imaging marker for assessment of response in new drug trials |

Two imaging patterns have been described for pulmonary tuberculosis on FDG PET: the lung and lymph node pattern. The lung pattern includes lesions involving lung parenchyma with mildly increased uptake. Cold lesions are also seen; however, these are mostly old healed lesions that stay the same over years. The cavitary lesions show heterogenous uptake depending on disease activity within the lesions. Calcification and satellite lesions are other features of tuberculosis. The lymph node pattern includes predominantly larger and more intense chest (hilar and mediastinal) nodes. Tuberculosis lesions reveal increase in uptake of SUV of 10 to 12.

**Challenging areas in tuberculosis**

[a] *$^{18}$F-FDG-PET/CT in prognostication of active disease*: It has been reported that the degree of FDG uptake (SUV lesion/SUV-liver ratio) directly correlates with size of lesion and this in turn is directly related to response according to World Health Organization (WHO) criteria.[20,25] The FDG uptake has been described as nearly independent of immune status of the patient.

[b] *Differentiating active tuberculosis from malignant lesions*: This is one of the most challenging areas especially in pulmonary involvement. With such techniques as dual time point imaging and using non-FDG tracers, response to antitubercular therapy has been used for this differentiation[26] but significant overlap exists.

[c] *Response to therapy*: Assessing response to therapy in tuberculosis is a challenging task. As a rule of thumb, response is accompanied by reduction in FDG uptake because of reduction of inflammation. Sputum culture at 2 months is the most widely accepted marker for predicting a favorable outcome, but it has limited use in predicting relapse (pooled sensitivity is 40%).

In assessing quantitative response to therapy in patients with multidrug-resistant tuberculosis using $^{18}$F-FDG PET/CT, it is observed that most responding subjects had at least a 50% decrease

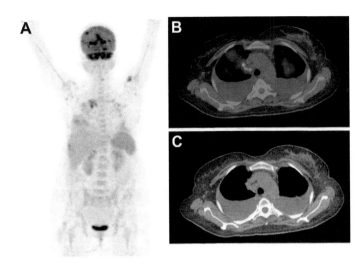

Fig. 8. A 45-year-old female patient on antitubercular treatment for the past 6 months came for follow-up FDG-PET/CT. The MIP (A) showed infective changes and multiple mediastinal nodes along with massive pleural effusion in bilateral lungs on axial PET (B) and CT (C).

in overall FDG avidity at 2 months with minimal changes on high-resolution (HR) CT parameters, with nonresponders showing increased or no change in glycolytic activity. Thus it was concluded that PET/CT performed better than liquid culture test. Sood and colleagues[27] recommend assessment of interim response at 3 to 4 months as a better predictor for clinical outcome.

**Nonfluorodeoxyglucose PET tracers for tuberculosis** Although fairly useful, the lack of specificity with FDG made it imperative for other radiotracers to be explored in tuberculosis.[18]F-Alfatide II PET/CT showed lower uptake in tuberculosis; this

was caused by poor expression of integrin. Chronic inflammation showed higher degrees of uptake, whereas sarcoidosis showed low degrees of uptake. [18]F-Alfatide II PET/CT has been postulated to be useful for differentiating tuberculosis from malignant lesions and nontubercular chronic inflammation but not from sarcoid lesions.[28] Tubercular lesions showed low uptake on [11]C-choline. [11]C-Choline uptake was found to be independent of size of the lesions vis-à-vis [18]F-FDG. The uptake of FDG was found to be proportionate to tumor size in malignant lesions and tubercular lesions; however, [11]C-choline uptake was constant for all sizes of tumors and tubercular lesions (around 3.5 and 2, respectively).[29]

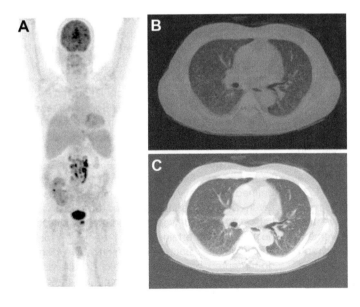

Fig. 9. A 50-year-old male patient who is diagnosed with miliary tuberculosis for 6 months with a history of renal transplant, came for 18F-FDG PET/CT for response assessment post antituberculosis treatment. Axial PET (B) and CT (C) images showed mildly FDG-avid multiple diffuse tiny nodules uniformly distributed in bilateral lungs. MIP (A) image also showed multiple FDG-avid abdominal lymph nodes.

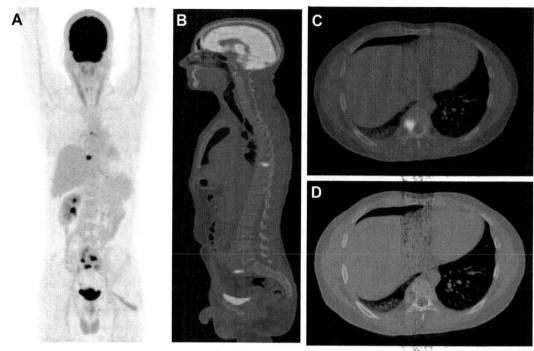

**Fig. 10.** A 33-year-old male patient diagnosed with vertebral tuberculosis underwent FDG-PET/CT for evaluation of disease status. MIP (*A*), fused sagittal (*B*), transaxial PET (*C*), and CT transaxial slice (*D*) showed FDG-avid lytic lesions with right paravertebral extraosseous soft tissue thickening involving the body and right pedicle of eighth thoracic vertebra.

A tumor-imaging agent, an earlier report showed that ratio between SUVmax of [18]F-fluorothymidine and [18]F-FDG was found to be of great potential in assessment of tuberculosis by its potential to separate subgroups of patients having malignancy, tuberculosis, and other benign lesions. Conversely, a recent analysis concluded that [18]F-fluorothymidine PET/CT could not reliably differentiate benign and malignant lesions; this area needs further studies.[30] A preliminary study using [68]Ga-citrate showed that by comparison [18]F-FDG detects more abnormal lesions in tuberculosis; the full potential of [68]Ga-citrate is not yet known.[31]

### Other infectious conditions

HIV/AIDS HIV/AIDS is associated with opportunistic infections and malignancies, and [18]F-FDG-PET/CT can play an essential role in evaluating disease burden and extent of involvement in various stages of the disease. Many of these have been defined in the recent years. [18]F-FDG-PET/CT has been observed to characterize midstages (Centers for Disease Control and Prevention stage B2) of the disease with active involvement stages of mediastinal, hilar, and axillary lymph node groups. CD4 counts and viral load need to be correlated while interpreting [18]F-FDG-PET/CT findings in patients with HIV. [18]F-FDG-PET/CT may be specifically useful in stage C1 to C3 for assessing infections and malignancies, although it is challenging to differentiate between the two.[32]

[18]F-FDG-PET/CT findings have been shown to correspond to viral load. Negative or suppressed patients (on highly active antiretroviral therapy) showed no abnormal FDG uptake except a rare mild axillary uptake, whereas patients with early or advanced disease or patients who stopped highly active antiretroviral therapy (when scanned after few days) showed uptake in lymph node groups and other regions as per the stage of disease.[33]

Most studies in the HIV population have been done with FDG. [68]Ga-Pentixafor has recently been investigated for its potential for evaluation of arterial inflammation in the setting of HIV.[34]

Fever of unknown origin or bacteremia of unknown origin Fever of unknown origin (FUO) is defined classically as an intermittent, unresolved fever, with temperatures higher than 38.3°C, and lasting at least 3 weeks without a definite diagnosis being ascertained after 1 week of in-patient investigations. Bacteremia of unknown origin is documented bacteremia on blood cultures with no localizing features. The commonest three etiologies are infection, malignancy, and noninfectious inflammatory diseases. [18]F-FDG-PET/CT may be used to localize or exclude a site as the potential cause for the fever.[35]

[18]F-FDG-PET/CT plays an important role in the search for potential diagnostic clues as a whole-body imaging tool (Fig. 11). [67]Ga, an important scintigraphic modality for assessment of FUO in the past, has lost to [18]F-FDG-PET/CT because of its shorter imaging times, better resolution, and even cost-effectiveness.[36] [18]F-FDG-PET/CT has been used as a guiding tool to hold antibiotic therapy in patients with staphylococcus bacteremia.[37]

Bharucha and colleagues[38] showed pooled diagnostic yield of 56% (95% confidence interval, 50%–61%; $I^2$ = 61%) from 18 studies and 905 patients for [18]F-FDG-PET/CT in FUO, a yield beyond conventional CT at 32% (95% confidence interval, 22%–44%; $I^2$ = 66%) was noted. Data suggest maximum usefulness of [18]F-FDG-PET/CT in FUO because of noninfectious inflammatory diseases, especially rheumatoid etiology and for guiding biopsy.[39] Pneumonias and tuberculosis along with large vessel vasculitis and sarcoidosis were the most common thoracic causes for FUO.

The most common involved site is lung for infection-related FUO and tuberculosis is the most common pathogen.[18]F-FDG-PET/CT made a diagnostic impact on nearly 90% of patients and helped guide site for biopsy for definitive diagnosis. The recommended indications for [18]F-FDG-PET/CT scan in FUO include postoperative fever and recurrent sepsis, immunodeficiency-related FUO, neutropenic fever, and isolated acute-phase inflammation markers (persistently raised C-reactive protein and/or erythrocyte sedimentation rate).[40]

No particular non-[18]F-FDG radiotracer has proven to be singularly effective in evaluation of FUO. However [18]F-FDG-labeled white blood cells may be explored for FUO. False-negative findings of [18]F-FDG white blood cell PET or PET/CT may arise because of poor host immune reaction, low virulence, or chronic infections; however, its full potential for FUO and bacteremia of unknown origin is yet to be explored.

## Benign Tumors of Thorax

### Characterization of thymic masses: thymoma and rebound thymic hyperplasia

Fluorodeoxyglucose PET/computed tomography Normally thymus is a triangular or bilobed structure with homogenous parenchyma and absence of any mass effects, which does not show uptake higher than background on [18]F-FDG-PET/CT. On any increase in thymic uptake commonly rebound thymic hyperplasia must be considered. Such factors as [18]F-FDG uptake, size, and CT characteristics have been found to be significantly different than in tumor infiltrative thymus and rebound thymic hyperplasia. A mean SUV of 2.8 and homogeneous soft tissue attenuation with convex margins is the usual finding in rebound thymic hyperplasia.

Thymic epithelial tumors are the most common adult anterior mediastinal tumors, with thymoma

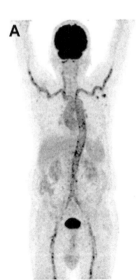
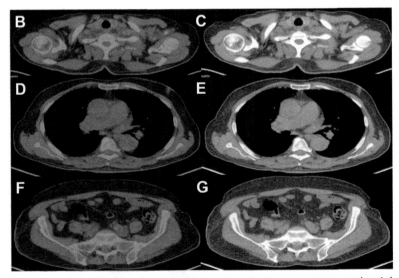

Fig. 11. A 77-year-old male patient presented with fever for 4 weeks, evening rise in temperature, and weight loss. He was diagnosed with pyrexia of unknown origin and underwent FDG-PET/CT to diagnose the underlying pathology. The MIP (A) and multiple axial PET (B, D, F) and CT (C, E, G) sections showed increased FDG uptake in multiple large- and medium-sized vessels throughout the body, suggestive of vasculitis.

comprising about 37.3%. Thymic tumors may be benign (thymomas) or malignant, which include all others, such as thymic carcinomas, neuroendocrine tumors, germ cell tumors, or lymphomas of the thymus. Kumar and colleagues[41] showed that [18]F-FDG-PET/CT could help to characterize thymic masses (seen on conventional modalities) into benign and malignant (Fig. 12). These findings were further consolidated by Ito and colleagues,[42] who showed that [18]F-FDG uptake on PET/CT has been found to correlate with grade of thymic tumors (WHO); enabled classification into low grade (eg, WHO A, AB), higher grades (B1, B2, B3), and carcinomas; and may even be able to predict WHO grades. FDG uptake was able to predict thymoma from carcinoma and graded thymomas from each other and from carcinomas. A cutoff of 5.4 was suggested for high- and low-grade thymomas and 7.4 for high-grade thymomas and thymic carcinomas; this was found to be reasonably accurate. Invasive thymic epithelial tumors were found to have higher cutoff of SUVs than noninvasive ones. Dual time point [18]F-FDG-PET/CT imaging has also been used for further characterization of thymic masses into benign or malignant.

Detecting ectopic thymomas in the mediastinum and establishing the diagnosis is essential from a prognostic point of view because they are completely resectable. Ectopic thymomas in middle mediastinum, although rare, may be detected on CT as paratracheal lymph nodes and may be further characterized by PET/CT. Usually thymomas are not considered as a differential in paratracheal nodules or middle mediastinal masses; however, their malignant potential and excellent prognosis on complete resection mandated them to be considered as an important differential. One must be aware of other sites of ectopic thymomas, such as lungs and thorax, which although rare, do exist.

**Non-fluorodeoxyglucose PET/computed tomography in thymoma and other thymic masses**
Thymoma has been shown to demonstrate an intensive choline uptake with a mean SUVmax of approximately 8.6. Higher uptake was noted in invasive thymomas of higher grade (eg, WHO B2).These findings have mostly been detected and reported incidentally while assessing choline PET ([11]C or [18]F) images for other established indications, such as prostate cancer. However, the potential of using these PET radiopharmaceuticals for thymic evaluation has been mentioned and needs to be examined. Similarly, [68]Ga-PSMA has also shown avidity in thymoma, although this agent was primarily used for assessment of prostate cancer imaging. [68]Ga-DOTA-TOC/NOC/TATE PET studies has potential to detect more lesions in thymic tumors with neuroendocrine component.[43,44]

*Other benign tumors: Castleman disease*
Castleman disease (CD), also known as angiofollicular or giant lymph node hyperplasia, is a benign complex lymphoproliferative disease found most commonly in the mediastinum, and is unicentric or multicentric (UCD or MCD) (Fig. 13). Most UCDs arise in the mediastinum. Other sites include hila, axillae, pleural space, chest wall, and extrapleural soft tissues. Radiologically UCD appear as well-defined highly enhancing masses. Differentials include masses of thyroid, paragangliomas, parathyroid adenomas, and hemangiomas (Figs. 14 and 15). UCD shows moderate uptake of [18]F-

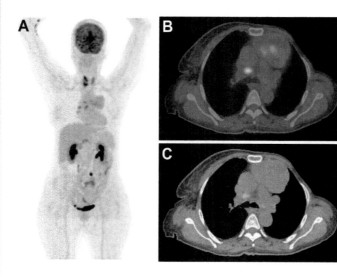

Fig. 12. A 69-year-old male patient was diagnosed with thymoma came for FDG-PET/CT postsurgery and postradiotherapy. MIP (*A*), transaxial PET (*B*), and CT (*C*) images showed lobulated soft tissue mass measuring 5.5 × 3.8 cm with heterogenous FDG uptake in the right lung paramediastinal region abutting ascending aorta and right atrium closely adherent to the pericardium along with mediastinal lymph node involvement.

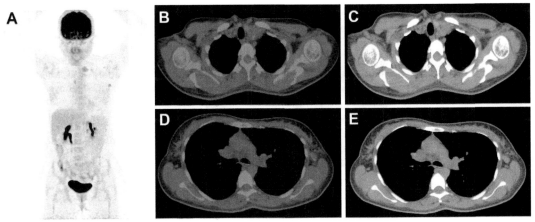

Fig. 13. A 40-year-old female patient was diagnosed with multicentric Castleman disease and was treated with steroids for 6 months. FDG PET/CT (*A*) demonstrates tracer-avid discrete lymph node in left supraclavicular location measuring 2.8 × 1.5 cm (*B, C*) and another left axillary level I lymph node measuring 2 × 1.2 cm (*D, E*) with significant FDG uptake.

FDG, similar to paragangliomas and other benign tumors. This helps exclude other high vascularity (enhancing pattern of these lesions) lesions, such as hemangiomas and thyroid goiters, which show mostly no [18]F-FDG uptake.[45] In MCD, diffuse pattern of hypermetabolic lymphadenopathy most pronounced in the axilla, neck, and mediastinum is noted and PET/CT is useful for response assessment (see **Fig. 13**).

Differentiation from paragangliomas may be made with [131]I-MIBG imaging. Differential diagnosis in anterior mediastinal UCD includes such tumors as Hodgkin lymphoma, germ cell tumors, and thymic epithelial neoplasms. In UCD of posterior mediastinum neurogenic and solitary fibrous tumors of pleura are differentials. UCDs have more pronounced enhancement on CT and more intense FDG uptake than benign peripheral nerve sheath tumors, such as schwannomas and neurofibromas. Solitary fibrous tumors of the pleura may mimic posterior mediastinal UCD but they are usually larger and heterogeneous in appearance, with areas of fluid attenuation or signal intensity that do not enhance secondary to necrosis or myxoid degeneration. These tumors show faint FDG uptake compared with UCD. However, malignant solitary fibrous tumors show high [18]F-FDG uptake.

**Non-fluorodeoxyglucose PET tracers in the setting of Castleman disease** [99m]Tc-HYNIC-TOC (SSTR imaging) has been used in CD. [68]Ga-DOTATATE may be used in conjunction with [18]F-FDG, especially in MCD of mediastinum, because both tracers have been demonstrated to be taken up by this tumor.

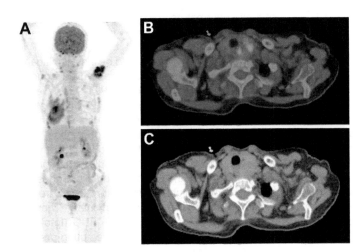

Fig. 14. A 60-year-old female patient with a known case of osteosarcoma left humerus visited for baseline staging FDG-PET/CT, which revealed lytic FDG-avid primary lesion on the left humerus with multiple other skeletal involvement. Incidentally a heterogenous lesion of 2.3 × 2.1 × 2.5 cm was noted in the posteroinferior region to the left lobe of thyroid with mild FDG uptake on MIP (*A*), transaxial PET (*B*), and CT (*C*) images. On biochemical evaluation parathyroid hormone and calcium were found to be elevated suggestive of parathyroid adenoma.

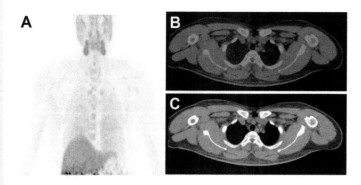

**Fig. 15.** A 28-year-old male patient with primary hyperthyroidism, intact para-thyroid hormone levels of 189.4 mg/dL, and serum calcium levels of 11.9 mg/dL came for 18F-fluorocholine PET/CT for further evaluation. The MIP (A) and transaxial images shows intense choline-avid soft tissue density lesion measuring 7.8 × 1.1 × 19 mm between the right brachiocephalic trunk just behind the medial end of right clavicle (B, C).

## Interstitial Lung Disease

Interstitial lung diseases (ILD) are a heterogeneous group of disorders that are characterized by a variable degree of fibrosis and inflammation in the pulmonary interstitium. They may occur as idiopathic diseases, or be associated with connective tissue disorders, or result from exposures to environmental agents and drugs.

For all descriptive purposes and to understand the pathologic processes, the pulmonary interstitium is divided into three zones: axial (hilum and bronchovascular tree); peripheral (the interlobular septa and pleura); and intralobular (connective tissue of the alveolar walls). The secondary pulmonary lobule is the smallest functional pulmonary unit that is surrounded by connective tissue (ie, interlobular septa and septal structures). These structures are important for imaging descriptions during PET/CT and HRCT.[46]

Imaging modalities include plain radiographs, CT scan, MR imaging, and PET/CT. Plain radiographs lack sensitivity and specificity. HRCT is highly sensitive and can form a firm base for guiding further diagnostic or interventional procedures, such as bronchoalveolar lavage and lung biopsies for final diagnosis. MR imaging is highly sensitive to recognize parenchymal changes associated with inflammatory changes and recognizes perfusion abnormalities associated with CT changes in ILD.

### *18F-Fluorodeoxyglucose PET/computed tomography and conventional imaging techniques in interstitial lung disease*

Idiopathic pulmonary fibrosis (IPF), also known as usual interstitial pneumonia, and nonspecific interstitial pneumonia (NSIP) are subtypes of ILD and although CT scan may describe extent of involvement is often unable to predict course of disease. PET/CT has been examined for prognostication of both these subtypes of ILD because they have an unpredictable disease course.[47]

IPF typically show enhanced FDG uptake including in patients with IPF showing normal patterns on chest CT. In NSIP, CT typically shows bilateral, symmetric ground glass opacities (GGOs) and predominant pattern of basal reticular opacities with traction bronchiectasis and associated volume loss. This is supported with histology. Diagnosis of NSIP is not challenging; however, its prognostication remains elusive with conventional modalities. 18F-FDG-PET/CT shows increased uptake in all areas of active inflammation in ILD. Areas found to be fibrotic as per HRCT but with active inflammatory component also show increased uptake on 18F-FDG-PET/CT, and therefore show potentially reversible lesions.

Prognostic correlation with PET/CT was found to be better than with HRCT (Fig. 16). Extent of involvement (ie, area of involvement) has been found to be directly related to prognosis because uptake and inflammation would respond to treatment and fibrotic areas (areas of no or low uptake) would not be amenable to response/improvement. Respiratory gating can help improve assessment of these parameters.

Among the two variants (ie, fibrotic and inflammatory), it is assumed that the role of PET in fibrotic-predominant ILD would be less significant, and we expect inflammatory-predominant conditions to be hypermetabolic on PET. However, it has been seen that areas of high 18F-FDG uptake are also seen even in fibrotic ILD on CT. This is less than expected and higher uptake has been seen in areas with reticulation and honeycombing when compared with ground glass regions.[48] There is evidence in some studies suggesting that areas with higher SUV in fibrotic ILD represented a poorer prognosis functionally. There is also suggestion of increased 18F-FDG uptake in areas with normal CT, probably depicting preclinical disease. This needs further clarifications. In a

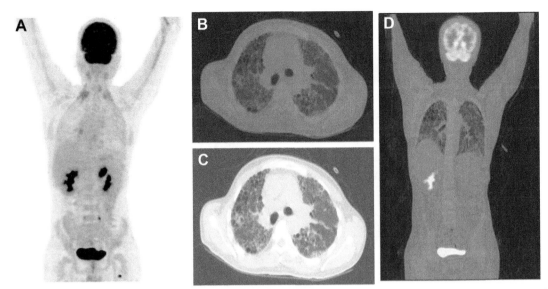

**Fig. 16.** A 40-year-old male patient who is a known smoker for 20 years and later on diagnosed with interstitial lung disease, came for FDG PET/CT before lung transplant as part of presurgical work-up to assess the level of involvement and the uptake of activity. MIP image (*A*) shows diffuse heterogenous lung uptake noted in bilateral lungs. Fused transaxial PET/CT (*B*) and CT (*C*) sections of thorax and fused coronal whole-body PET/CT (*D*) shows diffuse ground glass changes with interstitial thickening and superimposed reticular changes showing mild metabolic activity on FDG in bilateral lungs resulting in classic honeycombing appearance.

few studies, dual time point $^{18}$F-FDG-PET/CT showing positive retention index of $^{18}$F-FDG was associated with higher fibroblast activity and poorer prognosis.[49] Further studies in dual time point imaging are required to ascertain these preliminary findings.

## Nonfluorodeoxyglucose PET/computed tomography in interstitial lung disease

$^{18}$F-Fluorocholine has shown increased tracer uptake in nonmalignant inflammation in various situations. Patterns of physiologic uptake of choline (F-18 or C-11) in the thorax need to be understood along with common benign conditions showing significant uptake on choline PET. This may be used in assessment of ILDs.[50] In a study targeting activity-based probes targeting cysteine cathepsins, the $^{68}$Ga-BMV101 PET/CT probe showed exciting results in humans for differentiating interstitial lung disease (IPF variety) from unclassified fibrosis or normal control subjects.[51] Win and colleagues[52] demonstrated uptake of $^{68}$Ga-somatostatin-labeled compounds in diffuse parenchymal lung disease. They showed accumulation of $^{68}$Ga-DOTATATE and $^{18}$F-FDG. The distribution of parenchymal uptake was similar, with both tracers corresponding to the distribution of HRCT changes.

In a preclinical study by Bondue and colleagues[53] $^{18}$F-4-fluorobenzamido-N-ethylamino-maleimide ($^{18}$F-FBEM)–labelled leukocytes increased

localization of labeled leukocytes in early days when inflammation was induced and reduced over days when fibrosis took over. Human studies are yet to explore the potential of this imaging tool.

Similarly, Desogere and colleagues[54] used a peptide-based PET probe ($^{68}$Ga-CBP8) that targets collagen type I, which showed high specificity for pulmonary fibrosis and could have potential for monitoring response as demonstrated in animal models. Clinical proof-of-concept study using the potential of a novel F-18 folate-based agent (18F-AzaFol) as an imaging tool for the visualization of macrophage-driven fibrotic lung diseases opens up the potential of futuristic agents for imaging of this disease.[55]

## Sarcoidosis

Sarcoidosis is a granulomatous systemic disease with unknown cause. Varying degrees of inflammation of involved organs is the key feature (**Fig. 17**) with interpatient and intrapatient heterogeneity in disease severity and response to treatment.[56] Assessment is done with clinical features (eg, uveitis in the eye, granulomas in lungs); biochemistry (eg, serum calcium and ACE (Angiotensin-Converting Enzyme ) levels); conventional imaging modalities, such as radiography, CT, and MR imaging; and functional imaging, such as PET/CT to the extent of active inflammatory involvement and effects of postinflammatory sequelae.

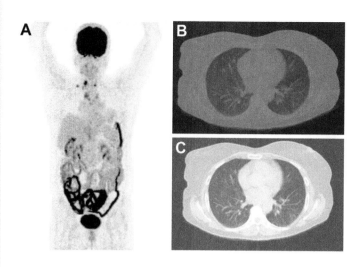

Fig. 17. A 59-year-old female patient who is a known case of sarcoidosis underwent FDG-PET/CT. The MIP display (A) showed FDG-avid supraclavicular lymph node along with multiple mediastinal lymph nodes. The transaxial PET (B) and CT (C) sections showed multiple tiny non-FDG-avid subpleural nodules in both lungs.

Sarcoid granulomas include GLUT-expressing CD4+ lymphocytes and activated macrophages. Thus, F-18 FDG uptake is high similar to tumors.

Various prospective and retrospective studies on [18]F-FDG-PET/CT in sarcoidosis comparing findings with histopathology as gold standard have shown that [18]F-FDG-PET/CT can be considered the gold standard of diagnosing active disease.[56,57] [18]F-FDG-PET/CT is helpful in alleviating the need for biopsy from critical organs, such as cardiac sarcoidosis or neurosarcoidosis, and guiding site for biopsy in thoracic involvement.[18]F-FDG-PET/CT has proven to be a better marker of active disease than biochemical markers and plain radiography.[58]

The follow-up PET/CT scans were also compared with lung functions to predict outcome of therapy. Differentiation between ongoing inflammation and burned out fibrosis is important because the former may be amenable to therapeutic benefits by changing or intensifying therapy.

Cardiac sarcoidosis can present as a heart block, ventricular arrhythmia, or cardiomyopathy. Varied physiologic uptakes of FDG in the myocardium make this challenging. Preparing with high-fat, high-protein, and low-carbohydrate diet, 12 hours fasting with added predose of unfractionated heparin may increment utility of FDG of cardiac sarcoid assessment by reducing physiologic uptake and enhancing areas with inflammatory involvement. Additionally, myocardial perfusion scan findings provide incremental information for assessment of cardiac sarcoidosis, such as presence of focal perfusion defect with FDG uptake was reported to be predictive of adverse cardiac events. Furthermore, reduction in myocardial FDG uptake corresponded to improvement in left ventricular ejection fraction, and extent of involvement on [18]F-FDG-PET/CT corresponded to prognosis.[59]

In their evidence-based review, Treglia and colleagues have suggested that [18]F-FDG-PET/CT is useful in assessing (1) extent of disease involvement, (2) severity of disease involvement or marker of active disease, (3) identification/selection of sites amenable to biopsy, (4) assessing response to established therapy, and (5) new drug evaluation.[60] Oberstein and colleagues[61] demonstrated that the severity of pulmonary involvement in patients with sarcoidosis, as assessed by HRCT parameters, is directly associated with FDG-PET activity. Mostard and colleagues[62] showed additional bone/bone marrow involvement detected by [18]F-FDG-PET/CT compared with CT images. Even in the absence of raised serum markers, [18]F-FDG-PET/CT could provide information on disease activity in symptomatic patients. Studies assessing FDG activity in response to steroid therapy revealed reduction in uptake in patients responding to therapy. The FDG uptake corresponded to clinical response and assisted in modifying treatment in patients including in assessment of tumor necrosis factor-$\alpha$ therapy. There are limited data presently on the minimum lesion size for detection specifically for sarcoid lesions, so a size of 8 to 10 mm considered standard for detection of malignant lesions on PET/CT may be considered for all practical purposes.

### Non-fluorodeoxyglucose PET/computed tomography in Sarcoidosis

[68]Ga-Citrate PET/CT along with [18]F-FDG-PET/CT has been examined and reported to provide information on sites of involvement especially

extrapulmonary sites with the advantage of lower radiation dose and better and faster images compared with [67]Ga-citrate for sarcoidosis. A [68]Ga-citrate-[18]F-FDG mismatch could lead to additional lesions indicating other disease process, such as malignancy, as shown by Tetikkurt and colleagues.[63] Lesions of sarcoidosis are SSTR-avid especially in thoracic involvement, and a fraction of 32% improved yield in diagnosis of lung lesions above CT scan has been seen on SSTR imaging. Nobashi and colleagues[64] showed superiority of [68]Ga-DOTATOC PET/CT to [67]Ga scintigraphy in detecting more lesions and also proposed potential to assess disease activity by quantitative analysis.

Yamada and colleagues[65] demonstrated corresponding uptake of [18]F-FDG and [11]C-methionine in hilar and mediastinal lymphadenopathy of sarcoid; however, lesions with [18]F-FDG had better prognosis than those with [11]C-methionine uptake. [18]F-FMT has been shown to help differentiate sarcoid lesions from malignancy when both coexist on [18]F-FDG-PET/CT because the malignant lesions show accumulation of [18]F-FMT and not sarcoidosis.[66]

[18]F-Fluoromisonidazole is a hypoxia PET tracer. However, because it does not accumulate in physiologic myocardium and has shown to concentrate in sarcoid lesions in one study it was proposed to be used for cardiac sarcoidosis.[67]

## Lung Transplant Evaluation

In the lungs, end-stage chronic disease in the settings of cystic fibrosis and chronic obstructive pulmonary disease may require transplantation. These patients require evaluation involving (1) posttransplant function; (2) development of failure; (3) inflammation; (4) malignancy; and (5) effects of immunosuppressive drugs, many of which may be subtle to detect in early stages. Because of its inherent property of high proliferating cells, inflammation, and cancers,[18]F-FDG may be potentially useful in detecting several posttransplant complications. Various authors studied effectiveness of [18]F-FDG in posttransplant patients.[68] [18]F-FDG-PET/CT was found to assist in detecting or ruling out malignancy, localizing sites of inflammation, and guiding sites of biopsy in these patients. Based on a patient-based analysis, the sensitivity, specificity, positive predictive value, and negative predictive value of FDG-PET/CT were 78%, 90%, 78%, and 90%, respectively, with a global accuracy of 86% for assessing post lung transplantation complications.

With regard to lung transplant recipients, chronic lung allograft dysfunction is one of the major factors that limit long-term survival in these patients. Chronic lung allograft dysfunction has been classified into two main types: an obstructive (bronchiolitis obliterans syndrome [BOS]) and a restrictive (restrictive allograft syndrome [RAS]). Both these types have prognostic significance, with the restrictive type (RAS) having a poorer prognosis. Although widely evaluated by the lung function criteria, there is further need for modalities to effectively establish RAS or BOS. The presence of parenchymal infiltrates in RAS and low-dose CT-based volumetry and CT-based anatomic modeling have been used but are not standard of care because of lack of larger data. Because [18]F-FDG has been shown to effectively help in ILD (discussed previously), its role has been studied for differentiating between RAS and BOS. Verleden and colleagues[69] showed [18]F-FDG-PET/CT is able to differentiate between RAS and BOS with 76% sensitivity and 87% specificity using the SUVmax cutoff of 2.2. Higher SUV favored RAS, whereas the lower values favored BOS and stable results. Higher degree of metabolism was associated with poorer outcome.

## COVID-19 Features

The pandemic of SAR-COV in 2019 brought the world to a near standstill and all modalities of medical science steered toward patient care for this disease. Detection of viral RNA remains the gold standard for diagnosis of COVID-19 infection; however, imaging modalities are required for assessment of disease involvement and response assessment. Commonly found CT features in COVID-19 are GGOs; reticular opacities; consolidations with or without GGOs; and rarely crazy paving pattern, defined as GGOs with superimposed intralobular lines and interlobular septal thickening. These lesions show FDG uptake on PET with SUVmax values ranging from 4.6 to 12.2. Other CT findings are adjacent pleural thickening, intralobular septal thickening, pulmonary vascular enlargement, subpleural lines, air bronchograms, and a reverse halo sign (**Fig. 18**). Joob and Wiwanitkit[70] commented that there is no definite established additional role of [18]F-FDG-PET/CT in COVID-19 pneumonia further to CT and it is considered to be a higher risk procedure for this indication. The appearance of COVID-19 lung on [18]F-FDG-PET/CT was described by Qin and colleagues.[71] They described COVID-19 lungs as showing peripheral GGOs and/or lung consolidations in more than two pulmonary lobes with, increased [18]F-FDG uptake and lymph node involvement as a regular feature. Initial reports have elucidated

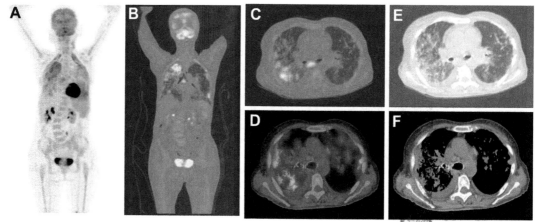

**Fig. 18.** A 72-year-old female patient who is a known case of angioimmunoblastic T-cell lymphoma came for FDG-PET/CT post-chemotherapy. She was also infected with COVID-19, around 2 months back. The FDG PET/CT MIP (*A*), coronal (*B*), and transaxial images show FDG-avid areas of consolidation with fibroparenchymal opacities (*C, D*) in bilateral lungs along with air bronchograms and bilateral pleural effusion (*E, F*).

that COVID-19 has pulmonary tropism, which highlights the need for more and more studies in this area.[70] It is imperative that FDG-PET/CT has a role in differential diagnosis of suspected or complex cases, and it may not be prudent to do away with the modality without further investigation. Zou and Zhu[72] reported a typical presentation noted in COVID-19 of [18]F-FDG-avid mass with [18]F-FDG-avid hilar lymphadenopathy, progressing over days to the contralateral side or more lobes, with likely recovery.

### Nonfluorodeoxyglucose tracers in COVID-19

[11]C-Choline and [68]Ga-PSMA have shown to accumulate in GGOs in addition to prostate lesions during imaging for the same in patients with COVID-19 lung involvement.[73] These tracers could be further explored for any advantage over CT or [18]F-FDG-PET/CT COVID imaging.

### Cardiomyopathy Evaluation: Current Status

The European classification on cardiomyopathies has defined five patterns of cardiomyopathy as follows: (1) dilated cardiomyopathy, (2) hypertrophic cardiomyopathy, (3) restrictive cardiomyopathy, (4) arrhythmogenic right ventricular cardiomyopathy, and (5) nonclassified cardiomyopathy (including left ventricular noncompaction and takotsubo cardiomyopathy). The multimodality approach includes involvement of the following modalities: transthoracic echocardiography, cardiac MR imaging, cardiac CT, and cardiac nuclear imaging. The strength of PET/CT lies in its ability to assess ischemia and metabolism. Among the

various types of cardiomyopathy involvement PET/CT has a role in assessing cardiac sarcoidosis. Currently, the role is to accurately detect myocardial inflammation, guide immunosuppressive therapy, assess prognosis, and monitor response to therapy in cardiac involvement of inflammatory cardiomyopathy. Considering the other modalities for evaluation of left ventricle, PET/CT is less effective compared with other modalities in volume assessment (cardiac MR imaging more preferred), spatial and temporal resolution of anatomy and coronary vessel morphology (invasive coronary angiogram), valves (transesophageal echocardiography), and tissue characterization (cardiac MR imaging).[74]

### FUTURE DIRECTIONS

It is evident that PET/CT has the potential to play a significant role in various nonmalignant disorders of the thorax. Undoubtedly the volume of data supports [18]F-FDG PET/CT in application of PET/CT for nonmalignant disorders of the thorax. The particularly effective role is emphasized in various infectious and noninfectious inflammatory disorders, such as invasive fungal infections, tuberculosis, FUO, sarcoidosis, and ILD. Limited data are presently available in non-FDG tracers. More prospective studies are required to further strengthen the role of PET/CT and place it at center stage for the decision-making algorithm while managing major medical dilemmas.

## CLINICS CARE POINTS

- Volume of data in the literature exists on application of $^{18}$F-FDG PET/CT in non-malignant disorders of the thorax, esp. in various infectious and non-infectious inflammatory disorders.

- Pyrexia of unknown origin (PUO), tuberculosis, sarcoidosis, invasive fungal infections, and ILD are the dominant entities that have been examined with FDG in a number of studies, with emphasis on its important role in the diagnosis of source of PUO, and assessing disease activity and monitoring therapy response are major areas.

- Limited data are presently available in non-FDG tracers, where evidence base needs to grow further before definitive conclusion on their role in non-malignant thoracic disorders.

## REFERENCES

1. Alavi A, Gupta N, Alberini JL, et al. Positron emission tomography imaging in non-malignant thoracic disorders. Semin Nucl Med 2002;32(4):293–321.

2. Basu S, Saboury B, Werner T, et al. Clinical utility of FDG-PET and PET-CT in non-malignant thoracic disorders. Mol Imaging Biol 2011;13(6):1051–60.

3. Carter BW, Betancourt SL, Viswanathan C, et al. Potential pitfalls in interpretation of positron emission tomography/computed tomography findings in the thorax. Semin Roentgenol 2015;50(3):210–6.

4. Zhao J, Day RM, Jin JY, et al. Thoracic radiation-induced pleural effusion and risk factors in patients with lung cancer. Oncotarget 2017;8(57):97623–32.

5. Iravani A, Turgeon GA, Akhurst T, et al. PET-detected pneumonitis following curative-intent chemoradiation in non-small cell lung cancer (NSCLC): recognizing patterns and assessing the impact on the predictive ability of FDG-PET-CT response assessment. Eur J Nucl Med Mol Imaging 2019;46(9): 1869–77.

6. Karanikas G, Beheshti M. $^{11}$C-acetate PET-CT imaging: physiologic uptake, variants, and pitfalls. PET Clin 2014;9(3):339–44.

7. Gray KR, Contractor KB, Kenny LM, et al. Kinetic filtering of [(18)F]Fluorothymidine in positron emission tomography studies. Phys Med Biol 2010; 55(3):695–709.

8. Chondrogiannis S, Marzola MC, Al-Nahhas A, et al. Normal biodistribution pattern and physiologic variants of 18F-DOPA PET imaging. Nucl Med Commun 2013;34(12):1141–9.

9. Sharma P, Mukherjee A, Karunanithi S, et al. Potential role of 18F-FDG PET-CT in patients with fungal infections. AJR Am J Roentgenol 2014;203(1): 180–9.

10. Bleeker-Rovers CP, Warris A, Drenth JP, et al. Diagnosis of *Candida* lung abscesses by 18F-fluorodeoxyglucose positron emission tomography. Clin Microbiol Infect 2005;11(6):493–5.

11. Pan Q, Luo Y, Cao X, et al. Pulmonary cryptococcosis accidently detected by 68Ga-pentixafor PET-CT in a patient with multiple myeloma. Clin Nucl Med 2020;45(5):423–5.

12. Parisien-La Salle S, Morency-Potvin P, Lord M, et al. The use of $^{18}$F-FDG PET-CT to guide management of adrenal histoplasmosis over time. Eur J Nucl Med Mol Imaging 2020. https://doi.org/10.1007/s00259-020-05016-1.

13. Bryant AS, Cerfolio RJ. The maximum standardized uptake values on integrated FDG-PET-CT is useful in differentiating benign from malignant pulmonary nodules. Ann Thorac Surg 2006;82(03):1016–20.

14. Ankrah AO, Span LFR, Klein HC, et al. Role of FDG PET-CT in monitoring treatment response in patients with invasive fungal infections. Eur J Nucl Med Mol Imaging 2019;46(1):174–83.

15. Rolle AM, Hasenberg M, Thornton CR, et al. ImmunoPET/MR imaging allows specific detection of *Aspergillus fumigatus* lung infection in vivo. Proc Natl Acad Sci U S A 2016;113(8):E1026–33.

16. Petrik M, Franssen GM, Haas H, et al. Preclinical evaluation of two 68Ga-siderophores as potential radiopharmaceuticals for *Aspergillus fumigatus* infection imaging. Eur J Nucl Med Mol Imaging 2012; 39:1175–83.

17. Batra P, Batra RS. Thoracic coccidioidomycosis. SeminRoentgenol 1996;31:28–44.

18. Chen JH, Zheng X, Liu XQ. Usefulness of positron emission tomography in patients with syphilis: a systematic review of observational studies. Chin Med J (Engl) 2017;130(9):1100–12.

19. Pelletier-Galarneau M, Martineau P, Zuckier LS, et al. 18F-FDG-PET-CT imaging of thoracic and extrathoracic tuberculosis in children. Semin Nucl Med 2017;47(3):304–18.

20. Sánchez-Montalvá A, Barios M, Salvador F, et al. Usefulness of FDG PET-CT in the management of tuberculosis. PLoS One 2019;14(8):e0221516.

21. Agarwal KK, Behera A, Kumar R, et al. 18F-Fluorodeoxyglucose-positron emission tomography/computed tomography in tuberculosis: spectrum of manifestations. Indian J Nucl Med 2017;32(4): 316–21.

22. Sharma SK, Mohan A, Sharma A. Challenges in the diagnosis and treatment of miliary tuberculosis. Indian J Med Res 2012;135:703–30.

23. Sun Y, Yu H, Ma J, et al. The role of 18F-FDG-PET-CT integrated imaging in distinguishing malignant from

benign pleural effusion. PLoS One 2016;11: e0161764.

24. Gratz S, Dörner J, Fischer U, et al. 18F-FDG hybrid PET in patients with suspected spondylitis. Eur J Nucl Med Mol Imaging 2002;29:516–24.

25. Davis SL, Nuermberger EL, Um PK, et al. Noninvasive pulmonary [18F]-2-fluoro-deoxy-D-glucose positron emission tomography correlates with bactericidal activity of tuberculosis drug treatment. Antimicrob Agents Chemother 2009;53:4879–84.

26. Matthies A, Hickeson M, Cuchiara A, et al. Dual time point 18F-FDG PET for the evaluation of pulmonary nodules. J Nucl Med 2002;43:871–5.

27. Sood A, Mittal BR, Modi M, et al. 18F-FDG PET-CT in tuberculosis: can interim PET-CT predict the clinical outcome of the patients? Clin Nucl Med 2020;45(4): 276–82.

28. Du X, Zhang Y, Chen L, et al. Comparing the differential diagnostic values of 18F-alfatide II PET-CT between tuberculosis and lung cancer patients. Contrast Media Mol Imaging 2018;2018:8194678.

29. Hara T, Kosaka N, Suzuki T, et al. Uptake rates of 18F-Fluorodeoxyglucose and 11C-Choline in lung cancer and pulmonary tuberculosis: a positron emission tomography study. Chest 2003;124(Issue 3):893–901.

30. Rayamajhi SJ, Mittal BR, Maturu VN, et al. 18)F-FDG and (18)F-FLT PET-CT imaging in the characterization of mediastinal lymph nodes. Ann Nucl Med 2016;30(3):207–16.

31. Ankrah AO, Lawal IO, Boshomane TMG, et al. Comparison of fluorine(18)-fluorodeoxyglucose and gallium(68)-citrate PET-CT in patients with tuberculosis. Nuklearmedizin 2019;58(5):371–8. English.

32. Goshen E, Davidson T, Avigdor A, et al. PET-CT in the evaluation of lymphoma in patients with HIV-1 with suppressed viral loads. Clin Nucl Med 2008; 33:610–4.

33. Brust D, Polis M, Davey R, et al. Fluorodeoxyglucose imaging in healthy subjects with HIV infection: impact of disease stage and therapy on pattern of nodal activation. AIDS 2006;20:985–93.

34. Lawal IO, Popoola GO, Mahapane J, et al. [68Ga] Ga-Pentixa for Pentax PET imaging of vascular expression of CXCR-4 as a marker of arterial inflammation in HIV-infected patients: a comparison with 18F [FDG] PET imaging. Biomolecules 2020;10(12):1629.

35. Keidar Z, Gurman-Balbir A, Gaitini D, et al. Fever of unknown origin: the role of 18FFDG PET-CT. J Nucl Med 2008;49:1980–5.

36. Meller J, Altenvoerde G, Lehmann K, et al. 19. Fever of unknown origin: prospective comparison of 18F-FDG imaging with a double head coincidence camera and 67Ga citrate SPECT. Nucl Med Commun 2001;22:1158–9.

37. Berrevoets MAH, Kouijzer IJE, Slieker K, et al. 18)F-FDG-PET-CT-guided treatment duration in patients with high-risk Staphylococcus aureus bacteremia: a proof of principle. J Nucl Med 2019;60:998–1002.

38. Bharucha T, Rutherford A, Skeoch S, et al. FDG-PET-CT in fever of unknown origin working group. Diagnostic yield of FDG-PET-CT in fever of unknown origin: a systematic review, meta-analysis, and Delphi exercise. Clin Radiol 2017;72:764–71.

39. Basu S, Pawaskar A. Individualized management of pyrexia of unknown origin: will fludeoxyglucose-positron emission tomography/computed tomography emerge as the imaging common-point in the algorithm? Indian J Nucl Med 2018;33(4):376–7.

40. Jamar F, Buscombe J, Chiti A, et al. EANM/SNMMI guideline for 18F-FDG use in inflammation and infection. J Nucl Med 2013;54(4):647–58.

41. Kumar A, Regmi SK, Dutta R, et al. Characterization of thymic masses using (18)F-FDG PET-CT. Ann Nucl Med 2009;23(6):569–77.

42. Ito T, Suzuki H, Sakairi Y, et al. 18F-FDG-PET-CT predicts grade of malignancy and invasive potential of thymic epithelial tumors. Gen Thorac Cardiovasc Surg 2020. https://doi.org/10.1007/s11748-020-01439-7.

43. Hephzibah J, Shanthly N, Oommen R. Diagnostic utility of PET CT in thymic tumours with emphasis on 68Ga-DOTATATE PET CT in thymic neuroendocrine tumour: experience at a tertiary level hospital in India. J Clin Diagn Res 2014;8(9):QC01-3.

44. Krishnaraju VS, Basher RK, Singh H, et al. Incidental detection of type B2 thymoma on 68Ga-labeled prostate-specific membrane antigen PET-CT imaging. Clin Nucl Med 2018;43(5):356–8.

45. Kligerman SJ, Auerbach A, Franks TJ, et al. Castleman disease of the thorax: clinical, radiologic, and pathologic correlation: from the radiologic pathology archives. Radiographics 2016;36(5):1309–32.

46. Neji H, Attia M, Affes M, et al. Interstitial lung diseases: imaging contribution to diagnosis and elementary radiological lesions. Semin Diagn Pathol 2018;35(5):297–303.

47. Jacquelin V, Mekinian A, Brillet PY, et al. FDG-PET-CT in the prediction of pulmonary function improvement in nonspecific interstitial pneumonia. Eur J Radiol 2016;85(12):2200–5.

48. Groves AM, Win T, Screaton NJ, et al. Idiopathic pulmonary fibrosis and diffuse parenchymal lung disease: implications from initial experience with 18F-FDG PET-CT. J Nucl Med 2009;50:538–45.

49. Umeda Y, Demura Y, Morikawa M, et al. Prognostic value of dual-time-point 18F-FDG PET for idiopathic pulmonary fibrosis. J Nucl Med 2015;56(12):1869–75.

50. Savelli G, Morassi M, Cobelli M, et al. 18F-Fluorocholine uptake by a head and neck meningeal inflammatory pseudotumor. Clin Nucl Med 2019; 44(8):657–9.

51. Withana NP, Ma X, McGuire HM, et al. Non-invasive imaging of idiopathic pulmonary fibrosis using cathepsin protease probes. Sci Rep 2016;6:19755.

52. Win T, Screaton NJ, Porter J, et al. Novel positron emission tomography/computed tomography of diffuse parenchymal lung disease combining a labeled somatostatin receptor analogue and 2-deoxy-2[18F]fluoro-D-glucose. Mol Imaging 2012;11(2):91–8.

53. Bondue B, Sherer F, Van Simaeys G, et al. PET-CT with 18F-FDG- and 18F-FBEM labeled leukocytes for metabolic activity and leukocyte recruitment monitoring in a mouse model of pulmonary fibrosis. J Nucl Med 2015;56:127–32.

54. Désogère P, Tapias LF, Hariri LP, et al. Type I collagen-targeted PET probe for pulmonary fibrosis detection and staging in preclinical models. Sci Transl Med 2017;9:eaaf4696.

55. Schniering J, Benešová M, Brunner M, et al. [18]F-AzaFol for detection of folate receptor-β positive macrophages in experimental interstitial lung disease: a proof-of-concept study. Front Immunol 2019;10:2724.

56. Keijsers RGM, Grutters JC. In which patients with sarcoidosis is FDG PET-CT indicated? J Clin Med 2020;9(3):890.

57. Guleria R, Jyothidasan A, Madan K, et al. Utility of FDG-PET-CT scanning in assessing the extent of disease activity and response to treatment in sarcoidosis. Lung India 2014;31:323–30.

58. Mostard RL, Verschakelen JA, van Kroonenburgh MJ, et al. Severity of pulmonary involvement and 18F-FDG PET activity in sarcoidosis. Respir Med 2013;107: 439–47.

59. Sperry BW, Tamarappoo BK, Oldan JD, et al. Prognostic impact of extent, severity, and heterogeneity of abnormalities on 18F-FDG PET scans for suspected cardiac sarcoidosis. JACC Cardiovasc Imaging 2018;11:336–45.

60. Treglia G, Annunziata S, Sobic-Saranovic D, et al. The role of 18F-FDG-PET and PET-CT in patients with sarcoidosis: an updated evidence-based review. Acad Radiol 2014;21(5):675–84.

61. Oberstein A, von Zitzewitz H, Schweden F, et al. Non invasive evaluation of the inflammatory activity in sarcoidosis with high-resolution computed tomography. Sarcoidosis Vasc Diffuse Lung Dis 1997;14(1): 65–72.

62. Mostard RL, Prompers L, Weijers RE, et al. F-18 FDG PET-CT for detecting bone and bone marrow involvement in sarcoidosis patients. Clin Nucl Med 2012; 37(1):21–5.

63. Tetikkurt C, Yanardag H, Sayman BH, et al. Diagnostic utility of 68Ga-citrate and 18FDG PET-CT in sarcoidosis patients. Monaldi Arch Chest Dis 2020; 90(4). https://doi.org/10.4081/monaldi.2020.1509.

64. Nobashi T, Nakamoto Y, Kubo T, et al. The utility of PET-CT with (68)Ga-DOTATOC in sarcoidosis: comparison with (67)Ga-scintigraphy. Ann Nucl Med 2016;30:544–52.

65. Yamada Y, Uchida Y, Tatsumi K, et al. Fluorine-18-fluorodeoxyglucose and carbon-11-methionine evaluation of lymphadenopathy in sarcoidosis. J Nucl Med 1998;39:1160–6.

66. Kaira K, Oriuchi N, Otani Y, et al. Diagnostic usefulness of fluorine-18- alpha-methyltyrosine positron emission tomography in combination with 18F-fluorodeoxyglucose in sarcoidosis patients. Chest 2007;131:1019–27.

67. Furuya S, Naya M, Manabe O, et al. [18]F-FMISO PET-CT detects hypoxic lesions of cardiac and extracardiac involvement in patients with sarcoidosis. J Nucl Cardiol 2019.

68. Muller N, Kessler R, Caillard S, et al. 18F-FDG PET-CT for the diagnosis of malignant and infectious complications after solid organ transplantation. Nucl Med Mol Imaging 2017;51(1):58–68.

69. Verleden SE, Gheysens O, Goffin KE, et al. Role of 18F-FDG PET-CT in restrictive allograft syndrome after lung transplantation. Transplantation 2019; 103(4):823–31.

70. Joob B, Wiwanitkit V. 18F-FDG PET-CT and COVID-19. Eur J Nucl Med Mol Imaging 2020;47(6):1348.

71. Qin C, Liu F, Yen TC, et al. [18]F-FDG PET-CT findings of COVID-19: a series of four highly suspected cases. Eur J Nucl Med Mol Imaging 2020 May; 47(5):1281–6. https://doi.org/10.1007/s00259-020-04734-w.

72. Zou S, Zhu X. FDG PET-CT of COVID-19. Radiology 2020;296(2):E118.

73. Scarlattei M, Baldari G, Silva M, et al. Unknown SARS-CoV-2 pneumonia detected by PET-CT in patients with cancer. Tumori 2020;106:325–32. https://doi.org/10.1177/0300891620935983.

74. Ederhy S, Mansencal N, Réant P, et al. Role of multimodality imaging in the diagnosis and management of cardiomyopathies. Arch Cardiovasc Dis 2019; 112(10):615–29.

# Fluorodeoxyglucose PET/ Computed Tomography in Evaluation of Prosthetic Joints and Diabetic Foot

## A Comparative Perspective with Other Functional Imaging Modalities

Swati Sodagar Rachh, MBBS, DRM, DNB, MNAMS[a,b],
Sandip Basu, MBBS, DRM, DNB, MNAMS[b,c],*,
Abass Alavi, MD, MD (Hon), PhD (Hon), DSc (Hon)[d]

## KEYWORDS

- FDG-PET/CT • Prosthetic joints • Diabetic foot • Infection • Charcot neuroarthropathy
- Combined leukocyte-marrow scintigraphy • Antigranulocyte antibody scintigraphy

## KEY POINTS

- PET with 18F fluorodeoxyglucose (18F FDG) can play a promising role in the setting of complicated orthopedic conditions and make this a pivotal investigational modality in patients with complicated prosthetic implants and diabetic foot.
- Location rather than intensity of 18F FDG uptake is critical in diagnosing hip and knee periprosthetic infection (PPI). 18F FDG uptake at the middle portion of the femoral component and at the bone-prosthesis interface can be considered positive criteria for PPI in hip and knee prostheses, respectively.
- The ability for quantification of the inflammatory process by 18F FDG-PET may drive clinical decisions in managing diabetic foot infection better than clinical criteria alone and could serve an invaluable adjunct to clinical assessment in difficult situations such as associated underlying neuroarthropathy.
- PET–MR imaging is an emerging technique and may offer specific advantages over PET-computed tomography in defining the different complications of the diabetic foot in the near future.

## INTRODUCTION

Infection imaging has been an important part of nuclear medicine practice. Infections in prosthetic joint and diabetic foot are most devastating complications encountered in the clinical practice, and a diagnosis of these infections remains a clinical challenge. For many years, conventional nuclear medicine techniques have been used to frame a painful joint arthroplasty or diabetic foot infection. Despite their proven utility, conventional nuclear medicine techniques have several practical shortcomings including cost and complexity of procedures. Over the last decade, fluorodeoxyglucose PET (FDG-PET)/computed tomography

[a] Department of Nuclear Medicie, Gujarat Cancer & Research Institute, Civil Hospital Campus, Asarwa, Ahmedabad 380016, India; [b] Radiation Medicine Centre (B.A.R.C), Tata Memorial Centre Annexe, Parel, Mumbai, India; [c] Homi Bhabha National Institute, Mumbai, India; [d] Department of Radiology, Hospital of the University of Pennsylvania, Philadelphia, PA, USA
* Corresponding author. Radiation Medicine Centre (B.A.R.C), Tata Memorial Hospital Annexe, Jerbai Wadia Road, Parel, Mumbai 400012, India.
E-mail address: drsanb@yahoo.com

PET Clin 17 (2022) 517–531
https://doi.org/10.1016/j.cpet.2022.02.002
1556-8598/22/

(CT) has evolved as a widely examined modality for diagnosing diverse group of infection and inflammatory processes, including its application in diagnosis of prosthetic joint and diabetic foot.

## IMAGING OF THE PROSTHETIC JOINTS

The current evidence shows that prosthetic implant failure is most commonly related to 2 reasons, aseptic loosening and infection, where both of them may significantly affect the patients' quality of life.[1] There is great importance of preoperative identification of the underlying process, as both complications are managed in different ways. The management of periprosthetic infection (PPI) involves multiple surgical interventions and prolonged courses of antimicrobial therapy. The surgical options for treatment of infection include debridement, antibiotics, and implant retention, single- or 2-stage revision surgery, and salvage procedures (eg, arthrodesis or amputation). The goals of treatment include both eradication of the infection and reestablishment of a pain-free and well-functioning joint. A 2-stage revision surgery is generally considered to be the gold-standard procedure. In contrast, an aseptic process manifesting as a failed joint arthroplasty requires single-stage surgery for the removal of the original loose prosthesis and reimplantation.[2] The recent consensus guidelines by Romano and colleagues[3] and Sconfienza and colleagues[4] have outlined algorithms for diagnosis of prosthetic joint infections. Despite these complex algorithms, differentiating between these 2 most common types of implant failure continues to be difficult. Current PPI definitions rely on 4 diagnostic classes of investigations: (1) clinical presentation, (2) serum and synovial markers, (3) imaging techniques, and (4) microbiological and histological findings.[3] With regard to the clinical presentation, the presence of a draining sinus or an exposed implant is considered as pathognomonic or highly specific; however, this sign may be totally absent in more than 70% of PPI, thus featuring a low sensitivity for the diagnosis. No single biomarker has been shown to be 100% accurate in diagnosing PPI. CT and MR imaging may be useful to document the extent of bone lesions as well as abnormalities in the articular space, and therefore, they may help the surgeon in planning the most appropriate strategy. Main drawback of cross-sectional imaging modalities are that they are distorted by artefacts produced by the metal implants. Moreover, ultrasound and CT are quite useful for performing fluid aspirations (when feasible), thus representing an important tool in the diagnostic workup of PPI. Joint aspiration has been reported to approach a specificity of 100%; however, the wide range of reported sensitivity (0%–100%) by different research groups has made it an unreliable diagnostic modality in differentiating septic and aseptic prosthesis loosening.[3] In addition, the aspiration of the joint is invasive, and the contamination of a noninfected joint always poses a major concern. Several nuclear medicine and molecular imaging techniques can be used to evaluate PPI including bone scintigraphy, radiolabeled white blood cell (WBC) scintigraphy (with or without combined bone marrow scintigraphy), antigranulocyte antibody scintigraphy, and PET with 18F fluorodeoxyglucose ([18]F FDG-PET). Both planar and tomographic acquisitions, with single photon emission tomography (SPECT), can be performed, and the use of hybrid modalities such as SPECT/CT or PET/CT increases the diagnostic accuracy in terms of the exacting the location and extent of the infectious process. Importantly, these functional imaging modalities are not affected by metallic hardware. However, due to inherent drawbacks of the traditional methods together with several other infectious and inflammatory diseases, there has been a shift in recent years from traditional modalities, that is, bone scintigraphy, leukocyte scintigraphy, and bone marrow scintigraphy, toward [18]F FDG-PET/CT.

## FLUORODEOXYGLUCOSE PET/COMPUTED TOMOGRAPHY FOR PROSTHETIC JOINT IMAGING

FDG-PET imaging has been examined for its potential as a useful imaging technique for the detection of both infectious and inflammatory processes. The advantages of FDG-PET/CT over conventional nuclear medicine techniques for imaging both infections and inflammations are its high sensitivity, high-resolution images, high target-to-background ratio, and faster technique, which is completed in one session (Box 1).[5] FDG-PET has established role in the diagnosis of infectious disorders, and developing role in

---

**Box 1**
**Advantages of fluorodeoxyglucose PET/computed tomography over conventional radionuclide studies in infection and inflammation**

High sensitivity

High-resolution images

High target-to-background ratio

Fast technique completed in one session

*From* Hess S, Hansson SH, Pedersen KT, et al. FDG-PET/CT in Infectious and Inflammatory Diseases. PET Clin 2014(9); 497–519.

the diagnosis of complicated orthopedic conditions makes this a likely main investigational modality for patients with complicated prosthetic implants.

Review of the literature by Chacko and colleagues[6] clearly delineates the current status of FDG-PET and FDG-PET/CT in the diagnosis and management of arthroplasty-associated infections. For diagnosing infection, 2 different criteria for FDG uptake at the bone-prosthesis interface and the intensity of FDG uptake around the head and neck of the prosthesis. The uptake was consistently located at the bone-prosthesis interface in patients with infection, whereas those patients with an uncomplicated prosthesis were found to have a greater intensity of uptake but it was located around the head and neck of the prosthesis (ie, not near the bone shaft).[6] As described by Zhuang and colleagues,[7] the nonspecific increase in FDG uptake around the head or neck portion of the prosthesis occurs frequently and can persist for many years, even in patients without any complications.[8] Defining these distinct uptake patterns illustrates that the site of tracer accumulation is an essential parameter for the accurate diagnosis of PPI and will aide in minimizing false-positive results in the future (Table 1).

Chacko and colleagues[9] compared the effectiveness of FDG-PET in the diagnosis of hip and knee prosthesis infection (Fig. 1). They reported equal sensitivity of FDG-PET in detecting hip and knee PPI (91.7% and 92.0%, respectively); however, specificity was shown to be higher in hip arthroplasty cases compared with knee cases. Manthey and colleagues[10] described the efficacy of FDG-PET not only in diagnosing infected prostheses but also in differentiating between synovitis, prosthetic loosening, and infection of hip and knee prostheses as 3 possible causes of lower limb pain following arthroplasty. They included both intensity and location of periprosthetic radiotracer uptake in their analysis. A visual quantitative scale to differentiate septic and aseptic loosening showed that high and intermediate levels of FDG uptakes at the bone-prosthesis interface were considered positive for infection and loosening, respectively. Any amount of uptake restricted to the synovium was interpreted as synovitis. Using this method, they reported an accuracy of 96% in differentiating these 3 entities by FDG-PET imaging. Despite the lower specificity of FDG described in earlier studies,[6,10] a retrospective study[11] showed added value of FDG-PET/CT in comparison to conventional tests in diagnosing hip PPI (cultures of joint fluid/periprosthetic tissues or clinical follow-up more than 6 months served as gold standard). Fukui and colleagues[12] used FDG-PET in order to make more appropriate decision-making in terms of retention of well-fixed uncemented femoral component in 2-stage total hip surgery that included delayed reimplantation of an acetabular component in 5 patients. FDG-PET was used to assess whether the infection had invaded the bone around femoral component. By a mean follow-up point of 4.2 years after the second-stage operation, none of the 5 patients experienced recurrence of PPI.

In a retrospective study by Wenter and colleagues,[13] infections were diagnosed clinically in 101 of the 215 patients. PET and PET/CT scans revealed 87 true-positive, 76 true-negative, 38 false-positive, and 14 false-negative results, indicating a sensitivity of 86%, a specificity of 67%, a positive predictive value (PPV) of 70%, a negative predictive value (NPV) of 84%, and an accuracy of 76%. The sensitivity of PET/CT was 88%, but specificity, PPV, NPV, and accuracy (76%, 76%, 89%, and 82%, respectively) were higher than those of stand-alone PET. They concluded, FDG-PET is able to identify with high sensitivity the presence of osteomyelitis in orthopedic surgery and implant-associated infections in patients with nonspecific clinical symptoms of infection.

Table 1
Proposed interpretation points for fluorodeoxyglucose uptake pattern in suspected hip prosthesis infection

|  | Infection | Nonspecific Inflammation |
|---|---|---|
| Acetabular component | − | − |
| Femoral neck | − | + |
| Femur stem in contact with bone (the tip) | ... | − |
| Tip of the femur stem | − | + |

+ indicates FDG uptake; − indicates no FDG uptake.
*From* Hess S, Hansson SH, Pedersen KT, et al. FDG-PET/CT in Infectious and Inflammatory Diseases. PET Clin 2014(9); 497–519.

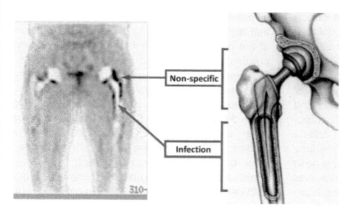

Fig. 1. (*Right*) Regions of FDG uptake corresponding to the site of nonspecific aseptic reaction and infection. (*Left*) Coronal image of a patient with bilateral painful hip prostheses. Focal uptake is noted around the neck region of prosthesis (*blue arrow*). There is also an intense uptake in the proximal upper femur in the interface between prosthesis and bone (*red arrow*), which represents infection (confirmed by further investigation). (*From* Chacko TK, Zhuang H, Stevenson K, et al. The importance of the location of fluorodeoxyglucose uptake in periprosthetic infection in painful hip prostheses. Nucl Med Commun 2002;23(9):851–5.)

Jin and colleagues calculated the diagnostic performance of FDG-PET or PET/CT in detecting prosthetic infection after arthroplasty and found a pooled sensitivity and specificity of 86% (95% confidence interval [CI]: 82–90) and 86% (95% CI: 83–89), respectively. Pooled sensitivity of FDG-PET or PET/CT in demonstrating hip and knee prosthetic infection was 88% (95% CI: 83–92) and 72% (95% CI: 58–84), respectively. Pooled specificity of FDG-PET or PET/CT in demonstrating hip and knee prosthetic infection was 88% (95% CI: 84–91) and 80% (95% CI: 71–88), respectively.[14,15]

A meta-analysis focused on PPI confirmed the good diagnostic accuracy of 18F FDG-PET or PET/CT in this setting with pooled sensitivity and specificity of 86% (95% CI: 80–90) and 93% (95% CI: 90–95), respectively, using increased 18F FDG uptake in the bone-prosthesis interface as the criterion for infection for the index test.[14,16] Another meta-analysis focused on periprosthetic knee infection demonstrated a not optimal diagnostic accuracy of [18]F FDG-PET or PET/CT in this setting with pooled sensitivity and specificity of 70% (95% CI: 56–81) and 84% (95% CI: 76–90).[14,17]

Some factors influencing the diagnostic performance of [18]F FDG-PET/CT in patients with osteomyelitis should be underlined: first of all, several interpretation criteria of [18]F FDG-PET have been used in the literature, by using visual and/or semiquantitative criteria, leading to different diagnostic accuracy values. Furthermore, continuous physiologic [18]F FDG activity around the prostheses may be the cause of false-positive [18]F FDG-PET/CT findings for PPI.[14–17] However, investigators have shown that standardized uptake value (SUV) measurements cannot differentiate between infection and aseptic loosening reliably. Knowledge of the typical patterns that are commonly observed following hip arthroplasty is required in interpreting the FDG-PET scans. 18F FDG uptake at the middle portion of the femoral component and 18F FDG uptake at the bone-prosthesis interface can be considered positive criteria for PPI in hip and knee prostheses, respectively.[18]

## COMPARISON OF FLUORODEOXYGLUCOSE PET/COMPUTED TOMOGRAPHY WITH OTHER FUNCTIONAL IMAGING MODALITIES
### Three-Phase Bone Scintigraphy

Three-phase bone scintigraphy (TPBS) is very sensitive to any bone remodeling (**Table 2**). When a joint is replaced, remodeling may proceed for a couple of years. A single study investigated this point, showing that at 21 months after surgery, 3-phase bone scintigraphy had 50% sensitivity and 71% specificity, concluding that this examination should be avoided in the first year after surgery.[19] However, the great advantage of 3-phase bone scan is that a negative examination allows excluding the diagnosis of PPI.[20] The overall accuracy of radionuclide bone imaging in the evaluation of the painful prosthetic joint is about 50% to 70%, too low to be clinically useful, except perhaps as a screening test or in conjunction with other radionuclide studies such as labeled leukocyte imaging. Previous studies with FDG-PET/CT show higher sensitivity, specificity, and accuracy than TPBS.[21–23]

### Radiolabeled Leukocyte Imaging

In vitro labeled autologous leukocyte scintigraphy (LLS) is a valuable imaging modality for the diagnosis of PPI. Labeled leukocytes do not accumulate at sites of increased bone turnover or remodeling in the absence of infection. The introduction of in vitro labeled WBC has improved the accuracy for the diagnosis of PPI.[24] Because neutrophils are predominantly labeled cells, and neutrophils are present in the infected prosthetic joint, WBC scintigraphy is considered the gold-

**Table 2**
Enumeration of comparison studies on periprosthetic joint infection

| Author | Primary Theme of the Study | No of Patients | Results |
|---|---|---|---|
| Van Acker et al,[33] 2001 | FDG-PET, [99m]Tc-HMPAO white blood cell SPECT, and bone scintigraphy in the evaluation of painful total knee arthroplasty | 29(K) | Both methods were reported to have a sensitivity of 100%; however, specificity was shown to be 73% and 93% for FDG-PET and combined leukocyte marrow scintigraphy, respectively |
| Vanquickenborne et al,[34] 2003 | FDG-PET, 99mtc-HMPAO white blood cell SPECT, and bone scintigraphy in the evaluation of painful total hip arthroplasty | 17(H) | FDG-PET alone has the same sensitivity as conventional combined leukocyte marrow scintigraphy in detecting periprosthetic hip infection; however, the specificity was shown to be suboptimal compared with those of combined leukocyte-marrow scintigraphy, 77.8% and 100%. |
| Pill et al,[36] 2006 | FDG-PET and combined leukocyte-marrow scintigraphy in diagnosing periprosthetic infection | 92(H) | A comparable specificity (93.0% and 95.1%, respectively); FDG-PET was shown to have a substantially higher sensitivity of 95.2% compared with 50.0% for combined leukocyte-marrow scintigraphy. |
| Love et al,[35] 2004 | FDG-PET and combined leukocyte marrow scintigraphy in diagnosing periprosthetic infection | 40(H)+ 19(K) | Accuracy 71% for the detection of infection, which was much lower than the 95% accuracy of combined leukocyte-marrow scintigraphy in their study population. |
| Reinartz et al,[21] 2005 | FDG-PET and TPBS | 92(H) | FDG-PET achieved sensitivity, specificity, and accuracy of 93.9%, 94.9%, and 94.6%, respectively, whereas values of 68%, 76%, and 74% were achieved by TPBS. |
| Stumpe et al,[22] 2004 | FDG-PET and TPBS | 35(H) | The sensitivities and specificities of FDG-PET, conventional radiography, and TPBS were 27.5%, 83.5%, and 50.0% and 83.0%, 57.5%, and 90.0%. |

(continued on next page)

| Table 2 (continued) | | | |
|---|---|---|---|
| Author | Primary Theme of the Study | No of Patients | Results |
| Mumme et al,[23] 2005 | FDG-PET and TPBS | 70(H) | The sensitivity/specificity of FDG-PET was 91%/92% (accuracy 91%) compared with 78%/70% (accuracy 74%) for TPBS. A high correlation could be proved between FDG-PET investigation and operative histopathological findings (r(Spear)> or = 0.9). |
| Basu et al,[37] (2014) | FDG-PET/CT vs combined 111In-labeled leukocyte/ 99mTc sulfur colloid bone marrow | 88(H + K) | The sensitivity, specificity, PPV, NPV, and AUC For hip prosthesis FDG-PET:81.8%, 93.1%, 79.4%, 94.0%, and 0.874, WBC/BM imaging: 38.5%, 95.7%, 71.4%, 84.6%, and 0.671, respectively For knee prosthesis FDG-PET: 94.7%, 88.2%, 69.2%, 98.4%, and 0.915. WBC/BM imaging:33.3%, 88.5%, 25.0%, 92.0%, and 0.609 |

*Abbreviations:* H, hip prosthesis; K, knee prosthesis.

standard radionuclide imaging technique for this purpose.

In the study by Blanc and colleagues,[25] the sensitivity, specificity, and PPV of LLS were 72%, 60%, and 80%, respectively. LLS performed better than antigranulocyte antibody scintigraphy. SPECT-CT revealed the accurate locations of infections. The sensitivity of LS was not significantly affected by the causative pathogen or the injected activity. No correlation was evident between the current antibiotic treatment and the LS value. The test was more sensitive for knee (84%) than hip arthroplasty (57%) but was less specific for knee (52% vs 75%). Sensitivity and specificity of LS varied by the location of infection. Bone scan provided no additional value in PPI diagnosis. Current antibiotic treatment had no influence on LS sensitivity as well as labeling leukocyte activity or pathogens responsible for chronic PPI. SPECT-CT to LS increased the specificity to 80%[26]; SPECT-CT is useful for differentiating soft tissue infection (STIs) from bone infections.

Leukocytes have also been labeled in vitro with 18F FDG, in an attempt to develop a more specific, positron-emitting radiopharmaceutical for PET or PET/CT imaging. Aksoy and colleagues[27] compared FDG-PET/CT and FDG-labeled leukocyte PET/CT in the diagnosis of PPI. FDG-PET/ CT was found to have a PPV of 28% (15/54). The sensitivity, specificity, and positive and NPVs of FDG-labeled leukocyte PET/CT were 93.3% (14/ 15), 97.4% (38/39), 93.3%, and 97.4%, respectively. However, there are some drawbacks to FDG-labeled leukocyte PET/CT, including the relatively long time needed for labeling leukocytes, longer time between injection and imaging (3 hours), and the necessity of higher injected FDG doses (double the doses used as compared with standard oncological imaging).[27]

99mTc-antigranulocyte scintigraphy uses radiolabeled monoclonal antibodies that target surface antigens of leukocytes in inflamed tissues.[28,29] In 2019, antigranulocyte scintigraphy was for the first time recommended as part of the diagnostic workup of PPI[30] and of peripheral bone infections,[31] although studies are still limited. These recent guidelines recommend antigranulocyte scintigraphy as part of the diagnostic workflow only in patients with late infections to confirm positive findings of a previous 3-phase bone scan or FDG-PET/CT. In the recent study by Plate and colleagues,[32] the overall sensitivity and specificity for the diagnosis of an infection were 77.8% and 94.1%, respectively. The PPV was 87.5% and the NPV 88.9%. Diagnostic accuracy was 88.5%. However, one important drawback of 99mTc-antigranulocyte SPECT/CT needs to be acknowledged: owing to the high physiologic population of granulocytes and granulocyte precursors in hematopoietic bone marrow, [99m]Tc-antigranulocyte SPECT/CT is of limited value in these regions. Hence, infections of the spine, shoulder, and hip joints should be examined with other methods.

## Combined Leukocyte/Marrow Imaging

The use of combined WBC scintigraphy (using either [99m]Tc-HMPAO-WBC or [111]In-oxine-WBC) and bone marrow scintigraphy (with radiolabeled colloids) has been studied by many investigators. This technique allows us to reduce the number of false-positive cases with WBC scintigraphy due to WBC accumulation in areas of expanded/displaced bone marrow by providing a map of bone marrow activity. It is particularly useful in cases of suspected PPI and in patients with a doubtful qualitative or semiquantitative analysis of WBC scintigraphy. Concordant findings between both techniques rule out an infectious process, whereas discordant findings (uptake on WBC scintigraphy without corresponding uptake on bone marrow scintigraphy) highly suggest an infection.

In a prospective study[33] in 221 prostheses and subgroup comparison with combined [111]In-labeled leukocyte/[99m]Tc sulfur colloid bone marrow imaging in 88 prostheses, the sensitivity, specificity, PPV, and NPV of FDG-PET in hip prostheses were 81.8%, 93.1%, 79.4%, and 94.0%, respectively, and in knee prostheses were 94.7%, 88.2%, 69.2%, and 98.4%, respectively. The sensitivity, specificity, PPV, and NPV of WBC/BM imaging in hip prostheses were 38.5%, 95.7%, 71.4%, and 84.6%, respectively, and in knee prostheses were 33.3%, 88.5%, 25.0%, and 92.0%, respectively. In those cases that underwent both FDG-PET and WBC/BM imaging, there was a trend ($P = .0625$) toward a higher sensitivity for FDG-PET, whereas other comparisons did not show any significant differences between the 2 imaging modalities. The correct interpretation criteria to be used have also been recently published by the EANM.[30] The combination of those modalities has been reported having accuracy ranging from 86% to 98% for both [99m]Tc-HMPAO-WBC and [111]In-oxine-WBC for both knee and hip PPI,[33] and comparison to FDG-PET/CT, combined leukocyte labeling, and marrow imaging show comparable sensitivity, specificity, and accuracy.[34–37]

## [18]F-Fluoride PET/Computed Tomography

[18]F-fluoride PET/CT provides a promising alternative to conventional skeletal scintigraphy. [18]F-fluoride is a radiopharmaceutical that shows a high affinity to bone and a rapid blood clearance with high bone-to-background ratio in a shorter time than for standard [99m]Tc-based tracers. In combination with PET and its excellent spatial resolution [18]F-fluoride PET/CT may offer highly valuable images for detecting loose components of total hip and knee arthroplasties.

A retrospective study[38] including 26 patients with 24 hip and 13 knee prostheses obtained sensitivity of 95.00%, specificity of 87.04%, and an accuracy of 89.19% for 18F-fluoride PET/CT. In a prospective study, Kobayashi and colleagues[39] described the effectiveness of 18F-fluoride PET imaging in differentiating septic from aseptic prosthesis loosening after THA. Based on the amount of bone prosthesis interface radiotracer uptake, they classified PET imaging into 3 types. Their result showed that the classification they used was significantly associated with the final diagnosis because the type 3 uptake pattern had the sensitivity and specificity of 95% and 98%, respectively, for the diagnosis of infection. Using SUVmax, they also reported a significant difference between SUVmax of septic and aseptic loosening because it was significantly higher in symptomatic patients than controls and was also significantly higher in septic joints compared with those that were not infected.

Choe and colleagues[40] used 18F-fluoride PET scanning in the preoperative planning of 23 patients scheduled for total hip arthroplasty revision surgery. They used the images to semiquantitatively determine those areas of the joint with the most 18F-fluoride uptake either on the acetabular or on the femoral side of the prosthesis. Samples for histopathologic examination, microbiological culture, and real-time polymerase chain reaction were taken from areas of increased uptake. All 17 patients as having areas of major uptake before surgery had definitive diagnosis of infection after surgery. The remaining 6 surgical patients had preoperative scans with only minor-uptake regions and were found to be aseptic when the acetabular and femoral spaces were sampled. A control group had no regions of major uptake and only 3 regions of mild uptake. Although the sample size was small, these data illustrate the potential role of F-18 PET imaging in perioperative planning in patients with complicated prostheses to ensure optimal tissue sampling and a reduction in false-negative results.

The primary role of nuclear medicine in the evaluation of the painful joint replacement is to differentiate aseptic loosening from infection. The current imaging modalities being used include TPBS, labeled leukocyte imaging, combined leukocyte/marrow scintigraphy, antigranulocyte antibodies scintigraphy, and FDG-PET/CT, yet no one method has proved to be highly sensitive and specific as well as safe and time-effective. Labeled leukocyte/marrow scintigraphy has some serious practical disadvantages, being complex, costly, and potential hazardous because of direct handling of blood products and involving a considerable radiation burden (with a spleen receiving radiation dose of ~5.5 mGy/MBq of 111In).[41]

FDG-PET in patients suspected of PPI has high sensitivity but lower specificity than WBC scintigraphy or antigranulocyte antibodies scintigraphy. However, in view of its high NPV and high-quality images with better interobserver agreement, FDG-PET can play an effective role in better assessment of patients with prosthesis implant where superimposed infection is suspected and is the best available imaging technique to exclude infection. Location rather than intensity of FDG uptake is important and critical in diagnosing hip and knee PPI.[18] The criterion is likely to further refine in the future years.

### Imaging in Diabetic Foot

Among the several complications of the diabetes, a systemic disease, diabetic foot infections (DFIs) are one of the challenging complications. The pathogenesis of diabetic foot involves a multifactorial mechanism and a complex pathophysiology (Fig. 2).[37] Imaging in diabetic foot has important role in 3 settings in clinical decision-making and will be most helpful to podiatrists if found accurate:

1. Diagnosis of deep STI and osteomyelitis,
2. Differentiating Charcot arthropathy from osteomyelitis, and
3. Evaluating the ischemia/atherogenesis component in a particular case.

Although both conventional WBC imaging and FDG-PET/CT have demonstrated equivalent results, the latter is emerging as the preferred modality because of several advantages: short acquisition time, preferential [18]F FDG accumulation in the infection site, facilitating the detection of osteomyelitis and the differential diagnosis from neuropathic osteoarthropathy, whole-body analysis, lack of metallic hardware artifacts, and high resolution enabling precise tracer recognition in small bones as the distal forefoot.[42]

A first meta-analysis focused on the diagnostic performance of [18]F FDG-PET or PET/CT in osteomyelitis related to diabetic foot reported a pooled sensitivity and specificity of 74% (95% CI: 60–85) and 91% (95% CI: 85–96), respectively.[43] Lauri and colleagues[44] in a systematic review and meta-analysis comparing MR imaging, WBC scintigraphy, and FDG-PET reported that 18F FDG-PET/CT as well as 99mTc-HMPAO–labeled leukocyte SPECT/CT offer the highest specificity of 92% (95% CI: 85–96) for diagnosing diabetic foot osteomyelitis while demonstrating comparable sensitivity of 89% (95% CI: 68–97) to the other imaging modalities (Table 3).

According to a meta-analysis undertaken by Dinh and colleagues,[45] the presence of exposed bone or a positive probe-to-bone test result is moderately predictive of osteomyelitis, and MR imaging is the most accurate imaging test for diagnosis of osteomyelitis. The combined PET-CT and PET–MR imaging fusion approaches offer unique tools for the diagnosis and management of the diabetic foot.

A study by Yang and colleagues[46] included 48 consecutive diabetic patients with a suspicion of pedal osteomyelitis out of which 21 patients had serum glucose levels less than 150 mg/dL and 27 had serum glucose levels greater than 150 mg/dL. The sensitivity of 18F FDG-PET imaging was 87.5% (7/8) in patients with serum glucose levels less than 150 mg/dL and 88.9% (8/9) in patients with serum glucose levels greater than 150 mg/dL. These results do not significantly differ from the overall sensitivity of 88.3%. The results have shown that mild-to-moderate hyperglycemia will not decrease the sensitivity of 18F FDG-PET imaging in the detection of pedal osteomyelitis in diabetic patients.

Rastogi and colleagues[47] compared the efficacy of PET/CT using 18F-fluoride (F-fluoride PET/CT)

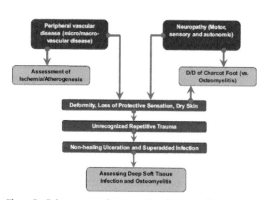

Fig. 2. Primary pathogenetic factors (*blue*), the further complicating factors (*brown*) in diabetic foot syndrome and diagnostic challenges where PET-CT/PET–MR imaging has a potential role (*green*). D/D, differential diagnosis. (*From* Basu S, Zhuang H, Alavi A, et al. FDG PET and PET/CT.Imaging in Complicated Diabetic Foot. PET Clin 2012(7); 151–160.)

**Table 3**
**Studies on fluorodeoxyglucose PET in diabetic foot infection**

| Author, Year | Modality | N | Charcot Arthropathy Separately Analyzed | Conclusion (Useful/Limited Accuracy) |
|---|---|---|---|---|
| Hopfner et al,[56] 2004 | PET alone | 16 | Yes | Useful |
| Keidar et al,[55] 2005 | PET/CT | 18 | No | Useful |
| Basu et al,[57] 2007 | PET alone | 63 | Yes | Useful |
| Schwegler et al,[54] 2008 | PET alone | 20 | No | Limited accuracy |
| Nawaz et al,[52] 2010 | PET alone | 110 | No | Useful |
| Familiari et al,[53] 2011 | PET/CT | 13 | No | Limited accuracy |
| Kagna et al,[51] 2012 | PET/CT | 39 | No | Useful |
| Ruotolo et al,[50] 2013 | PET/CT | 25 | Yes | Useful |
| Shagos et al,[49] 2015 | PET/CT | 79 | Yes | Useful |
| Lauri et al,[48] 2020 | PET/CT | 251 | Yes | Useful |

and 18F FDG–labeled autologous leukocytes (F-FDG-LL PET/CT) in comparison with contrast-enhanced MR imaging (CE-MR imaging) for the detection of diabetic foot osteomyelitis in patients with Charcot neuroarthropathy. Twenty-three patients were included in the study. Bone culture suggested diabetic foot osteomyelitis in 12 patients. CE-MR imaging identified 10 of the 12 cases of osteomyelitis. F-fluoride PET/CT and F-FDG-LL PET/CT showed increased tracer uptake (SUVmax = 22.7 ± 18.1 and 8.4 ± 4.7, respectively) at the clinically involved site in 10 of the 12 patients (TP). Among 11 biopsy-negative patients, CE-MR imaging reported diabetic foot osteomyelitis in 4 (false positive); there were no false positives with FDG-LL PET/CT. The sensitivity and specificity of FDG-LL PET/CT was 83.3% and 100% compared with 83.3% and 63.6% for CE-MR imaging, respectively; for the diagnosis of diabetic foot osteomyelitis in the background of Charcot neuroarthropathy, FDG-LL PET/CT has high specificity for the diagnosis of DFI in complicated diabetic foot. The $^{18}$F-fluoride PET/CT helps in the characterization the extent of underlying Charcot neuroarthropathy. An early and accurate diagnosis with FDG-LL PET/CT was proposed to aid the rational initiation of antibiotics for diabetic foot osteomyelitis.

## COMPARISON OF FLUORODEOXYGLUCOSE PET/COMPUTED TOMOGRAPHY WITH OTHER FUNCTIONAL IMAGING MODALITIES

On literature view of comparison of FDG-PET/CT with other functional imaging modalities,[48–57] all recent studies were based on combined PET/CT imaging; however, few studies were based on only PET imaging. Most of the studies have shown useful role of FDG-PET/CT in comparison to other nuclear medicine studies except few studies,[53,54] which concluded no useful role of FDG-PET/CT imaging; however, these 2 studies have included less number of patients in the analysis.

The recent large retrospective multicenter study by Lauri and colleagues,[48] for comparison of WBC scintigraphy, FDG-PET/CT, and MR imaging in suspected diabetic foot infection, images and clinical data from 251 patients enrolled by 5 centers were collected in order to calculate the sensitivity, specificity, and accuracy of WBC, FDG, and MR imaging in diagnosing osteomyelitis (OM), STI, and Charcot osteoarthropathy. In OM, WBC acquired following the European Society of Nuclear Medicine (EANM) guidelines was more specific and accurate than MR imaging (91.9% vs 70.7% and 86.2% vs 67.1%, respectively). In STI, both FDG and WBC achieved a significantly higher specificity than MR imaging (97.9% and 95.7% vs 83.6%, respectively). In Charcot, both MR imaging and WBC demonstrated a significantly higher specificity and accuracy than FDG (88.2% and 89.3% vs 62.5%; 80.3% and 87.9% vs 62.1%, respectively). Moreover, in Charcot, WBC was more specific than MR imaging (89.3% vs 88.2%). Given the limitations of a retrospective study, WBC using EANM guidelines was shown to be the most reliable imaging modality to differentiate between OM, STI, and Charcot in patients with suspected DFI.

In a study by Shagos and colleagues,[49] 79 patients with complicated diabetic foot (osteomyelitis/cellulitis, Charcot's neuropathy) were prospectively investigated. TPBS followed by FDG-PET within 5 days were performed in all patients. Based on referral indication, patients were grouped into osteomyelitis/cellulitis and Charcot neuropathy. The sensitivity, specificity, PPV, and NPV of FDG-PET were 87.5%, 71%, 87.5%, and 71% and 81.25%, 28.5%, 72%, and 40% for TPBS, respectively, in osteomyelitis group. In the Charcot neuroarthropathy group, TPBS identified more patients of Charcot and cellulitis than FDG-PET/CT. FDG-PET/CT has a higher specificity and NPV than TPBS in diagnosing pedal osteomyelitis. TPBS, being highly sensitive, is more useful than FDG-PET in detecting Charcot neuropathy.

Ruotolo and colleagues[50] selected 25 out of 40 diabetic patients with an acute Charcot foot Charcot neuropathic osteoarthropathy (CNO), without any bone involvement on radiograph (stage 0 CNO). Diagnostic criteria were inflammatory clinical signs of the affected foot and skin temperature difference greater than 2°C compared with the contralateral foot (ΔT). All patients underwent radiography, MR imaging, and 18F FDG-PET/CT scanning (expressed as SUVmax) at baseline (T0). All patients underwent another 18F FDG-PET/CT within 1 month after ΔT was less than 2°C (clinical recovery [T1]) and again every 3 months until SUVmax was less than 2 (final recovery [T2]); at this time, MR imaging confirmed the end of the inflammatory condition. T0 ΔT was 3.04 ± 1.65°C. All patients showed T0 SUVmax of the affected foot higher than the contralateral one (3.83 ± 1.087 vs 1.24 ± 0.3; $P < .001$). At clinical recovery (T1), defined by ΔT less than 2°C, the inflammatory signs were no longer present (T0 vs T1 ΔT = 3.04 ± 1.65 vs 0.9 ± 0.55°C; $P < .0001$). At T1, SUVmax was unchanged from T0 (3.80 ± 1.69 vs 3.83 ± 1.09; P = ns). At final recovery (T2), ΔT was 0.74 ± 0.29°C (similar to T1 ΔT), whereas the SUVmax dropped from T1 to T2 (3.8 ± 1.69 vs 1.72 ± 0.52; $P < .0001$). Standard therapy was total contact cast and removable cast walker until T2 (15.12 ± 5.45 mo). No patient developed foot bone fractures nor had relapses during follow-up (21.75 ± 16.7 mo). The investigators concluded that PET/CT scan allows the quantification of the inflammatory process; therefore, it may drive clinical decisions in the management of acute CNO better than clinical criteria.

Kagna and colleagues[51] basing the final diagnosis on histopathological and microbiologic examination of bone specimens, imaging, or clinical follow-up, evaluated the role of 18F FDG-PET/CT in the diagnosis of osteomyelitis in 39 diabetics with 46 sites suspicious for infections. In this study, the sensitivity, specificity, and accuracy, using lesion analysis, were 100%, 93%, and 96%, respectively; using patient-based analysis,

the sensitivity, specificity, and accuracy were 100%, 92%, and 95%, respectively. Nawaz and colleagues,[52] in a prospective study, using visual analysis, reported a sensitivity, specificity, and accuracy of 81%, 93%, and 90%, respectively, for diagnosing pedal osteomyelitis, but no information about the number of patients with foot ulcers was provided. By contrast, several studies have reported 18F FDG-PET/CT to be less useful and less sensitive in diagnosing diabetes-related osteomyelitis. Familiari and colleagues,[53] using visual and semiquantitative analysis, and bone biopsy or tissue culture for final diagnosis, conducted a study on 13 patients with very high pretest probability of osteomyelitis (7 with ulcers, 6 with exposed bone). Patients were examined with sequentially performed [99m]Tc-exametazime leukocyte scan and 18F FDG-PET/CT. The investigators found FDG-PET/CT to have a lower diagnostic accuracy (54%–62%) for osteomyelitis compared with 99mTc-exametazime–labeled leukocyte scintigraphy (92%). Schwegler and colleagues[54] conducted a prospective study in 20 diabetic patients with a chronic foot ulcer without antibiotic pretreatment and without clinical signs for osteomyelitis, to assess the prevalence of clinically unsuspected osteomyelitis and to compare the value of MR imaging, FDG-PET/CT, and [99m]Tc-labeled monoclonal antigranulocyte antibody scintigraphy. MR imaging resulted superior to the other 2 imaging modalities in detecting biopsy-proven osteomyelitis. FDG-PET sensitivity was 29%, and its accuracy in detecting osteomyelitis was similar to that of [99m]Tc-labeled monoclonal antigranulocyte antibody scintigraphy.

In one of the earliest reports with PET-CT, Keidar and colleagues[55] evaluated 14 diabetic patients with 18 clinically suspected sites of infection; PET, CT, and hybrid images were independently evaluated for the diagnosis and localization of an infectious process. Open wounds or ulcers were present in 12 of the 18 sites. PET/CT correctly localized 8 foci in 4 patients to bone, indicating osteomyelitis, whereas it correctly excluded osteomyelitis in 5 foci in 5 patients, with the abnormal FDG uptake limited to infected soft tissues only. The accuracy of FDG-PET/CT in this investigation was about 94%. The mean SUVmax in infectious foci was 5.7 (range, 1.7–11.1) for both osseous and soft tissue sites of infection. The investigators found no relationship between the patients' glycemic state and the degree of FDG uptake. They recommended FDG-PET for the diagnosis of diabetes-related infection and concluded that precise anatomic localization of increased FDG uptake provided by PET/CT enables accurate differentiation between osteomyelitis and STI.

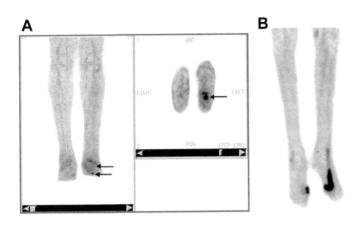

Fig. 3. (A) FDG-PET in a patient with diabetes mellitus demonstrating focal uptake in the ulcer (arrows) in the transaxial images and the relatively low-grade diffuse uptake in the neuropathic osteoarthropathy (arrows) are clearly distinguishable from the uptake observed on the unaffected contralateral limb by visual inspection. (B) High-grade FDG uptake clearly distinctive from that of Charcot neuroarthropathy. (From Basu S, Chryssikos T, Houseni M, et al. Potential role of FDG-PET in the setting of diabetic neuro-osteoarthropathy: can it differentiate uncomplicated Charcot's neuroarthropathy from osteomyelitis and soft-tissue infection? Nucl Med Commun. 2007;28(6):465-72.)

Hopfner and colleagues[56] evaluated 39 lesions of Charcot osteoarthropathy confirmed at surgery in 16 patients and noted that FDG-PET with a dedicated full-ring PET scanner accurately diagnosed this disorder in 37 lesions, with a sensitivity of 95%. In contrast, the coincidence PET camera provided a sensitivity of 77%, and MR imaging had a sensitivity of 79%. The mean SUVmax in the Charcot arthropathy lesions was 1.8 (range, 0.5–4.1). Those investigators concluded that FDG-PET can correctly distinguish osteomyelitis from Charcot osteoarthropathy and may be preferable to radiography and MR imaging in the preoperative evaluation of patients with Charcot neuroarthropathy of the foot.

Another analysis from a prospective research study by Basu and colleagues[57] also demonstrated promising results in diagnosing osteomyelitis and differentiating it from Charcot foot. In this study, a total of 63 patients in 4 groups were evaluated. A low degree of diffuse FDG uptake that was clearly distinguishable from that of normal

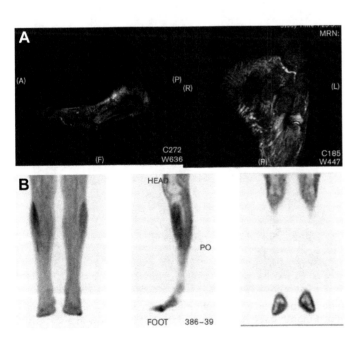

Fig. 4. A 60-year-old man presented with plantar left fifth metatarsal head region ulcer. The initial clinical impression was of osteomyelitis of the fifth metatarsal head versus Charcot neuroarthropathy of fifth metatarsophalangeal joint.(A) MR images consistent with early osteomyelitis of fifth metatarsal head and proximal phalanx. Mild intramuscular edema of midfoot was also observed in keeping with diabetic changes. (B) FDG-PET images demonstrate a tiny focus of moderately increased uptake in the left distal foot in the inferolateral aspect corresponding to the ulcer consistent with soft tissue involvement. However, there is no abnormal uptake characteristic of osteomyelitis of the feet as noted in the coronal image. The patient improved on oral antibiotic treatment (cephalexin, 250 mg, for 10 days) during the follow-up evaluation period. After 15 days post-imaging procedures, the wound had healed and was clean. No evidence of cellulitis. Clinical diagnosis was refined to Charcot neuroarthropathy. (From Basu S, Chryssikos T, Houseni M, et al. Potential role of FDG PET in the setting of diabetic neuro-osteoarthropathy: can it differentiate uncomplicated Charcot's neuroarthropathy from osteomyelitis and soft-tissue infection? Nucl Med Commun. 2007;28(6):465-72.)

joints was observed in joints of patients with Charcot osteoarthropathy (**Figs. 3** and **4**). The SUVmax in lesions of patients with Charcot osteoarthropathy varied from 0.7 to 2.4 (mean, 1.3 ± 0.4), whereas those of the midfoot of the healthy control subjects and the uncomplicated diabetic foot ranged from 0.2 to 0.7 (mean, 0.42 ± 0.12) and 0.2 to 0.8 (mean, 0.5 ± 0.16), respectively. The only patient with Charcot osteoarthropathy with superimposed osteomyelitis in this series had an SUVmax of 6.5. The SUVmax of the sites of osteomyelitis as a complication of diabetic foot ranged from 2.9 to 6.2 (mean,

4.38). A unifactorial analysis of variance test yielded a statistical significance in the SUVmax among the 4 groups (P.05). Although the presence of an underlying neuroarthropathy makes the diagnosis of osteomyelitis difficult, high accuracy and specificity rates have been reported using FDG-PET/CT for the differentiation of osteomyelitis from neuroarthropathy.

In summary, a precise diagnosis of osteomyelitis versus STI with better anatomic localization (**Fig. 5**), superior image quality, and faster imaging is possible with PET/CT than gamma camera–based techniques. PET/CT scan allows the

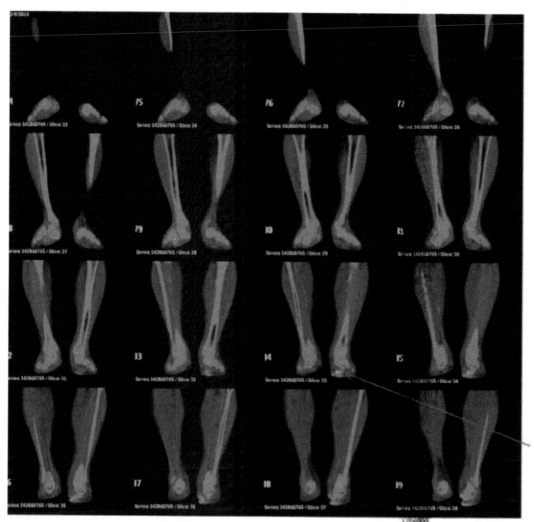

**Fig. 5.** A 54-year-old man is a known case of type 2 diabetes on antidiabetic medication since the age of 12 years. He had a nonhealing ulcer in the left foot about 1 month back. Radiograph of the left foot showed a soft tissue swelling in the left foot and predominantly around the ankle posteriorly. He was referred for FDG-PET/CT to look for any bony involvement. Coronal PET-CT images shows intense FDG uptake, primarily in the ulcer and soft tissue of the left foot (*arrows*) with the bone uninvolved ruling out osteomyelitis. (*From* Basu S, Ranade R. 18-Fluorodeoxyglucose-PET/Computed Tomography in Infection and Aseptic Inflammatory Disorders: Value to Patient Management. PET Clin. 2015 Jul;10(3):431-9.)

quantification of the inflammatory process; therefore, it may drive clinical decisions in the management of diabetic foot better than clinical criteria. Furthermore, PET/CT has been found to be superior to leukocyte-labeled and antigranulocyte monoclonal antibody fragment techniques in the diagnosis of chronic osteomyelitis.[58,59] In patients with medical implants, which can cause distortion in MR imaging, PET/CT is a good alternative. This technique might also be preferred in the postoperative assessment of these patients.

## SUMMARY

Evidence seems to be evolving in a positive direction for the use of FDG-PET/CT for imaging of prosthesis imaging. With high resolution and capability of functional assessment such as spectroscopy, MR imaging is a good choice for combination with PET. PET/MR imaging is an emerging technique and may offer some advantages over PET/CT. Chiefly, PET/MR imaging has lower radiation dose and better coregistration with PET data. PET/MR imaging may gain an important role in defining the different complications of the diabetic foot in the near future, and it is hoped to solve these challenging clinical scenarios.

## CLINICS CARE POINTS

- Advantages of FDG-PET/CT compared to conventional gamma camera based imaging: (a) Higher resolution of PET-CT, (b) less complexity, less technically demanding and patient-friendly. Issues with FDG-PET/CT: evolution of more specific and reliable diagnostic criterion in each of the conditions.

- PET/MR imaging may resolve the challenging clinical scenarios encountered with PET-CT and likely to assume an important role in defining the different complications of the diabetic foot in the near future.

- Increased 18F-FDG uptake at the middle portion of the femoral component bone-prosthesis interface at the shaft region as the as the positive criteria for peri-prosthetic infection in hip and knee prostheses, respectively yields the best diagnostic accuracy of 18F FDG-PET or PET/CT.

- FDG uptake at the (a) femoral neck and (b) tip of the femur stem are non-specific and cannot be considered as infection in a given setting.

## DISCLOSURE

The authors have nothing to disclose.

## REFERENCES

1. Lohmann CH, Rampal S, Lohrengel M, et al. Imaging in peri-prosthetic assessment:an orthopaedic perspective. EFORT Open Rev 2017;2(5):117–25.
2. Kini SG, Gabr A, Das R, et al. Two-stage revision for periprosthetic hip and knee joint infections. Open Orthop J 2016;10(Suppl-2):579–88. M2).
3. Romanò CL, Petrosillo N, Argento G, et al. The role of imaging techniques to define aperi-prosthetic hip and knee joint infection:multidisciplinary consensus statements. J Clin Med 2020;9(8):2548.
4. Sconfienza LM, Signore A, Cassar-Pullicino V, et al. Diagnosis of peripheral bone and prosthetic joint infections: overview on the consensus documents by the EANM,EBJIS, and ESR (with ESCMID endorsement). Eur Radiol 2019;(29):6425–38.
5. Hess S, Hansson SH, Pedersen KT, et al. FDG-PET/CT in infectious and inflammatory diseases. PET Clin 2014;9(4):497–519.
6. Saboury B, Ziai P, Parsons M, et al. Promising Roles of PET in Management of Arthroplasty Associated Infection. PET Clin 2012;7:139–50.
7. Zhuang H, Duarte PS, Pourdehnad M, et al. The promising role of 18F-FDG PET in detecting infected lower limb prosthesis implants. J Nucl Med 2001;42(1):44–8.
8. Zhuang H, Chacko TK, Hickeson M, et al. Persistent non-specific FDG uptake on PET imaging following hip arthroplasty. Eur J Nucl Med Mol Imaging 2002;29(10):1328–33.
9. Chacko TK, Zhuang H, Nakhoda KZ, et al. Applications of fluorodeoxyglucose positron emission tomography in the diagnosis of infection. Nucl Med Commun 2003;24(6):615–24.
10. Manthey N, Reinhard P, Moog F, et al. The use of [18 F]fluorodeoxyglucose positron emission tomography to differentiate between synovitis, loosening and infection of hip and knee prostheses. Nucl Med Commun 2002;23(7):645–53.
11. Kwee RM, Broos WA, Brans B, et al. Added value of 18F–FDG PET/CT in diagnosing infected hip prosthesis. Acta Radiol 2018;59:569–76.
12. Fukui K, Kaneuji A, Ueda S, et al. Should well–fixed uncemented femoral components be revised in infected hip arthroplasty? Report of five trial cases. J Orthop 2016;13(4):437–42.
13. Wenter V, Müller JP, Albert NL, et al. The diagnostic value of [(18)F]FDG PET for the detection of chronic osteomyelitisand implant-associated infection. Eur J Nucl Med Mol Imaging 2016;43:749–61.
14. Treglia G. Diagnostic Performance of (18)F-FDG PET/CT in Infectious and inflammatory diseases

according to published meta-analyses. Contrast Media Mol Imaging 2019;3018349.

15. Jin H, Yuan L, Li C. Diagnostic performance of FDG PET or PET/CT in prosthetic infection after arthroplasty: a meta-analysis. Q J Nucl Med Mol Imaging 2014;58(1):85–93.

16. VerberneS J, Raijmakers PG, Temmerman OPP. Accuracy of imaging techniques in the assessment of periprosthetic hip infection. J Bone Joint Surg 2016;98(19):1638–45.

17. VerberneS J, SonnegaR JA, Temmerman OP, et al. What is the accuracy of nuclear imaging in the assessment of periprosthetic knee infection? a metaanalysis. Clin Orthop Relat Res 2017;475(5): 1395–410.

18. Kwee RM, Kwee TC. 1 8F-FDG PET for diagnosing infections in prosthetic joints. PET Clin 2020;15: 197–205.

19. Wong MY, Beadsmoore C, Toms A, et al. Does 99mTc-MDP bonescintigraphy add to the investigation of patients with symptomatic unicompartmental knee replacement? Knee 2012;19:592–6.

20. Trevail C, Reddy RP, Sulkin T, et al. An evaluation of the role of nuclear medicine imaging in the diagnosis of periprosthetic infections of the hip. Clin Radiol 2016;(71):211–9.

21. Reinartz P. FDG-PET in patients with painful hip and knee arthroplasty: technical breakthrough or just more of the same. Q J Nucl Med Mol Imaging 2009;53(1):41–50.

22. Stumpe KD, Nö tzli HP, Zanetti M, et al. FDG PET for differentiation of infection and aseptic loosening in total hip replacements: comparison with conventionalradiography and three-phase bone scintigraphy. Radiology 2004;231(2):333–41.

23. Mumme T, Reinartz P, Alfer J, et al. Diagnostic values of positron emission tomography versus triple-phase bone scan in hip arthroplasty loosening. Arch Orthop Trauma Surg 2005;125(5):322–9.

24. Love C, Marwin SE, Palestro CJ, et al. Nuclear medicine and the infected joint replacement. Seminnucl Med 2009;39:66–78.

25. Blanc P, Bonnet E, Giordano G, et al. The use of labelled leucocyte scintigraphy to evaluate chronic periprosthetic joint infections: a retrospective multicentre study on 168 patients. Eur J Clin Microbiol Infect Dis 2019;(38):1625–31.

26. Weon YC, Yang SO, Choi YY, et al. Use of Tc-99m HMPAO leukocyte scans to evaluate bone infection: incremental value of additional SPECT images. Clin Nucl Med 2000;25(7):519–26.

27. Aksoy SY, Asa S, Ozhan M, et al. FDG and FDG-labelled leucocyte PET/CT in the imaging of prosthetic joint infection. Eur J Nucl Med Molimaging 2014;41(3):556–64.

28. Graute V, Feist M, Lehner S, et al. Detection of low-grade prosthetic joint infections using 99mTc-antigranulocyte SPECT/CT: initial clinical results. Eur J Nucl Med Mol Imaging 2010;37(9):1751–9.

29. Navalkissoor S, Nowosinska E, Gnanasegaran G, et al. Single-photon emission computed tomography-computed tomography in imaging infection. Nucl Med Commun 2013;34(4):283–90.

30. Signore A, Sconfienza LM, Borens O, et al. Consensus document for the diagnosis of prosthetic joint infections: a joint paper by the EANM, EBJIS, and ESR (with ESCMID endorsement). Eur J Nucl Med Mol Imaging 2019;46(4):971–88.

31. Glaudemans AWJM, Jutte PC, Cataldo MA, et al. Consensus document for the diagnosis of peripheral bone infection in adults: a joint paper by the EANM, EBJIS, and ESR (with ESCMID endorsement). Eur J Nucl Med Mol Imaging 2019;46(4):957–70.

32. Plate A, Weichselbaumer V, Schüpbach R, et al. Diagnostic accuracy of 99mTc-antigranulocyte SPECT/CT in patients with osteomyelitis and orthopaedic device-related infections: a retrospective analysis. Int J Infect Dis 2020;91:79–86.

33. Van Acker F, Nuyts J, Maes A, et al. FDG-PET,m99mtc-HMPAO white blood cell SPECTand bone scintigraphyin the evaluation of painful total knee arthroplasti. Eur J Nucl Med 2001;28(10): 1496–504.

34. Vanquickenborne B, Maes A, Nuyts J, et al. The value of (18)FDG-PET for the detection of infected hip prosthesis. Eur J Nucl Med Mol Imaging 2003; 30(5):705–15.

35. Love C, Marwin SE, Tomas MB, et al. Diagnosing infection in the failed joint replacement: a comparison of coincidence detection 18F-FDG and 111Inlabeled leukocyte/99mTc-sulfur colloid marrowimaging. J Nucl Med 2004;45(11):1864–71.

36. Pill SG, Parvizi J, Tang PH, et al. Comparison of fluorodeoxyglucose positron emission tomography and (111)indium-white blood cell imaging in the diagnosis of periprosthetic infection of the hip. J Arthroplasty 2006;21(6 Suppl 2):91–7.

37. Basu S, Zhuang H, Alavi A, et al. FDG PET and PET/CT.imaging in complicated diabetic foot. PET Clin 2012;(7):151–60.

38. Koob S, Gaertner FC, Jansen TR, et al. Diagnosis of peri-prosthetic loosening of total hip and knee arthroplasty using 18F-Fluoride PET/CT. Oncotarget 2019;10(No. 22):2203–11.

39. Kobayashi N, Inaba Y, Choe H, et al. Use of F-18 Fluoride PET to differentiate septic from aseptic loosening in total hip arthroplasty patients. Clinnucl Med 2011;36(11):e156–61.

40. Choe H, Inaba Y, Kobayashi N, et al. Use of 18F-fluoride PET to determine the appropriate tissue sampling region for improved sensitivity of tissue examinations in cases of suspected periprosthetic infection after total hip arthroplasty. Acta Orthop 2011;82(4):427–33.

41. Kwee TC, Basu S, Torigian DA, et al. FDG PET imaging for diagnosing prosthetic joint infection: discussing the facts, rectifying the unsupported claims and call for evidence-based and scientific approach. Eur J Nucl Med Mol Imaging 2013;40: 464–6.

42. Palestro CJ, Love C. Nuclear medicine and diabetic foot infections. Seminnucl Med 2009;39:52–65.

43. Treglia G, Sadeghi R, Annunziata S, et al. Diagnostic performance of Fluorine-18-Fluorodeoxyglucose positron emission tomography for the diagnosis of osteomyelitis related to diabetic foot: a systematic review and a meta-analysis. Foot 2013;23(4):140–8.

44. Lauri C, Tamminga M, Glaudemans AWJM, et al. Detection of osteomyelitis in the diabetic foot by imaging techniques: a systematic review and meta-analysis comparing MRI, white blood cell scintigraphy, and FDG-PET. Diabetes Care 2017;(40):1111–20.

45. Dinh MT, Abad CL, Safdar N. Diagnostic accuracy of physical examination and imaging tests for osteomyelitis underlying diabetic foot ulcers: meta analysis. Clin Infect Dis 2008;47(4):519–27.

46. Yang H, Zhuang H, Rubello D, et al. Mild to- moderate hyperglycemia will not decrease the sensitivity of 18F-FDG PET imaging in the detection of pedal osteomyelitis in diabetic patients. Nucl Med Commun 2016;37:259–62.

47. Rastogi A, Bhattacharya A, Prakash M, et al. Utility of PET/CT with fluorine-18-fluorodeoxyglucose-labeled autologous leukocytes for diagnosing diabetic foot osteomyelitis in patients with Charcot's neuroarthropathy. Nucl Med Commun 2016;37(12): 1253–9.

48. Lauri C, Glaudemans A, Campagna G, et al. Comparison of White Blood Cell Scintigraphy, FDG PET/CT and MRI in suspected diabetic foot infection: results of a large retrospective multicenter study. J Clin Med 2020;9:1645.

49. Shagos GS, Shanmugasundaram P, Varma AK, et al. 18-F fluorodeoxy glucose positron emission tomography-computed tomography imaging: a viable alternative to three phase bone scan in evaluating diabetic foot complications? Indian J Nucl Med 2015;30:97–103.

50. Ruotolo V, Pietro BD, Giurato L, et al. A new natural history of Charcot foot: clinical evolution and final outcome of stage 0 Charcot neuroarthropathy in a tertiary referral diabetic foot clinic. Clinnucl Med 2013;38(7):506–9.

51. Kagna O, Srour S, Melamed E, et al. FDG PET/CT imaging in the diagnosis of osteomyelitis in the diabetic foot. Eur J Nucl Med Mol Imaging 2012;39(10): 1545–50.

52. Nawaz A, Torigian DA, Siegelman ES, et al. Diagnostic performance of FDG-PET, MRI, and plain flm radiography (PFR) for the diagnosis of osteomyelitis in the diabetic foot. Mol Imaging Biol 2010;12(3): 335–42.

53. Familiari D, Glaudemans AW, Vitale V, et al. Can sequential 18FFDG PET/CT replace WBC imaging in the diabetic foot? J Nucl Med 2011;52(7):1012–9.

54. Schwegler B, Stumpe KD, Weishaupt D, et al. Unsuspected osteomyelitis is frequent in persistent diabetic foot ulcer and better diagnosed by MRI than by 18F-FDG PET or 99mTc-MOAB. J Intern Med 2008;263:99–106.

55. Keidar Z, Militianu D, Melamed E, et al. The diabetic foot: initial experience with 18F-FDG-PET/CT. J Nucl Med 2005;46:444–9.

56. Hopfner S, Krolak C, Kessler S, et al. Preoperative imaging of Charcot neuroarthropathy in diabetic patients: comparison of ring PET, hybrid PET, and magnetic resonance imaging. Foot Ankle Int 2004;25:890–5, 15.

57. Basu S, Chryssikos T, Houseni M, et al. Potential role of FDG-PET in the setting of diabetic neuroosteoarthropathy: can it differentiate uncomplicated Charcot's neuropathy from osteomyelitis and soft tissue infection? Nucl Med Commun 2007;28:465–72.

58. Kumar R, Basu S, Torigian D, et al. Role of modern imaging techniques for diagnosis of infection in the era of 18F-fluorodeoxyglucose positron emission tomography. Clin Microbiol Rev 2008;21:20924.

59. Basu S, Ranade R. 18-Fluoro-deoxyglucose-PET/computed tomography in infection and aseptic inflammatory disorders: value to patient management. PET Clin 2015;10(3):431–9.

# Utility of PET/Computed Tomography in Infection and Inflammation Imaging

Jasim Jaleel, MD[a], Sambit Sagar, MD[a],
Rakesh Kumar, MBBS, DRM, DNB, MNAMS, PhD[b],*

## KEYWORDS

• Infections • Inflammation • PET/CT • FDG

## KEY POINTS

- Metabolic uptake of 18F-fluorodeoxyglucose (FDG) is known to be upregulated in all the three phases of inflammation by different molecular mechanism.
- Dual time-point imaging with 18F FDG-PET/computed tomography (CT) can distinguish between malignant lesion and tuberculoma; also, 18F FDG-PET/CT at specific intervals of treatment is useful for response assessment of both pulmonary and extrapulmonary tuberculosis.
- For evaluation of cardiac sarcoidosis, adequate myocardial suppression with monitored diet planning to suppress physiologic myocardial glucose uptake is highly recommended to improve the sensitivity and specificity of the study.
- FDG-PET/CT has high specificity to rule out osteomyelitis with caveats such as postsurgical inflammatory changes and posttraumatic bone healing as false-positive findings.
- 18F FDG-PET/CT can be used for evaluation of post-coronavirus disease 2019 sequalae such as mucormycosis, neurologic pathologies, and so forth.

## INTRODUCTION

Nuclear medicine plays an important role in assessment of infection and inflammation. Gamma imaging with Gallium 67 (Ga-67) citrate and 99mTc-labeled white blood cells (WBCs) is being done for a long period of time. Limitations of these tracers such as poor spatial resolution and long imaging time were circumvented to an extend with the introduction of 18F-flurodeoxyglucose (FDG). 18F FDG is widely used for oncological imaging, but recently we have visualized a large number of nononcological indications where they were being used with literature supporting them. Inherent spatial resolution of PET tracers also provides a good image quality as compared with the previously used SPECT tracers.

In this article, the authors discuss the utility of 18F FDG in infection and inflammation imaging.

## Molecular Basis of 18F FDG in Inflammation and Infection Imaging

Findings of 18F FDG accumulation in inflammatory processes during routine scans done in patients with cancer led to the exploration of its clinical utility to image infection and inflammation. Further studies showed that cells involved in infection and inflammation were able to express high levels of glucose transporters, especially GLUT1 and GLUT3, and hexokinase activity.[1]

Inflammation process can be temporally divided into 3 phases: early vascular phase, acute cellular phase, and healing phase. The early vascular phase includes tissue hyperemia, increased vascular permeability, and release of inflammatory mediators. Increased tissue perfusion can result in greater FDG delivery to affected sites.[2] Cellular phase includes active cell recruitment, migration,

[a] Department of Nuclear Medicine, All India Institute of Medical Sciences, New Delhi 110029, India; [b] Division of Diagnostic Nuclear Medicine, Department of Nuclear Medicine, All India Institute of Medical Sciences, New Delhi 110029, India
* Corresponding author.
E-mail address: rkphulia@yahoo.com

PET Clin 17 (2022) 533–542
https://doi.org/10.1016/j.cpet.2022.02.004

and proliferation at the site of inflammation and release of several cytokines and other mediators. These mediators can lead to upregulation of GLUT-1 and GLUT-3 transporters, an increase in hexokinase activity, and an amplified affinity of GLUT for its substrates (ie, glucose and FDG).[3,4] In the phase of healing, the cellular milieu changes from polymorphonuclear leukocytes to macrophages and monocytes along with tissue healing. Increased expression of GLUT-3 in macrophages can lead to increased FDG uptake in tissues.[5]

## Tuberculosis

Tuberculosis is continuing to affect almost every part of the world, despite being both curable and preventable, with disproportionately increased incidence in developing and underdeveloped countries. It may infect people of any age and can affect any organ system, whereas its diagnosis in children with extrapulmonary tuberculosis (TB) and human immunodeficiency virus (HIV)-associated TB may be challenging. Drug-resistant TB further adds to the challenges in managing this infection. Newer diagnostic tools are the need of the hour for more comprehensive management of this deadly infection. Imaging techniques such as whole-body imaging with PET/computed tomography (CT) may help to address some of the challenges encountered in the management of TB by detecting sites of extrapulmonary involvement, biopsy sites, treatment response assessment, determining the extent of disease involvement, and possibly predicting individuals who are more likely to develop drug-resistant TB or to progress from latent to active TB.[6] For diagnosing TB, treating physician should be knowledgeable about the role and limitations of clinical evaluation, laboratory testing, and imaging. Cross-sectional imaging can help in identifying active, inactive, and latent disease. Newer technological advancement in the diagnostic imaging and microbiological techniques will assist in early diagnosis and follow-up of the patients.

### Pulmonary tuberculosis

Pulmonary TB can be of 2 types: primary pulmonary TB and postprimary reactivation. Primary TB is due to initial exposure to the *mycobacterium bacillus* that may result in multilobar consolidation that may result in either of the 3 outcomes: complete resolution, scar formation, or tuberculoma. Postprimary TB typically present as consolidation in the upper lobes or superior segments of the lower lobes with associated cavitation.[7]

Differential hypermetabolism of glucose in inflamed tissue, as opposed to the normal cells, is the pathophysiological basis for the use of 18F FDG-PET/CT in TB. The typical lung findings are mildly metabolically active areas of lung consolidation with or without cavities. Mediastinal and extrapulmonary lymphadenopathy along with other extrapulmonary FDG uptake may also be seen. Pulmonary-only findings may be seen in immunocompetent patients, whereas diffuse lesions may be seen in immunocompromised patients.[8]

As compared with CT alone, FDG-PET/CT could find as many as lung lesions and almost double the number of lymph nodal lesions in a study published by Sathekge and colleagues in 7 patients.[9] Also, some of these missed lymph nodal lesions were the only tubercular lesions in these patients. Missing these often-overlooked sites of CT may have a detrimental effect on treatment. So FDG-PET/CT with its enhanced field of view can help to detect distant extrapulmonary lesions, thereby altering treatment duration.

Dual time-point imaging with FDG-PET/CT is a useful method to differentiate between malignant and inflammatory processes in settings where such a distinction is essential for optimal patient management; this is based on the observation that standardized uptake values (SUVs) of inflammatory and nonneoplastic lesions tend to remain stable or decrease, whereas those of the malignant lesions tend to increase over time.[10] Kim and colleagues investigated the usefulness of 18F FDG dual time-point imaging in differentiating active from inactive pulmonary tuberculosis lesions in 25 patients, who were imaged at 60 and 120 min posttracer injection. Early and delayed SUVmax values were determined and found that active TB could be differentiated from inactive TB with 100% sensitivity and 100% specificity when using an early SUVmax cut-off value of 1.05, whereas the delayed SUVmax cut-off value of 0.97 yielded a sensitivity of 92.8%, and specificity of 100%.[11] Chen and colleagues studied the utility of 18F FDG dual time-point imaging in a total of 31 lesions to differentiate between malignant and benign lung lesions and found to have a sensitivity and specificity of 62% and 40%, respectively, when a retention index of greater than 10% for malignancy was used and no statistical difference were observed between the retention indexes of the benign versus malignant pulmonary nodules.[12] Another study by Sathekge and colleagues in 30 patients concluded that 18F FDG dual time-point imaging could not differentiate between malignant nodules from those due to tuberculoma. Using an SUVmax cutoff of 2.5, 18F FDG-PET only yielded a sensitivity and specificity of 85.7% and 25%, respectively, whereas using a change in SUVmax of greater than 10% yielded a sensitivity and specificity of 85.7% and 50%, respectively. They also found that rate of increase of SUVmax did not vary significantly between malignant lesions and tuberculoma.[13]

FDG-PET/CT plays an important role in evaluation of treatment response in patients with tuberculosis and undergoing antitubercular therapy. Davis and colleagues compared FDG-PET imaging–based outcomes with standard outcome measures of lung colony-forming unit counts and culture-positive relapse after treatment completion. FDG-PET could differentiate the bactericidal regimens from the bacteriostatic regimen in a time frame similar to that of the standard regimen (2 weeks). These findings suggested that FDG-PET imaging may be useful for monitoring TB treatment response. In a meta-analysis by Sjö-lander and colleagues, estimated overall percentage change in SUVmax was found to be −54.38% (95% confidence interval [CI]; −57.81 to −50.96), and there was a trend toward usefulness of FDG-PET or FDG-PET/CT for evaluation of antitubercular therapy response.[14]

### Extrapulmonary tuberculosis

Extrapulmonary tuberculosis (EPTB) is tuberculosis outside of the lungs. EPTB includes tuberculosis meningitis, abdominal tuberculosis (usually with ascites), skeletal tuberculosis, Pott disease (spine), scrofula (lymphadenitis), and genitourinary (renal) tuberculosis. Disseminated or miliary tuberculosis often includes pulmonary and extrapulmonary sites.

TB meningitis can occur as a consequence of dissemination of tuberculous bacilli during hematogenous spread or following its release from a focus of infection into the subarachnoid space. FDG-PET/CT is useful in these cases for identifying the foci of infection and the disease burden, which in turn guides the course of treatment. Gambhir and colleagues, in their study comprising 10 patients, showed that FDG-PET/CT could identify additional lesions in vertebrae, spinal cords, and lymph nodes, which were missed by conventional imaging. They concluded that FDG-PET/CT was complementary to MR imaging for detecting cranial lesions and is more sensitive in detecting the extracranial tuberculosis burden in the patients with TB meningitis.[15] Modi and colleagues analyzed 70 cases of patients with TB meningitis (definite [n = 26] or probable [n = 44]) using FDG-PET/CT and found evidence of pulmonary involvement in 62 (88.6%) and lymph nodal involvement in 61 (87.1%) patients, thus clearly delineating the disease burden.[16] Also, FDG-PET/CT can be used for response evaluation after antitubercular therapy. Newer studies are being conducted with 11C-Rifampicin in TB meningitis with an aim to optimize treatment.[17]

### Sarcoidosis

Sarcoidosis is a multisystem disorder of unknown cause, characterized by the accumulation of T lymphocytes, mononuclear phagocytes, and non-caseating granulomas in involved tissues. Lungs are most common site of involvement, followed by skin, lymph nodes, and eyes.[18] The clinical course is extremely variable, and the imaging features are diverse and depends on site of involvement, degree of inflammation, and treatment the patient receives. Atypical manifestations and imaging findings can further make diagnosis and management difficult.[19] In the last decades, PET/CT has demonstrated an important role in assessment of disease extent and activity, treatment planning, and monitoring response to therapy, with a crucial role in the management of cardiac sarcoidosis.[20]

Thoracic sarcoidosis encompassing both lungs and mediastinal lymph node involvement is the most location of disease involvement. Chest radiograph is usually the first line of investigation. Based on chest radiograph findings, 4 stages of pulmonary sarcoidosis have been described. Stage 1 consists bilateral hilar lymphadenopathy without infiltration. Stage 2 is represented by bilateral hilar lymphadenopathy with infiltration. Stage 3 consists of exclusive pulmonary parenchymal infiltration, and stage 4 consists of pulmonary fibrosis with either of fibrotic bands, bullae, hilar retraction, bronchiectasis, and diaphragmatic tenting.[21] CT findings range from normal lung findings to interstitial involvement with reticulonodular syndrome, septal and nonseptal thickenings, ground glass opacites, fibrosis (bronchiectasis and bronchial distortion, honeycombing, emphysema), and mediastinal lymphadenopathies.[22]

FDG-PET/CT is not indicated in routine first-line evaluation of pulmonary sarcoidosis. They are useful in patients showing atypical presentations. FDG-PET/CT is more sensitive than other imaging modalities in detecting inflammatory activity within lungs and thoracic lymph nodes. Yamada and colleagues studied uptake of 18F FDG in mediastinum and hilar lymph nodes in 31 patients with sarcoidosis and found that there was FDG accumulation in 30 patients (97%).[23] Braun and colleagues evaluated FDG-PET/CT for diagnosis and therapeutic follow-up of 20 patients with biopsy-proven sarcoidosis. Sensitivity was found to be 100%, 100%, and 80%, respectively, for thoracic, sinonasal, and pharyngo-laryngeal locations.[24] Keijsers and colleagues, in their retrospective study including 36 newly diagnosed, symptomatic sarcoidosis patients, found that

FDG-PET was positive in 34 of 36 patients, thereby showing 94% sensitivity.[25] Teirstein and colleagues performed 18F FDG-PET scans in 137 patients with proven sarcoidosis, of which 139 had positive findings. The most common positive sites were mediastinal lymph nodes (n = 54), extrathoracic lymph nodes (n = 30), and lungs (n = 24). The SUV ranged from 2.0 to 15.8. Twenty occult disease sites were identified. Eleven repeat scans showed a decrease in SUV in response to corticosteroid therapy. FDG-PET scan findings were found in two-thirds of patients with radiographic stage II and III sarcoidosis. Negative pulmonary FDG-PET scan findings were common in patients with radiographic stage 0, I, and IV sarcoidosis.[26]

Ambrosini and colleagues prospectively investigated role of FDG-PET/CT in assessment of disease activity and extension of sarcoidosis in comparison with high-resolution CT (HRCT) and evaluates the potential clinical impact of PET/CT findings in 35 patients. PET/CT was found to be concordant with HRCT in 45.7% (n = 16), detecting active disease in 10 patients and no signs of activity in 4 patients. PET/CT findings had a direct impact on management in 4 patients. In 54.3% (n = 19) discordant cases, PET/CT was positive in 14 and negative in 5 of them. PET/CT findings influenced the clinical management in 18/19 patients. Considering all scans, PET/CT information influenced the clinical management of 63% (n = 23) patients. They concluded that FDG-PET/CT was useful in assessing disease activity and disease extent in patients with sarcoidosis and provided valuable information for the clinical management in a single-step examination.[27] Treglia and colleagues, in their systematic review, concluded that FDG-PET is useful in staging, evaluating disease activity, and monitoring treatment response in patients with sarcoidosis and have a higher diagnostic accuracy as compared with Ga-67 citrate scintigraphy.[28] FDG-PET/CT can also guide as a suitable tool for identifying which lymph node should be sampled to help in diagnosis.

Heart is the most notorious site of sarcoid involvement, as it can cause severe morbidity and mortality. Antemortem diagnosis of cardiac sarcoidosis remains challenging because of broad and nonspecific sets of signs and symptoms ranging from asymptomatic electrocardiogram findings to sudden death and progressively worsening heart failure and arrhythmias.[29] It has been reported in some cases as heart as the only site of involvement.[30] Granulomatous inflammation of myocardial tissue can lead to myocardial tissue scarring (fibrosis), which in turn triggers an arrhythmic event or abnormal conduction, thereby causing sudden cardiac death.

Imaging of cardiac sarcoidosis involves both perfusion imaging and metabolism imaging. Perfusion imaging shows metabolic defects except in the early stage, which can be picked up by FDG imaging.[29] Whole-body FDG-PET/CT is useful in identifying extracardiac disease also. Yamagishi and colleagues compared 13N-ammonia/18F FDG-PET imaging, Ga-67, and Thallium-201 scintigraphy in 17 patients with pathology-proven systemic sarcoidosis and cardiac involvement. Fifteen of seventeen of these patients had increased myocardial 18F FDG uptake, 6 patients had perfusion defects on Thallium-201 scintigraphy, and only 3 patients showed Ga-67 uptake.[31] Seven of these patients were treated with steroid and underwent follow-up cardiac PET after 1 month. Perfusion defects exhibited no significant change after steroid therapy, whereas FDG uptake was markedly diminished in size and intensity in 5 patients and disappeared completely in 2 patients, which underlines the role of FDG-PET in monitoring response to treatment.[31]

Langah and colleagues retrospectively reviewed 76 patients and found that FDG-PET showed 85% sensitivity and 90% specificity with a diagnostic accuracy of 86.7%.[32] Okumura and colleagues compared diagnostic accuracy of 18F FDG-PET with 99mTc- MIBI perfusion imaging and Ga-67 citrate scintigraphy. FDG-PET/CT had 100% sensitivity as compared with 63.6% and 36.3% of 99mTc- MIBI perfusion imaging and Ga-67 citrate scintigraphy, respectively. They also suggested that FDG-PET can detect the early stage of cardiac sarcoidosis, in which fewer perfusion abnormalities and high inflammatory activity were noted, before advanced myocardial impairment.[33] Ohira and colleagues compared FDG-PET and MR imaging in the assessment of cardiac sarcoidosis in 21 patients. Sensitivity and specificity for diagnosing cardiac sarcoidosis were 87.5% and 38.5%, respectively, for 18F FDG-PET, and 75% and 76.9%, respectively, for MRI.[34]

The main limitation of FDG imaging is patient preparation to suppress myocardial glucose uptake. It is absolutely necessary to ensure that patients are compliant with the appropriate diet, as inadequate suppression of 18F FDG uptake will reduce the test specificity.[35] Here comes the importance of 68Ga-DOTANOC PET/CT in cardiac sarcoidosis, as it does not need any patient preparation. DOTANOC binds to somatostatin receptors on inflammatory cells in sarcoid granulomas. Gormsen and colleagues performed FDG-PET/CT and DOTANOC PET/CT in 19 patients with suspected cardiac sarcoidosis. Diagnostic accuracy of FDG was 79%, where as that of DOTANOC was 100%.[36] Kaushik and colleagues compared 68Ga-DOTANOC PET/CT with cardiac MR imaging in 17 patients with clinical suspicion of cardiac sarcoidosis. PET and CMR were concordant in 13 (76.5%) patients and discordant in 4 (23.5%). They concluded that cardiac MR imaging is superior to 68Ga-DOTANOC PET/CT for detecting cardiac involvement in sarcoidosis; however, 68Ga-DOTANOC PET/CT may be better than cardiac MR imaging in identifying patients with active inflammation, as they directly target inflammatory cells and can have a complementary role to MR imaging.[37]

In neurosarcoidosis, PET detection of neurologic involvement may be affected by physiologic intense FDG uptake in the brain, which may mask potential lesions, and by the usual small size of neurologic lesions, which are often inferior to PET resolution with possible false negative due to partial volume effect. But, FDG-PET/CT may be useful in determining potential sites extraneurologic involvement to help diagnose multisystem sarcoidosis and guide biopsy site.[21] Chan and colleagues demonstrated utility of 18F-fluoroethyl tyrosine (FET) PET/CT in a case of neurosarcoidosis, which showed FET uptake. 18F-FET is a promising radiolabeled amino acid tracer due to its high uptake in biologically active tumor tissue and low uptake in normal brain tissue.[38]

In cutaneous sarcoidosis, FDG-PET is useful in assessing extent of disease involvement, monitoring response to therapy, and guiding site of biopsy. Various case reports have been published showing utility of FDG-PET/CT in cutaneous sarcoidosis Fig. 1.[39–42]

## Osteomyelitis

Osteomyelitis can be categorized as acute, subacute, and chronic. Acute osteomyelitis develops within 2 weeks after disease-onset, subacute osteomyelitis within 1 to several months and chronic osteomyelitis after a few months. Three-phase bone scintigraphy is the most widely used nuclear imaging procedure for the evaluation of osseous infections owing to its widespread availability and low cost. Even though bone scintigraphy is extremely sensitive (exceeding 90%), it has a limited specificity (around 50%), which may be explained by uptake of radiotracer at all sites of increased osteoblastic activity irrespective of the underlying cause.[43]

18F FDG-PET/CT imaging can accurately differentiate chronic osteomyelitis from the normal postsurgical or posttraumatic healing process as compared with bone scintigraphy, which may be positive in both active disease and healing bone.[44] Meta-analysis by Termaat and colleagues showed a pooled sensitivity of 96% (95% CI, 88%–99%) for 18F FDG-PET/CT as compared with 82% (95% CI, 70%–89%) for bone scintigraphy, 61% (95% CI, 43%–76%) for leukocyte scintigraphy, 78% (95% CI, 72%–83%) for combined bone and leukocyte scintigraphy, and 84% (95% CI, 69%–92%) for MR imaging. Pooled specificity demonstrated that bone scintigraphy had the lowest specificity, with a specificity of 25% (95% CI, 16%–36%) compared with 60% (95% CI, 38%–78%) for MR imaging, 77% (95% CI, 63%–87%) for leukocyte scintigraphy, 84% (95% CI, 75%–90%) for combined bone and leukocyte scintigraphy, and 91% (95% CI, 81%–95%) for FDG-PET.[45]

On 18F FDG-PET/CT, fracture or surgical trauma is less likely to cause false-positive results in the evaluation for chronic osteomyelitis. Compared with other isotope imaging techniques, 18F FDG-PET/CT is superior for distinguishing soft tissue infection from osteomyelitis.[43] FDG-PET may have limited value in a diagnosis of uncomplicated cases of acute osteomyelitis compared with the combination of physical examination, evaluation of biochemical marker alteration (WBC count, serum C-reactive protein, and serum erythrocyte sedimentation rate), and 3-phase bone scanning or MR imaging.[46]

False-positive results in FDG-PET imaging can be caused by postsurgical inflammatory changes for as long as 6 months after the procedure. Thus, it has been proposed that an interval of 3 to 6 months should be allowed before FDG-PET imaging to minimize the risk of false-positive results during stages of postsurgical and traumatic bone healing. However, a negative FDG-PET scan can virtually eliminate the possibility of chronic osteomyelitis Fig. 2.[43]

## Vasculitis

Vasculitis is a heterogeneous group of pathologies characterized by inflammation of vessels. The clinical and pathologic features are variable and depend on the site and type of blood vessels affected. Vasculitis may occur as a primary process or may also be secondary to another underlying disease.[47]

18F FDG-PET/CT has become increasingly recognized as an important tool for rheumatologists in the assessment of large vessel vasculitis. 18F FDG is taken up by the inflammatory cells that migrate and reside in the inflamed arterial wall.[48] 18F FDG-PET/CT is not suitable for evaluating small- and medium-sized arteries. But they

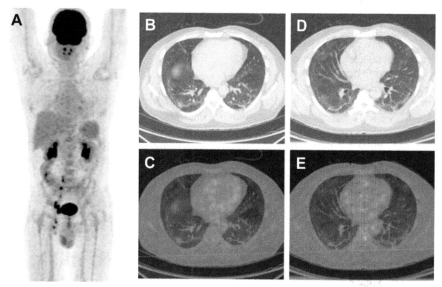

**Fig. 1.** A 38-year-old man with known COVID-19 history, showing bilateral basal ground glass and reticular opacities, showing mildly increased 18F FDG activity in maximum intensity projection images (*A*) and axial CT and fused PET/CT images (*B–E*).

are well established in use in case of large vessel vasculitis. Because of its helpfulness, PET/CT has been strongly recommended as a tool for the early diagnosis of vasculitis by both the American College of Rheumatology and the European League Against Rheumatism.[48,49] Meta-analysis by Lee and colleagues showed pooled sensitivity and specificity of 18F FDG-PET or PET/CT were 75.9% (95% CI, 68.7–82.1) and 93.0% (95% CI 88.9–96.0), respectively. The positive likelihood ratio, negative likelihood ratio, and diagnostic odds ratio were 7.267 (95% CI 3.707–14.24), 0.303 (95% CI 0.229–0.400), and 32.04 (95% CI 13.08–78.45), respectively.[50] Another meta-analysis by Geest and colleagues [51] showed 18F FDG-PET/CT may detect relapsing/refractory disease with a sensitivity of 77% (95% CI, 57%–90%) and specificity of 71% (95% CI, 47%–87%).

Other than detection of large vessel vasculitis, 18F FDG-PET/CT may also play an important

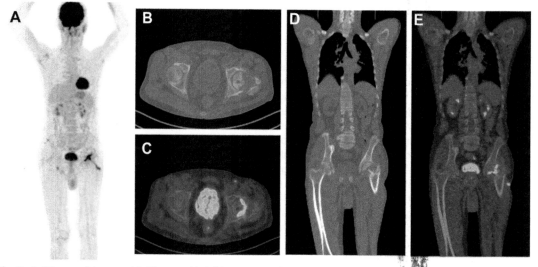

**Fig. 2.** A 45-year-old man with history of left hip osteomyelitis showing increased FDG uptake in the left hip region in MIP image (*A*). It is seen as lytic lesion with increased FDG uptake with destruction of neck region in axial (*B, C*) and coronal (*D, E*) CT and fused PET/CT images. MIP, maximum intensity projection.

role in therapeutic response assessment. Also, FDG-PET/CT can be used for prognostication of patients. Another important use of 18F FDG-PET/CT is helping to identify the site of biopsy **Fig. 3**.

## Immunoglobulin G4–Related Diseases

Immunoglobulin G4–related disease (IgG4-RD) is a recently defined emerging clinical entity characterized by tissue infiltration by IgG4-positive plasma cells, tissue fibrosclerosis, and elevated serum IgG4 concentration. The most important feature of IgG4-RD is chronic inflammation with multiple organ involvement. IgG4-RD has been found in multiple organs/tissues, including the pancreas (also known as autoimmune pancreatitis), pancreatobiliary tract, lacrimal gland, salivary gland, lung, retroperitoneal region, and kidney.[52] Clinically, more than half of the patients have elevated serum IgG4 levels, and the initial response to corticosteroid-based treatment is usually good, although relapses are frequent.[53] The clinical diagnosis of IgG4-RD remains difficult because most patients present with only mild symptoms and the clinical spectrum is extremely diverse; this makes it important to further establish the role of various noninvasive imaging techniques in the differential diagnosis of suspected IgG4-RD.[54]

18F FDG-PET/CT is useful in patients with IgG4-RD, as it can identify the disease distribution in the whole body. Zhang and colleagues demonstrated specific image characteristics and pattern of IgG4-RD in 29 patients, including diffusely elevated 18F FDG uptake in the pancreas and salivary glands, patchy lesions in the retroperitoneal region and vascular wall, and multiorgan involvement that cannot be interpreted as metastasis. After 2 to 4 weeks of steroid-based therapy at 40 mg to 50 mg prednisone per day, 72.4% of the patients showed complete remission, whereas the others exhibited greater than 81.8% decrease in 18F FDG uptake. Mittal and colleagues showed in their study that the most commonly affected sites were the lymph nodes followed by submandibular salivary glands. The least common sites of involvement were spleen, lacrimal glands, retroperitoneum, and chest nodules.[55] Ozaki and colleagues in their study showed that 18F FDG-PET/CT is useful in selecting a biopsy site for the pathologic examination of tissue that is necessary to diagnose or exclude IgG4-RD, which in turn can increase the diagnostic yield.[56] Khosroshahi and colleagues in their study showed that in their study comprising 20 patients, 7 had 18F FDG uptake in organs not suspected of involvement on a clinical basis alone, which included retroperitoneum, lymph nodes, thoracic aorta, lung, lacrimal glands, and nasopharynx.

## Coronavirus Disease 2019 Infection

Coronavirus disease 2019 (COVID-19) is a highly contagious infectious disease caused by severe acute respiratory syndrome coronavirus 2.

HRCT scan of chest could identify various patterns in COVID infection. Those abnormalities with highest incidence are ground-glass opacities, vascular enlargement, bilateral abnormalities, lower lobe involvement, and posterior predilection. Findings such as consolidation, linear opacity, septal thickening and/or reticulation, crazy-paving pattern, air bronchogram, pleural thickening, halo sign, bronchiectasis, nodules, bronchial wall thickening, and reversed halo sign are also consistent with intermediate chance of infection.[57] Based on HRCT chest, a scoring system called CT severity score was developed by Yang and colleagues with maximum score of

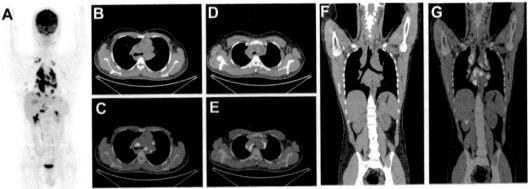

Fig. 3. A 27-year-old man with diagnosis of sarcoidosis showing multiple cervical, mediastinal, and abdominal lymph nodes in the 18F FDG MIP image (*A*). Multiple FDG avid discrete lower cervical, bilateral paratracheal, prevascular, subcarinal, and bilateral hilar lymph nodes are noted in the axial (*B–E*) and coronal (*F, G*) CT and fused PET/CT images.

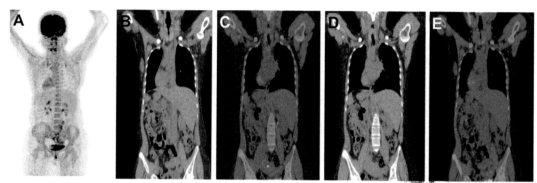

Fig. 4. A 20-year-old man with diagnosis of fever of unknown origin was referred for 18F FDG-PET/CT. MIP image (A) shows increased FDG uptake over bilateral carotid arteries. Coronal CT and fused PET/CT images (B-E) show increased FDG uptake along the walls of ascending aorta and bilateral carotid arteries, consistent with vasculitis.

25.[58] Saeed and colleagues in their study with 902 patients showed that CT severity scoring system aided in predicting COVID-19 disease outcome and significantly correlated with laboratory tests and oxygen requirements.[59] But the limitation of HRCT is the absence of certainty with which they can tell the presence of active infection.

18F FDG-PET/CT on the other hand shows increased FDG uptake in the active lesions. Those lesions with typical presentations of COVID-19 in HRCT chest and no significant FDG uptake usually represent a past infection. Metabolic parameters in these cases can guide us in these situations. A systematic review by Rafiee and colleagues showed that SUVmax in pulmonary lesions ranged from 2.2 to 18 in various case reports that have been published previously with a mean value of 4.9.[59]

More literature is yet to come on the use of 18F FDG-PET/CT IN COVID infection. Also, it may be possible to identify long-term sequalae such as mucormycosis and COVID-19–associated neurologic disorders in further studies Fig. 4.

## DISCLOSURE

The authors have nothing to disclose. They have no conflict of interest. No financial aid was provided for this project.

## CLINICS CARE POINTS

**Pearls:**

- In patients with pulmonary TB, 18F-FDG PET/CT can determine extra-pulmonary involvement, biopsy sites, treatment response assessment, determining the extent of disease involvement, and possibly predicting individuals who are more likely to develop drugresistant TB or to progress from latent to active TB.

- In patients with diagnosis of sarcoidosis, 18F-FDG PET/CT has demonstrated an important role in assessment of disease extent and activity, treatmentplanning, and monitoring response to therapy.

- 18F-FDG PET/CT has high negative predictive value in determining response to therapy in chronic osteomyelitis.

**Pitfalls:**

- 18F-FDG PET/CT cannot accurately differentiate between malignancies and inflammatory processes. Dual time-point imaging with 18F-FDG PET/CT can be a use as a method to differentiate between malignant and inflammatory processes.

- Urinary excretion of 18F-FDG may mask some lesions in genitourinary areas, especially in genitourinary tuberculosis.

- The role of FDG PET/CT in intracranial lesions are challengingowing to physiological uptake of FDG in the brain parenchyma.

- Physiological gut activity may obscure some lesions, especially in ileo-caecal tuberculosis. Special techniques like PET/CT enteroclysis can be useful in these cases.

## REFERENCES

1. Jamar F, Buscombe J, Chiti A, et al. EANM/SNMMI guideline for 18F-FDG use in inflammation and infection. J Nucl Med 2013;54(4):647–58.
2. Ohba K, Sasaki S, Oki Y, et al. Factors associated with fluorine-18-fluorodeoxyglucose uptake in benign thyroid nodules. Endocr J 2013;60(8):985–90.
3. Mochizuki T, Tsukamoto E, Kuge Y, et al. FDG uptake and glucose transporter subtype expressions in

experimental tumor and inflammation models. J Nucl Med 2001;42(10):1551–5.

4. O'Neill LAJ, Hardie DG. Metabolism of inflammation limited by AMPK and pseudo-starvation. Nature 2013;493(7432):346–55.

5. Wang ZG, Yu MM, Han Y, et al. Correlation of Glut-1 and Glut-3 expression with F-18 FDG uptake in pulmonary inflammatory lesions. Medicine (Baltimore) 2016;95(48). Available from. https://www.ncbi.nlm.nih.gov/pmc/articles/PMC5134797/ [cited 2021 Apr 14].

6. Mokoala KMG, Ankrah AO. Tuberculosis: a general overview. In: Sobic Saranovic D, Vorster M, Gambhir S, et al, editors. PET/CT in tuberculosis [internet]. Cham: Springer International Publishing; 2020. p. 1–7. https://doi.org/10.1007/978-3-030-47009-8_1. Available from.

7. Bomanji JB, Gupta N, Gulati P, et al. Imaging in tuberculosis. Cold Spring Harb Perspect Med 2015;5(6).

8. Soussan M, Brillet P-Y, Mekinian A, et al. Patterns of pulmonary tuberculosis on FDG-PET/CT. Eur J Radiol 2012;81(10):2872–6.

9. Sathekge M, Maes A, Kgomo M, et al. Impact of FDG PET on the management of TBC treatment: a pilot study. Nuklearmedizin 2010;49(1):35–40.

10. Kumar R, Basu S, Torigian D, et al. Role of modern imaging techniques for diagnosis of infection in the era of 18f-fluorodeoxyglucose positron emission tomography. Clin Microbiol Rev 2008;21(1):209–24.

11. Kim I-J, Lee JS, Kim S-J, et al. Double-phase 18F-FDG PET-CT for determination of pulmonary tuberculoma activity. Eur J Nucl Med Mol Imaging 2008;35(4):808–14.

12. Chen C-J, Lee B-F, Yao W-J, et al. Dual-phase 18F-FDG PET in the diagnosis of pulmonary nodules with an initial standard uptake value less than 2.5. AJR Am J Roentgenol 2008;191(2):475–9.

13. Sathekge MM, Maes A, Pottel H, et al. Dual time-point FDG PET-CT for differentiating benign from malignant solitary pulmonary nodules in a TB endemic area. S Afr Med J 2010;100(9):598–601.

14. Sjölander H, Strømsnes T, Gerke O, et al. Value of FDG-PET/CT for treatment response in tuberculosis: a systematic review and meta-analysis. Clin Transl Imaging 2018;6(1):19–29.

15. Gambhir S, Kumar M, Ravina M, et al. Role of 18F-FDG PET in demonstrating disease burden in patients with tuberculous meningitis. J Neurol Sci 2016;370:196–200.

16. Modi M, Goyal MK, Jain A, et al. Tuberculous meningitis: challenges in diagnosis and management: lessons learnt from Prof. Dastur's article published in 1970. Neurol India 2018;66(6):1550.

17. Tucker EW, Guglieri-Lopez B, Ordonez AA, et al. Noninvasive 11C-rifampin positron emission tomography reveals drug biodistribution in tuberculous meningitis. Sci Transl Med 2018;10(470): eaau0965.

18. Baughman RP, Lower EE, du Bois RM. Sarcoidosis. Lancet 2003;361(9363):1111–8.

19. Akaike G, Itani M, Shah H, et al. PET/CT in the diagnosis and workup of sarcoidosis: focus on atypical manifestations. RadioGraphics 2018;38(5):1536–49.

20. Larici AR, Glaudemans AW, Del Ciello A, et al. Radiological and nuclear medicine imaging of sarcoidosis. Q J Nucl Med Mol Imaging 2018; 62(1):14–33.

21. Piekarski E, Benali K, Rouzet F. Nuclear imaging in sarcoidosis. Semin Nucl Med 2018;48(3):246–60.

22. Zhou Y, Lower EE, Li H, et al. Clinical management of pulmonary sarcoidosis. Expert Rev Respir Med 2016;10(5):577–91.

23. Yamada Y, Uchida Y, Tatsumi K, et al. Fluorine-18-fluorodeoxyglucose and carbon-11-methionine evaluation of lymphadenopathy in sarcoidosis. J Nucl Med 1998;39(7):1160–6.

24. Braun JJ, Kessler R, Constantinesco A, et al. 18F-FDG PET/CT in sarcoidosis management: review and report of 20 cases. Eur J Nucl Med Mol Imaging 2008;35(8):1537–43.

25. Keijsers RG, Verzijlbergen FJ, Oyen WJ, et al. 18F-FDG PET, genotype-corrected ACE and sIL-2R in newly diagnosed sarcoidosis. Eur J Nucl Med Mol Imaging 2009;36(7):1131–7.

26. Teirstein AS, Machac J, Almeida O, et al. Results of 188 whole-body fluorodeoxyglucose positron emission tomography scans in 137 patients with sarcoidosis. Chest 2007;132(6):1949–53.

27. Ambrosini V, Zompatori M, Fasano L, et al. 18)F-FDG PET/CT for the assessment of disease extension and activity in patients with sarcoidosis: results of a preliminary prospective study. Clin Nucl Med 2013; 38(4):e171–7.

28. Treglia G, Annunziata S, Sobic-Saranovic D, et al. The role of 18F-FDG-PET and PET/CT in patients with sarcoidosis: an updated evidence-based review. Acad Radiol 2014;21(5):675–84.

29. Skali H, Schulman AR, Dorbala S. 18F-FDG PET/CT for the assessment of myocardial sarcoidosis. Curr Cardiol Rep 2013;15(4):352.

30. Okada DR, Bravo PE, Vita T, et al. Isolated cardiac sarcoidosis: a focused review of an under-recognized entity. J Nucl Cardiol 2018;25(4): 1136–46.

31. Yamagishi H, Shirai N, Takagi M, et al. Identification of cardiac sarcoidosis with (13)N-NH(3)/(18)F-FDG PET. J Nucl Med 2003;44(7):1030–6.

32. Langah R, Spicer K, Gebregziabher M, et al. Effectiveness of prolonged fasting 18f-FDG PET-CT in the detection of cardiac sarcoidosis. J Nucl Cardiol 2009;16(5):801–10.

33. Okumura W, Iwasaki T, Toyama T, et al. Usefulness of fasting 18F-FDG PET in identification of cardiac sarcoidosis. J Nucl Med 2004;45(12):1989–98.

34. Ohira H, Tsujino I, Ishimaru S, et al. Myocardial imaging with 18F-fluoro-2-deoxyglucose positron emission tomography and magnetic resonance imaging in sarcoidosis. Eur J Nucl Med Mol Imaging 2008;35(5):933–41.

35. Dweck MR, Jones C, Joshi NV, et al. Assessment of valvular calcification and inflammation by positron emission tomography in patients with aortic stenosis. Circulation 2012;125(1):76–86.

36. Gormsen LC, Haraldsen A, Kramer S, et al. A dual tracer 68Ga-DOTANOC PET/CT and 18F-FDG PET/CT pilot study for detection of cardiac sarcoidosis. EJNMMI Res 2016;6:52.

37. Kaushik P, Patel C, Gulati GS, et al. Comparison of 68Ga-DOTANOC PET/CT with cardiac MRI in patients with clinical suspicion of cardiac sarcoidosis. Ann Nucl Med 2021;35(9):1058–65.

38. Chan M, Hsiao E. Neurosarcoidosis on FET and FDG PET/CT. Clin Nucl Med 2017;42(3):197–9.

39. Arora S, Damle NA, Passah A, et al. Scar sarcoidosis on 18F-FDG PET/CT. Asia Ocean J Nucl Med Biol 2019;7(2):185–7.

40. Vidal M, Alvarado A, López J, et al. Scar sarcoidosis: a rare entity found by 18F-FDG-PET/CT. Radiol Case Rep 2018;13(6):1216–9.

41. Pruthi A, Kirtani P, Joshi P, et al. Tiger man Sign-F-18 FDG PET CT scan pattern in muscular and cutaneous sarcoidosis: a case report and literature survey. Indian J Nucl Med 2020;35(3):232.

42. Li Y, Berenji GR. Cutaneous sarcoidosis evaluated by FDG PET. Clin Nucl Med 2011;36(7):584–6.

43. Dioguardi P, Gaddam SR, Zhuang H, et al. FDG PET assessment of osteomyelitis: a review. PET Clin 2012;7(2):161–79.

44. Koort JK, Mäkinen TJ, Knuuti J, et al. Comparative 18F-FDG PET of experimental Staphylococcus aureus osteomyelitis and normal bone healing. J Nucl Med 2004;45(8):1406–11.

45. Termaat MF, Raijmakers PGHM, Scholten HJ, et al. The accuracy of diagnostic imaging for the assessment of chronic osteomyelitis: a systematic review and meta-analysis. J Bone Joint Surg Am 2005; 87(11):2464–71.

46. Basu S, Chryssikos T, Moghadam-Kia S, et al. Positron emission tomography as a diagnostic tool in infection: present role and future possibilities. Semin Nucl Med 2009;39(1):36–51.

47. Sangolli PM, Lakshmi DV. Vasculitis: a checklist to approach and treatment update for dermatologists. Indian Dermatol Online J 2019;10(6):617.

48. Ben Shimol J, Amital H, Lidar M, et al. The utility of PET/CT in large vessel vasculitis. Sci Rep 2020; 10(1):17709.

49. Dejaco C, Ramiro S, Duftner C, et al. EULAR recommendations for the use of imaging in large vessel vasculitis in clinical practice. Ann Rheum Dis 2018; 77(5):636–43.

50. Lee YH, Choi SJ, Ji JD, et al. Diagnostic accuracy of 18F-FDG PET or PET/CT for large vessel vasculitis : a meta-analysis. Z Rheumatol 2016;75(9):924–31.

51. van der Geest KSM, Treglia G, Glaudemans AWJM, et al. Diagnostic value of [18F]FDG-PET/CT for treatment monitoring in large vessel vasculitis: a systematic review and meta-analysis. Eur J Nucl Med Mol Imaging 2021;48(12):3886–902.

52. Stone JH, Khosroshahi A, Deshpande V, et al. Recommendations for the nomenclature of IgG4-related disease and its individual organ system manifestations. Arthritis Rheum 2012;64(10):3061–7.

53. Kamisawa T, Zen Y, Pillai S, et al. IgG4-related disease. Lancet 2015;385(9976):1460–71.

54. Mitamura K, Arai-Okuda H, Yamamoto Y, et al. Disease activity and response to therapy monitored by [18F]FDG PET/CT using volume-based indices in IgG4-related disease. EJNMMI Res 2020;10(1): 153.

55. Mittal B, Parihar A, Kumar R, et al. IgG4 related disease spectrum and 18F-FDG PET/CT: where does it fit in the management algorithm? J Nucl Med 2018; 59(supplement 1):603.

56. Ozaki H, Dobashi H, Susaki K, et al. FRI0240 usefulness of Fdg-Pet/Ct imaging in Igg4-related disease. Ann Rheum Dis 2014;73(Suppl 2):469–70.

57. Kwee TC, Kwee RM. Chest CT in COVID-19: what the radiologist needs to know. RadioGraphics 2020;40(7):1848–65.

58. Yang R, Li X, Liu H, et al. Chest CT severity score: an imaging tool for assessing severe COVID-19. Radiol Cardiothorac Imaging 2020;2(2):e200047.

59. Rafiee F, Keshavarz P, Katal S, et al. Coronavirus disease 2019 (COVID-19) in molecular imaging: a systematic review of incidental detection of SARS-CoV-2 pneumonia on PET studies. Semin Nucl Med 2021;51(2):178–91.

# Role of Fluorodeoxyglucose-PET in Interventional Radiology

Alireza Zandifar, MD[a], Joey Saucedo, BS[b], Arastoo Vossough, MD, PhD[a,b], Abass Alavi, MD[b], Stephen J. Hunt, MD, PhD[b,c,*]

KEYWORDS

• FDG-PET • Interventional radiology • Malignancy • Inflammation • Infection

KEY POINTS

• Fluorodeoxyglucose (FDG)-PET is an important tool for the interventional radiologist in the diagnosis and evaluation of treatment response in malignancies.
• FDG-PET can be applied to select the appropriate candidate for interventional procedures, including ablation and embolization techniques.
• FDG-PET can be a helpful tool for interventional radiologists in the management of infectious and inflammatory conditions.

## INTRODUCTION

Fluorodeoxyglucose (FDG)-PET plays an extensive role in modern personalized medicine. FDG is taken up by cells via glucose transporters (GLUTs) and undergoes phosphorylation by hexokinase.[1] However, unlike glucose, phosphorylated FDG cannot be further metabolized and therefore is not able to leave the cell, except through dephosphorylation by glucose-6-phosphatase. Reduced levels of glucose-6-phosphatase in neoplastic cells result in deposition of FDG-phosphate in malignant cells.[2] FDG can also be trapped in immune cells in the setting of inflammation or infection, and in cells with high turnover of glucose.[1]

Interventional radiology (IR) plays an important role in the diagnosis of inflammatory conditions, diagnosis, and treatment of localized infections, and in diagnosis and treatment of malignancy.[3–6] Interventional radiologists use direct tumor injection, ablation, and embolization techniques for treatment of a variety of malignancies.[7–9] IR techniques for infection management include aspiration or drainage of suspected infectious collections as well as venous access for systemic antimicrobial therapy.[10] In addition, interventional radiologists are playing an increasing role in diagnosis and endovascular management of vasculitis, arthropathies, and other inflammatory conditions.[11,12] FDG-PET can assist the interventional radiologist in selecting the best treatment option, in providing specificity in targeting of pathologic conditions, and in measuring treatment response.[13] In this article, the authors aim to review the role of FDG-PET in assisting the interventional radiologist in the management of malignancies, inflammatory conditions, and infection.

## MALIGNANCIES

Most neoplastic conditions show increased FDG uptake. The degree of uptake is dependent on

A. Zandifar and J. Saucedo contributed equally to this article.
[a] Department of Radiology, Division of Neuroradiology, The Children's Hospital of Philadelphia, Philadelphia, PA, USA; [b] Department of Radiology, Perelman School of Medicine, University of Pennsylvania, Philadelphia, PA, USA; [c] Penn Image-Guided Interventions Lab, University of Pennsylvania, Philadelphia, PA, USA
* Corresponding author. Department of Radiology, Hospital of University of Pennsylvania, Perelman School of Medicine, 3400 Spruce Street, Philadelphia, PA 19104.
E-mail address: stephen.hunt@pennmedicine.upenn.edu

PET Clin 17 (2022) 543–553
https://doi.org/10.1016/j.cpet.2022.03.003

many factors, including type of tumor, grade of neoplasia, prior treatments, and many other patient-related physiologic and pathophysiologic states.[14] Use of FDG-PET–derived information can guide image-guided biopsy and facilitate early and more accurate diagnosis and staging.[15] Because not all neoplasms show high FDG uptake, knowledge of the various forms of tumor and their typical FDG avidity,[16] along with the biological significance of various quantitative FDG uptake measures, is important in interpretation and guiding management. Various causes of potential false-positive interpretation and false-negative results should be entertained, including effects of tumor type, tumor size, and posttreatment changes, including confounders such as posttreatment inflammation.[17] Discussions between interventional radiologists and nuclear medicine specialists may be crucial for guiding the next steps in the management of these patients.

## Hepatocellular Carcinoma

Hepatocellular carcinoma (HCC) is the most common primary malignancy of the liver, and the second leading cause of cancer death worldwide.[18] Although FDG-PET is not a part of the standard workup of HCC, the standard uptake value (SUV) and SUV ratios of the tumor to normal liver SUVs can be helpful as quantitative measures to predict the aggressiveness of the tumor and response to locoregional treatments.[19–21] For instance, increased FDG uptake is correlated with the level of VEGF, $\alpha$-fetoprotein, and p-glycoprotein expression.[22] Specifically, in high-grade HCCs, FDG uptake is increased and can provide more details about the underlying tumor biology.[23] IR can benefit patients with inoperable HCC through several treatment options, including direct tumor injection, thermal ablation, transarterial chemoembolization (TACE), and transarterial radioembolization (TARE).[24] TARE with Yttrium-90 microspheres is a particularly useful therapy for those patients with portal vein thrombosis in which TACE represents a high risk for ischemic complication.[25] In a prospective study, Jreige and colleagues[26] showed $SUV_{max}$ and tumor-to-liver uptake ratio derived from FGD-PET can be a predictor of survival in patients with HCC who undergo TARE. However, global assessment of tumor burden using quantitative parameters, including total lesion glycolysis and metabolic tumor volume, have been demonstrated to be much more predictive of tumor response and overall survival after TARE than conventional FDG-PET parameters.[27] Combining FDG-PET and 11C-acetate can increase the accuracy of HCC diagnosis with PET,

specifically for lesions larger than 2 cm.[28] Using dual-tracer PET with FDG and 11C-acetate tracers can help physicians in risk stratification of patients with HCC, along with appropriate candidate selection for personalized Y90-TARE.[24] In addition, FDG and 11C-acetate PET/CT can predict both treatment response and recurrence after TACE, which can help the interventionalist in tailoring a more individualized treatment plan.[29] Similarly, Song and colleagues[30] showed that high SUV ratio (maximal tumor SUV/mean liver SUV > 1.70) has a significant correlation with $\alpha$-fetoprotein level and size of the tumor in patients undergoing TACE. The response to treatment, time to progression, and survival rate were significantly different in patients with high SUV ratio in comparison with those with a low SUV ratio.

## Colorectal Cancer

Colorectal cancer (CRC) is the fourth most commonly diagnosed malignancy and is the second leading cause of cancer death in the United States, second only to lung cancer.[31] Roughly 20% of patients diagnosed with CRC will have liver metastases by the time of diagnosis.[32] The liver is the most common organ for CRC to metastasize to, with lung metastasis being the second most common site.[33] In the setting of surgically unresectable or multiple CRC metastatic foci, interventional radiologists can use local ablative techniques for the treatment of oligometastatic disease. Typically, an ablation probe is placed in or near the target using ultrasound (US), computed tomography (CT), or MR imaging guidance. However, this target may sometimes have the same echogenicity, attenuation, or signal intensity as the surrounding tissue. In such scenarios, these lesions may be better visualized by FDG-PET (Fig. 1). During ablation, the zone of tissue destruction is not well visualized by US owing to the hyperechogenicity induced by gas in the treatment zone. Similarly, assessment for residual tumor with CT or MR imaging is often difficult because of posttreatment tissue changes and hyperemia.[34] FDG-PET has shown significant potential as a viable tool to detect residual tumor immediately after ablation.[9] 18F-FDG administered immediately before an ablation will remain in the tumor following ablation, which can obscure assessment of treatment adequacy. Using a split-dose technique can provide immediate and accurate confirmation of ablation success.[35] In this technique, an initial targeting dose is used, which is followed by a larger posttreatment dose to detect residual tumor.[35]

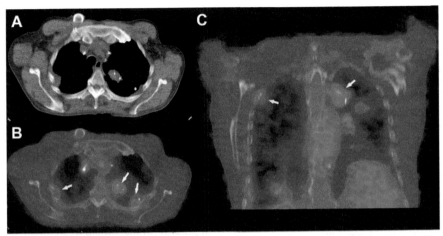

Fig. 1. FDG-PET in malignancy: A 67-year-old man presented with metastatic CRC to both lungs with rising carci-noembryonic antigen despite prior intervention. Axial CT image (*A*), corresponding axial fused FDG-PET (*B*), and (*C*) coronal fused FDG-PET of chest show increased FDG uptake in the left apical metastasis (*white arrows*), whereas the right apical metastasis does not show an increased uptake (*yellow arrows*). The left metastatic lesions were subsequently treated with cryoablation.

## Non–Small Cell Lung Cancer

Lung cancer is both the most commonly diagnosed cancer in the world and the cancer with the highest overall mortality, of which non–small cell lung cancer (NSCLC) makes up 85%.[36] Although surgery or radiation can provide a cure for isolated tumors, many patients are not appropriate surgical candidates because of comorbidities and are better suited for locoregional treatments, such as radiofrequency ablation (RFA), microwave ablation, and cryoablation. In addition, ablation provides an alternative therapy for recurrent tumors and metachronous tumors and is included in the NSCLC National Comprehensive Cancer Network guidelines for these indications.[37] FDG-PET has utility in NSCLC in the staging of NSCLC[38] and in determining tumor response, and predicting prognosis after treatment.[39,40] A negative FDG-PET study, although with consideration of lesion size, may allow for a more conservative surveillance approach and avoid unnecessary interventional procedures, whereas positive studies often imply that biopsies or interventions are justified.[41] Furthermore, evidence suggests that using FDG-PET in the management of NSCLC is cost-effective.[42,43] For follow-up and surveillance of NSCLC that has been treated nonoperatively with ablation, CT is the imaging modality of choice.[44] However, FDG-PET is more sensitive for the detection of tumor recurrence after ablation.[45] Much like radiation, the specificity immediately after ablation is low because of postablation inflammatory effects, and FDG-PET in this period can suffer from a

high false-positive rate.[45,46] After this inflammatory period has subsided (estimated at 3 months), however, FDG-PET is a useful tool for restaging.[47] Aside from FDG uptake values, FDG uptake patterns (classified as diffuse, focal, heterogeneous, rim, and rim plus focal uptake) are also predictive of treatment success or failure.[46] According to the mRECIST (modified response evaluation criteria in solid tumors) guidelines, FDG-PET, in combination with CT, is regarded as the most appropriate imaging modality for postablation follow-up and assessment.[48]

## Renal Cell Carcinoma

Renal cell carcinoma (RCC) comprises 3% of all malignancies and has the highest mortality among genitourinary neoplasms.[49–51] CT is the standard modality of choice for diagnosing and staging of RCC. FDG-PET can serve as a complementary tool in equivocal cases on CT.[51] The role of FDG-PET is more prominent in detecting recurrence after treatment with a comparable accuracy to abdominal CT.[52] In addition, FDG-PET can be very useful for early evaluation of response to treatments through both qualitative and quantitative assessments.[53] Ablation-based methods can be considered alternatives of surgical intervention for small RCCs.[54] These methods include RFA, cryoablation, and microwave ablation, which can be applied based on the size and location of tumor.[55] For tumors larger than 5 cm and tumors located in the central part of the kidney, embolization can be used to decrease the risk of hemorrhage and increase the efficacy of subsequent ablation.[56,57] Wagner and colleagues[58] reported that FDG-PET detects RCC recurrence earlier than routine CT after cryoablation. Lagerveld and colleagues[59] demonstrated that FDG-PET uptake was present in all renal tumors before ablation, and it is a very useful tool for predicting tumor response in patients with poor renal function in which contrast-enhanced CT or MR imaging is contraindicated.

### Thyroid Cancer

Thyroid cancer is the most prevalent endocrine-related malignancy and the third most rapidly increasing diagnosed cancer in the United States.[60,61] FDG-PET plays an important role in the follow-up of patients with differentiated thyroid carcinoma when their 131-Iodine whole-body scan is negative after thyroidectomy despite high thyroglobulin levels.[62–64] FDG-PET also can be applied as a part of the papillary thyroid carcinoma patient's workup and for evaluating the treatment response of non-iodine-avid cancers.[65] Although surgery is considered the standard treatment of several thyroid malignancies, some patients prefer minimally invasive options, including thermal ablation, to avoid the possible complications of surgery.[66,67] Combining FDG-PET with standard US can help differentiate benign from malignant thyroid nodules to prevent unnecessary resection.[68] Thyroid nodules having $SUV_{max}$ less than 5 on FDG-PET scan can be considered low risk for malignancy.[69] Lin and colleagues[68] demonstrated that FDG-PET can be applied to select low-risk candidates for RFA, and they concluded that RFA is an efficient and low-risk procedure for follicular neoplasms of thyroid with $SUV_{max}$ less than 5.

### Breast Cancer

Breast cancer is the most prevalent and second leading cause of cancer death among women.[31,70] TNM staging is a crucial part of the breast cancer workup in order to predict prognosis and to plan the best treatment method.[71] Recently, several studies evaluated the role of FDG-PET in clinical staging of pataients with breast cancer.[72,73] In a systematic review and meta-analysis by Han and Choi,[72] initial staging of breast cancer with FDG-PET, FDG-PET/CT, and FDG-PET/MR imaging resulted in changes of staging in 25% of patients and modification of management in 18% of patients. Another meta-analysis by Lu and colleagues[73] demonstrated that FDG PET/MR imaging has a high diagnostic accuracy for TNM staging of breast cancer. For example, they reported FDG PET/MR imaging can detect the M

stage of TNM with 98% sensitivity and 96% specificity.[73] Although surgery is the most common therapeutic modality for patients with breast cancer, ablation provides an effective alternative for early-stage small lesions ($\leq 2$ cm).[74] Ablation techniques, including cryoablation, microwave ablation, RFA, laser ablation, and high-intensity focused US, are particularly useful for lesions less than 3 cm diameter.[75–77]

## INFECTIOUS PROCESSES

In recent years, the value of FDG-PET with CT in the diagnosis, management, and therapeutic monitoring of infectious processes has become apparent.[6] In the setting of infection, activated inflammatory cells not only increase their expression of GLUTs but also demonstrate a greater affinity for deoxyglucose.[78] In this way, much like malignant lesions, sites of infection and inflammation are FDG-avid. Primary indications for using FDG-PET in suspected infection are peripheral bone osteomyelitis, in spondylodiscitis, and in the evaluation of a fever of unknown origin.[79]

Specific to IR, FDG-PET can be used in the evaluation of suspected infection of intravascular devices (**Fig. 2**), and the assessment of metabolic activity in suspected infectious collections.[79] It has also shown utility in detecting occult infectious foci in patients with bacteremia, ultimately reducing mortality by allowing for early diagnosis and intervention[80] (see **Fig. 2**). FDG-PET can also be helpful in infectious workup following endovascular interventions. Rottenstreich and colleagues[81] used FDG-PET to confirm the diagnosis of vascular infection after inferior vena cava (IVC) filter placement and concluded that FDG-PET is a valuable tool in these challenging cases. In a prospective study of patients with suspected vascular graft infections, Husmann and colleagues[82] showed that FDG-PET impacted the management in 76% of the patients, allowing for tailoring of antibiotic regimen specificity and length of treatment as well as diagnosing occult infections not related to the graft. Invasive fungal infections (IFI) in the cancer population represent a therapeutic challenge and often require interventional management after failed systemic antifungal therapy.[83] FDG-PET can provide earlier detection treatment failure in IFI patients allowing for a change in management to more effective treatment strategies.[84] FDG-PET has been described in the evaluation of potentially infected liver and kidney cysts, and it may help distinguish between sterile and infected abscesses.[79,85] For example, FDG-PET is a useful tool for evaluation of suspected infection in patients with autosomal dominant

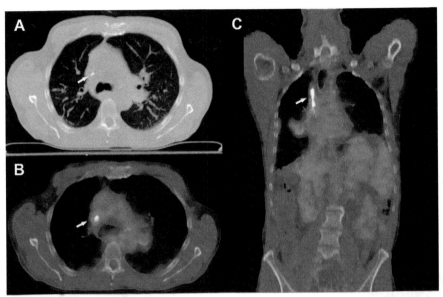

Fig. 2. FDG-PET in infection: Axial CT images (*A*) of a 67-year-old man with a history of colon cancer and long-standing chest port (*arrow*) for chemotherapy, presenting with recurrent fevers and rigors of unknown origin with negative blood cultures, unresponsive to antibiotics. Axial (*B*) and coronal (*C*) fused FDG-PET scans demonstrate metabolic uptake (*arrow*) along the catheter fibrin sheath. Explant of the port revealed colonization by *Stenotrophomonas maltophilia*, a multidrug-resistant organism known to colonize medical devices. Patient symptoms resolved after removing the port.

polycystic kidney disease.[86,87] FDG-PET is superior to conventional modalities in diagnosing infected cysts, which enables earlier drainage.[88–90] Wan and colleagues[91] showed that a focal uptake pattern in FDG-PET imaging of acute complicated pyelonephritis is associated with a higher frequency of abscess formation, and there should be a lower threshold for drainage in these patients.

## INFLAMMATORY CONDITIONS

Interventional radiologists can assist with diagnosis and management of several types of inflammatory conditions, including vasculitis, venous thromboembolism (VTE), and inflammatory arthropathies.[4,92] Large-vessel vasculitis (LVV) is a group of inflammatory vascular disorders that can cause symptomatic vascular stenoses and occlusions.[93] Takayasu arteritis (TA) and giant cell arteritis are the most common causes of LVV, which differ in their distribution.[93] In patients with suspected vasculitis, CT angiography or MR angiography may not have enough resolution to detect the vessel's abnormalities.[94,95] In these cases, more sensitive modalities may be required, such as catheter angiography.[95] Catheter angiography remains the gold standard for imaging diagnosis of vasculitis.[96] Patients with symptomatic stenoses and occlusions in the setting of LVV

can be considered for percutaneous transluminal angioplasty or surgical bypass.[12] TA also can be associated with aneurysms, which may benefit from endovascular management.[12] Raynaud syndrome is a peripheral vascular abnormality comprising pallor, cyanosis, and erythema induced by cold or stress. Diagnosis is typically made by clinical history and diagnostic exclusion of alternative causes; however, arteriography and noninvasive vascular laboratory assessment can help differentiate fixed arterial obstruction from vasospasm, as well as quantitating the severity of vascular pathologic condition.[97,98] Interventional treatments, such as botulinum toxin injection and sympathetic blocks, have been demonstrated to improve pain and healing of ulcers in small series.[97,98] Angiography remains the gold standard for diagnosis of polyarteritis nodosa (PAN), as conventional vascular imaging may lack adequate diagnostic resolution.[96] Classic angiographic findings include segmental arterial narrowing and microaneurysms.[96] However, the imperative for rapid diagnosis must be balanced with the risks of contrast-induced nephropathy in those patients with reduced renal function.[96] Buerger disease is a vasculitis affecting the small- and medium-sized peripheral vessels in the setting of substantial tobacco exposure. Angiographic findings include segmental arterial occlusions with bridging or corkscrew collaterals in the absence of calcific

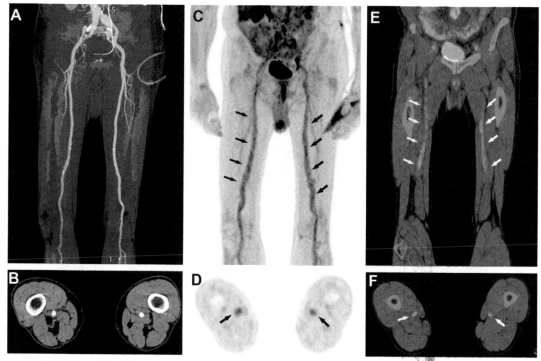

**Fig. 3.** FDG-PET scan in inflammation: A 64-year-old man with a history of skin cancer who underwent FDG-PET. No conventional angiography was performed; however, CT angiogram reported no significant abnormalities (*A*, *B*). Corresponding PET (*C*, *D*) and fused FDG-PET (*E*, *F*) scans demonstrate diffuse bilateral uptake (*arrow*) in the large vessels of the lower extremities, consistent with active vasculitis. The patient was subsequently diagnosed with PAN.

atherosclerosis.[99,100] Both catheter-directed thrombolysis and endovascular recanalization have been demonstrated to be effective in limb salvage.[101,102]

In inflammatory conditions, leukocytes and other inflammatory cells become activated, causing high-glucose metabolism, which can be detected by high FDG uptake in PET.[103] The role of FDG-PET has been shown in the evaluation of several inflammatory conditions, such as sarcoidosis, atherosclerosis, vasculitis, inflammatory bowel disease, and polymyalgia rheumatica.[104–106] Arauz and colleagues[107] demonstrated that there is a strong correlation between degree of atherosclerotic carotid artery stenosis measured on angiography and focal FDG uptake in FDG-PET. In addition, they revealed that high uptake of FDG-PET can be associated with poor prognosis after performing interventional procedures, such as carotid stenting or endarterectomy.[107] This supports pretreatment FDG-PET in evaluating active atherosclerotic plaque inflammation to select the most appropriate candidates for endovascular treatment.[107] In a recent meta-analysis, van der Geest and colleagues[108] demonstrated value of FDG-PET for treatment monitoring

in LVV. Specifically, FDG-PET can be applied for early diagnosis and treatment response monitoring of LVV, which may obviate the role of more invasive angiography.[109] FDG-PET can be useful in diagnosis of PAN, particularly in those patients with renal impairment, thus saving the patient those risks of catheter angiography (**Fig. 3**).[110] However, FDG-PET may not be sensitive in assessment of all vasculitis. Only 2 out of 17 patients had positive FDG-PET findings in a series of Buerger disease patients.[111] FDG-PET/CT was also unable to detect a difference in aortic vessel wall FDG uptake between rheumatoid arthritis patients and healthy controls.[112]

Inflammation can play an important role in pathogenesis of VTE.[113] Kaghazchi and colleagues[114] demonstrated that FDG-PET can detect thrombosis in patients with cancer before clinical presentations arise. They found that the IVC and lower-extremity veins are the most common sites for thrombi in these patients. Radiologists should also be attentive when reviewing the FDG-PET images of patients with cancer for evidence of vascular thrombosis.[114] Early detection of VTE in this patient population may enable interventional radiologists an earlier treatment window for catheter-directed thrombolysis and percutaneous mechanical thrombectomy, if needed.[115]

## SUMMARY

FDG-PET has expanding applications in the field of IR. FDG-PET provides both qualitative and quantitative assessments of malignancy, infection, and inflammation. These assessments can assist interventional radiologists in selecting the most appropriate treatment options for their oncology patients. FDG-PET is also useful for evaluating the response to interventional treatments and in predicting the prognosis of oncology patients. Finally, FDG-PET can assist the interventional radiologist in diagnosing and monitoring response to treatment of infection and inflammation. Nevertheless, there is a need for additional prospective studies to further establish the role of FDG-PET in these applications.

## CLINICS CARE POINTS

- FDG-PET imaging can be used by the treating interventional oncologist for monitoring for occult sites of recurrent malignancy.
- Local FDG uptake by tumors in the setting of treatment by the interventional oncologist can be difficult to distiguish from post-treatment inflammation.

## CONFLICT OF INTEREST

None.

## REFERENCES

1. Basu S, Hess S, Nielsen Braad P-E, et al. The basic principles of FDG-PET/CT imaging. PET Clin 2014; 9(4):355–70, v.
2. Nelson CA, Wang JQ, Leav I, et al. The interaction among glucose transport, hexokinase, and glucose-6-phosphatase with respect to 3H-2-deoxyglucose retention in murine tumor models. Nucl Med Biol 1996;23(4):533–41.
3. O'Neill SB, O'Connor OJ, Ryan MF, et al. Interventional radiology and the care of the oncology patient. Radiol Res Pract 2011;2011:160867.
4. Sharma AM, Singh S, Lewis JE. Diagnostic approach in patients with suspected vasculitis. Tech Vasc Interv Radiol 2014;17(4):226–33.
5. Edgell RC, Sarhan AE, Soomro J, et al. The role of catheter angiography in the diagnosis of central nervous system vasculitis. Interv Neurol 2016;5(3–4):194–208.
6. Kung BT, Seraj SM, Zadeh MZ, et al. An update on the role of 18F-FDG-PET/CT in major infectious and inflammatory diseases. Am J Nucl Med Mol Imaging 2019;9(6):255–73.
7. Winokur RS, Pua BB, Madoff DC. Role of combined embolization and ablation in management of renal masses. Semin Intervent Radiol 2014;31(1):82–5.
8. Ahmed M, Brace CL, Lee FT, et al. Principles of and advances in percutaneous ablation. Radiology 2011;258(2):351–69.
9. Seraj SM, Ayubcha C, Zadeh MZ, et al. The evolving role of PET-based novel quantitative techniques in the interventional radiology procedures of the liver. PET Clin 2019;14(4):419–25.
10. Hynes D, Aghajafari P. Janne d'Othée B. Role of interventional radiology in the management of infection. Semin Ultrasound CT MR 2020;41(1):20–32.
11. Chianca V, Orlandi D, Messina C, et al. Interventional therapeutic procedures to treat degenerative and inflammatory musculoskeletal conditions: state of the art. Radiol Med 2019;124(11):1112–20.
12. Angle JF, Nida BA, Matsumoto AH. Endovascular treatment of large vessel arteritis. Tech Vasc Interv Radiol 2014;17(4):252–7.
13. Lam MGEH, Hunt SJ, El-Haddad GE, et al. Evolving role of PET in interventional radiology-based oncology procedures. PET Clin 2019;14(4):xiii–xiv.
14. Hustinx R, Bénard F, Alavi A. Whole-body FDG-PET imaging in the management of patients with cancer. Semin Nucl Med 2002;32(1):35–46.
15. Cerci JJ, Tabacchi E, Bogoni M. Fluorodeoxyglucose-PET/computed tomography-guided biopsy. PET Clin 2016;11(1):57–64.
16. Vasireddi A, Nguyen NC. PET/CT limitations and pitfalls in urogenital cancers. Semin Nucl Med 2021. https://doi.org/10.1053/j.semnuclmed.2021.06.013.
17. Kikano EG, Avril S, Marshall H, et al. PET/CT variants and pitfalls in breast cancers. Semin Nucl Med 2021;51(5):474–84.
18. Fong ZV, Tanabe KK. The clinical management of hepatocellular carcinoma in the United States, Europe, and Asia: a comprehensive and evidence-based comparison and review. Cancer 2014; 120(18):2824–38.
19. Sun D-W, An L, Wei F, et al. Prognostic significance of parameters from pretreatment (18)F-FDG PET in hepatocellular carcinoma: a meta-analysis. Abdom Radiol (NY) 2016;41(1):33–41.
20. Benson AB, D'Angelica MI, Abbott DE, et al. Guidelines insights: hepatobiliary cancers, version

2.2019. J Natl Compr Canc Netw 2019;17(4): 302–10.

21. Schobert I, Chapiro J, Pucar D, et al. Fluorodeoxy-glucose PET for monitoring response to embolo-therapy (transarterial chemoembolization) in primary and metastatic liver tumors. PET Clin 2019;14(4):437–45.

22. Kornberg A, Schernhammer M, Friess H. 18F-FDG-PET for assessing biological viability and prognosis in liver transplant patients with hepatocellular carci-noma. J Clin Transl Hepatol 2017;5(3):224–34.

23. Ronot M, Clift AK, Vilgrain V, et al. Functional imag-ing in liver tumours. J Hepatol 2016;65(5):1017–30.

24. Ho CL, Chen S, Cheung SK, et al. Significant value of 11C-acetate and 18F-fluorodeoxyglucose PET/computed tomography on 90Y microsphere radio-embolization for hepatocellular carcinoma. PET Clin 2019;14(4):459–67.

25. Lau W-Y, Sangro B, Chen P-J, et al. Treatment for hepatocellular carcinoma with portal vein tumor thrombosis: the emerging role for radioemboliza-tion using yttrium-90. Oncology 2013;84(5):311–8.

26. Jreige M, Mitsakis P, Van Der Gucht A, et al. 18F-FDG PET/CT predicts survival after 90Y trans-arterial radioembolization in unresectable hepato-cellular carcinoma. Eur J Nucl Med Mol Imaging 2017;44(7):1215–22.

27. Seraj SM, Zadeh MZ, Werner TJ, et al. Pretreatment volumetric parameters of FDG-PET predict the sur-vival after Yttrium-90 radio-embolization in metasta-tic liver disease. Am J Nucl Med Mol Imaging 2019; 9(5):248–54.

28. Park J-W, Kim JH, Kim SK, et al. A prospective evaluation of 18F-FDG and 11C-acetate PET/CT for detection of primary and metastatic hepatocel-lular carcinoma. J Nucl Med 2008;49(12):1912–21.

29. Park S, Kim T-S, Kang SH, et al. 11C-acetate and 18F-fluorodeoxyglucose positron emission tomog-raphy/computed tomography dual imaging for the prediction of response and prognosis after transar-terial chemoembolization. Medicine (Baltimore) 2018;97(37):e12311.

30. Song MJ, Bae SH, Lee SW, et al. 18F-fluorodeoxy-glucose PET/CT predicts tumour progression after transarterial chemoembolization in hepatocellular carcinoma. Eur J Nucl Med Mol Imaging 2013; 40(6):865–73.

31. Bray F, Ferlay J, Soerjomataram I, et al. Global can-cer statistics 2018: GLOBOCAN estimates of inci-dence and mortality worldwide for 36 cancers in 185 countries. CA Cancer J Clin 2018;68(6): 394–424.

32. Vera R, González-Flores E, Rubio C, et al. Multidis-ciplinary management of liver metastases in pa-tients with colorectal cancer: a consensus of SEOM, AEC, SEOR, SERVEI, and SEMNIM. Clin Transl Oncol 2020;22:647–62.

33. Mitry E, Guiu B, Cosconea S, et al. Epidemiology, management and prognosis of colorectal cancer with lung metastases: a 30-year population-based study. Gut 2010;59(10):1383–8.

34. Antoch G, Vogt FM, Veit P, et al. Assessment of liver tissue after radiofrequency ablation: findings with different imaging procedures. J Nucl Med 2005; 46(3):520–5.

35. Ryan ER, Sofocleous CT, Schöder H, et al. Split-dose technique for FDG PET/CT-guided percuta-neous ablation: a method to facilitate lesion targeting and to provide immediate assessment of treatment effectiveness. Radiology 2013; 268(1):288–95.

36. Zappa C, Mousa SA. Non-small cell lung cancer: current treatment and future advances. Transl Lung Cancer Res 2016;5(3):288–300.

37. Ettinger DS, Wood DE, Aisner DL, et al. NCCN guidelines insights: non-small cell lung cancer, version 2.2021. J Natl Compr Canc Netw 2021; 19(3):254–66.

38. Kligerman S, Digumarthy S. Staging of non-small cell lung cancer using integrated PET/CT. AJR Am J Roentgenol 2009;193(5):1203–11.

39. Zhao H, Steinke K. Long-term outcome following microwave ablation of early-stage non-small cell lung cancer. J Med Imaging Radiat Oncol 2020; 64(6):787–93.

40. Acksteiner C, Steinke K. Percutaneous microwave ablation for early-stage non-small cell lung cancer (NSCLC) in the elderly: a promising outlook. J Med Imaging Radiat Oncol 2015;59(1):82–90.

41. Hashimoto Y, Tsujikawa T, Kondo C, et al. Accuracy of PET for diagnosis of solid pulmonary lesions with 18F-FDG uptake below the standardized uptake value of 2.5. J Nucl Med 2006;47(3):426–31.

42. Keith CJ, Miles KA, Griffiths MR, et al. Solitary pul-monary nodules: accuracy and cost-effectiveness of sodium iodide FDG-PET using Australian data. Eur J Nucl Med Mol Imaging 2002;29(8):1016–23.

43. Lejeune C, Al Zahouri K, Woronoff-Lemsi M-C, et al. Use of a decision analysis model to assess the medicoeconomic implications of FDG PET imaging in diagnosing a solitary pulmonary nodule. Eur J Health Econ 2005;6(3):203–14.

44. Lee W-K, Lau EWF, Chin K, et al. Modern diag-nostic and therapeutic interventional radiology in lung cancer. J Thorac Dis 2013;5(Suppl 5): S511–23.

45. Yoo DC, Dupuy DE, Hillman SL, et al. Radiofre-quency ablation of medically inoperable stage IA non-small cell lung cancer: are early posttreatment PET findings predictive of treatment outcome? AJR Am J Roentgenol 2011;197(2):334–40.

46. Singnurkar A, Solomon SB, Gönen M, et al. 18F-FDG PET/CT for the prediction and detection of

local recurrence after radiofrequency ablation of malignant lung lesions. J Nucl Med 2010;51(12):1833–40.

47. Alafate A, Shinya T, Okumura Y, et al. The maximum standardized uptake value is more reliable than size measurement in early follow-up to evaluate potential pulmonary malignancies following radiofrequency ablation. Acta Med Okayama 2013;67(2):105–12.

48. Herrera LJ, Fernando HC, Perry Y, et al. Radiofrequency ablation of pulmonary malignant tumors in nonsurgical candidates. J Thorac Cardiovasc Surg 2003;125(4):929–37.

49. Cairns P. Renal cell carcinoma. Cancer Biomark 2010;9(1–6):461–73.

50. Oh JJ, Lee JK, Do Song B, et al. Accurate risk assessment of patients with pathologic T3aN0M0 renal cell carcinoma. Sci Rep 2018;8(1):13914.

51. Schöder H, Larson SM. Positron emission tomography for prostate, bladder, and renal cancer. Semin Nucl Med 2004;34(4):274–92.

52. Park S, Lee H-Y, Lee S. Role of F-18 FDG PET/CT in the follow-up of asymptomatic renal cell carcinoma patients for postoperative surveillance: based on conditional survival analysis. J Cancer Res Clin Oncol 2021. https://doi.org/10.1007/s00432-021-03688-2.

53. Ranieri G, Marech I, Niccoli Asabella A, et al. Tyrosine-kinase inhibitors therapies with mainly anti-angiogenic activity in advanced renal cell carcinoma: value of PET/CT in response evaluation. Int J Mol Sci 2017;(9):18. https://doi.org/10.3390/ijms18091937.

54. Mueller-Lisse UG, Mueller-Lisse UL, Meindl T, et al. Staging of renal cell carcinoma. Eur Radiol 2007;17(9):2268–77.

55. Abdelsalam ME, Ahrar K. Ablation of small renal masses. Tech Vasc Interv Radiol 2020;23(2):100674.

56. Yamakado K, Nakatsuka A, Kobayashi S, et al. Radiofrequency ablation combined with renal arterial embolization for the treatment of unresectable renal cell carcinoma larger than 3.5 cm: initial experience. Cardiovasc Intervent Radiol 2006;29(3):389–94.

57. Woodrum DA, Atwell TD, Farrell MA, et al. Role of intraarterial embolization before cryoablation of large renal tumors: a pilot study. J Vasc Interv Radiol 2010;21(6):930–6.

58. Wagner AA, Solomon SB, Kavoussi LR. Imaging following cryoablation of a renal lesion. Nat Clin Pract Urol 2005;2(1):52–7 [quiz: 58].

59. Lagerveld BW, Sivro F, van der Zee JA, et al. 18F-FDG PET-CT findings before and after laparoscopic cryoablation of small renal mass: an initial report. J Kidney Cancer VHL 2015;2(4):174–86.

60. Brown RL, de Souza JA, Cohen EE. Thyroid cancer: burden of illness and management of disease. J Cancer 2011;2:193–9.

61. Morris LGT, Sikora AG, Tosteson TD, et al. The increasing incidence of thyroid cancer: the influence of access to care. Thyroid 2013;23(7):885–91.

62. Schlüter B, Bohuslavizki KH, Beyer W, et al. Impact of FDG PET on patients with differentiated thyroid cancer who present with elevated thyroglobulin and negative 131I scan. J Nucl Med 2001;42(1):71–6.

63. Chung JK, So Y, Lee JS, et al. Value of FDG PET in papillary thyroid carcinoma with negative 131I whole-body scan. J Nucl Med 1999;40(6):986–92.

64. Helal BO, Merlet P, Toubert ME, et al. Clinical impact of (18)F-FDG PET in thyroid carcinoma patients with elevated thyroglobulin levels and negative (131)I scanning results after therapy. J Nucl Med 2001;42(10):1464–9.

65. Abraham T, Schöder H. Thyroid cancer–indications and opportunities for positron emission tomography/computed tomography imaging. Semin Nucl Med 2011;41(2):121–38.

66. Ha SM, Sung JY, Baek JH, et al. Radiofrequency ablation of small follicular neoplasms: initial clinical outcomes. Int J Hyperthermia 2017;33(8):931–7.

67. Xiao J, Zhang Y, Zhang M, et al. Ultrasonography-guided radiofrequency ablation vs. surgery for the treatment of solitary T1bN0M0 papillary thyroid carcinoma: a comparative study. Clin Endocrinol (Oxf) 2021;94(4):684–91.

68. Lin W-C, Tung Y-C, Chang Y-H, et al. Radiofrequency ablation for treatment of thyroid follicular neoplasm with low SUV in PET/CT study. Int J Hyperthermia 2021;38(1):963–9.

69. Castellana M, Trimboli P, Piccardo A, et al. Performance of 18F-FDG PET/CT in selecting thyroid nodules with indeterminate fine-needle aspiration cytology for surgery. A systematic review and a meta-analysis. J Clin Med 2019;8(9). https://doi.org/10.3390/jcm8091333.

70. Momenimovahed Z, Salehiniya H. Epidemiological characteristics of and risk factors for breast cancer in the world. Breast Cancer (Dove Med Press) 2019;11:151–64.

71. Giuliano AE, Connolly JL, Edge SB, et al. Breast cancer-major changes in the American Joint Committee on Cancer eighth edition cancer staging manual. CA Cancer J Clin 2017;67(4):290–303.

72. Han S, Choi JY. Impact of 18F-FDG PET, PET/CT, and PET/MRI on staging and management as an initial staging modality in breast cancer: a systematic review and meta-analysis. Clin Nucl Med 2021;46(4):271–82.

73. Lu X-R, Qu M-M, Zhai Y-N, et al. Diagnostic role of 18F-FDG PET/MRI in the TNM staging of breast cancer: a systematic review and meta-analysis. Ann Palliat Med 2021;10(4):4328–37.

74. van de Voort EMF, Struik GM, Birnie E, et al. Thermal ablation as an alternative for surgical resection of small (≤2 cm) breast cancers: a meta-analysis. Clin Breast Cancer 2021. https://doi.org/10.1016/j.clbc.2021.03.004.

75. Kinoshita T. RFA experiences, indications and clinical outcomes. Int J Clin Oncol 2019;24(6):603–7.

76. Simmons RM, Ballman KV, Cox C, et al. A phase II trial exploring the success of cryoablation therapy in the treatment of invasive breast carcinoma: results from ACOSOG (Alliance) Z1072. Ann Surg Oncol 2016;23(8):2438–45.

77. Ahmed M, Goldberg SN. Basic science research in thermal ablation. Surg Oncol Clin N Am 2011;20(2):237–58, vii.

78. Zhuang H, Alavi A. 18-Fluorodeoxyglucose positron emission tomographic imaging in the detection and monitoring of infection and inflammation. Semin Nucl Med 2002;32(1):47–59.

79. Jamar F, Buscombe J, Chiti A, et al. EANM/SNMMI guideline for 18F-FDG use in inflammation and infection. J Nucl Med 2013;54(4):647–58.

80. Berrevoets MAH, Kouijzer IJE, Aarntzen EHJG, et al. 18F-FDG PET/CT optimizes treatment in Staphylococcus aureus bacteremia and is associated with reduced mortality. J Nucl Med 2017;58(9):1504–10.

81. Rottenstreich A, Bar-Shalom R, Bloom AI, et al. Endovascular infection following inferior vena cava (IVC) filter insertion. J Thromb Thrombolysis 2015;40(4):452–7.

82. Husmann L, Sah B-R, Scherrer A, et al. 18F-FDG PET/CT for therapy control in vascular graft infections: a first feasibility study. J Nucl Med 2015;56(7):1024–9.

83. Böhme A, Ruhnke M, Buchheidt D, et al. Treatment of fungal infections in hematology and oncology–guidelines of the infectious diseases working party (AGIHO) of the German Society of Hematology and Oncology (DGHO). Ann Hematol 2003;82(Suppl 2):S133–40.

84. Sathekge MM, Ankrah AO, Lawal I, et al. Monitoring response to therapy. Semin Nucl Med 2018;48(2):166–81.

85. Ertay T, Sencan Eren M, Karaman M, et al. 18F-FDG-PET/CT in initiation and progression of inflammation and infection. Mol Imaging Radionucl Ther 2017;26(2):47–52.

86. Jouret F, Lhommel R, Beguin C, et al. Positron-emission computed tomography in cyst infection diagnosis in patients with autosomal dominant polycystic kidney disease. Clin J Am Soc Nephrol 2011;6(7):1644–50.

87. Bleeker-Rovers CP, de Sévaux RGL, van Hamersvelt HW, et al. Diagnosis of renal and hepatic cyst infections by 18-F-fluorodeoxyglucose positron emission tomography in autosomal dominant polycystic kidney disease. Am J Kidney Dis 2003;41(6):E18–21.

88. Piccoli GB, Arena V, Consiglio V, et al. Positron emission tomography in the diagnostic pathway for intracystic infection in ADPKD and "cystic" kidneys. A case series. BMC Nephrol 2011;12:48.

89. Soussan M, Sberro R, Wartski M, et al. Diagnosis and localization of renal cyst infection by 18F-fluorodeoxyglucose PET/CT in polycystic kidney disease. Ann Nucl Med 2008;22(6):529–31.

90. Jiménez-Bonilla JF, Quirce R, Calabia ER, et al. Hepatorenal polycystic disease and fever: diagnostic contribution of gallium citrate Ga 67 scan and fluorine F 18 FDG-PET/CT. Eur Urol 2011;59(2):297–9.

91. Wan C-H, Tseng J-R, Lee M-H, et al. Clinical utility of FDG PET/CT in acute complicated pyelonephritis-results from an observational study. Eur J Nucl Med Mol Imaging 2018;45(3):462–70.

92. Goldman DT, Piechowiak R, Nissman D, et al. Current concepts and future directions of minimally invasive treatment for knee pain. Curr Rheumatol Rep 2018;20(9):54.

93. Miller DV, Maleszewski JJ. The pathology of large-vessel vasculitides. Clin Exp Rheumatol 2011;29(1 Suppl 64):S92–8.

94. Abdel Razek AAK, Alvarez H, Bagg S, et al. Imaging spectrum of CNS vasculitis. Radiographics 2014;34(4):873–94.

95. Guggenberger KV, Bley TA. Imaging in vasculitis. Curr Rheumatol Rep 2020;22(8):34.

96. Howard T, Ahmad K, Swanson JAA, et al. Polyarteritis nodosa. Tech Vasc Interv Radiol 2014;17(4):247–51.

97. Valdovinos ST, Landry GJ. Raynaud syndrome. Tech Vasc Interv Radiol 2014;17(4):241–6.

98. Motegi S-I, Sekiguchi A, Saito S, et al. Successful treatment of Raynaud's phenomenon and digital ulcers in systemic sclerosis patients with botulinum toxin B injection: assessment of peripheral vascular disorder by angiography and dermoscopic image of nail fold capillary. J Dermatol 2018;45(3):349–52.

99. Del Conde I, Peña C. Buerger disease (thromboangiitis obliterans). Tech Vasc Interv Radiol 2014;17(4):234–40.

100. Hida N, Ohta T. Current status of patients with Buerger disease in Japan. Ann Vasc Dis 2013;6(3):617–23.

101. Hussein EA, el Dorri A. Intra-arterial streptokinase as adjuvant therapy for complicated Buerger's disease: early trials. Int Surg 1993;78(1):54–8.

102. Graziani L, Morelli L, Parini F, et al. Clinical outcome after extended endovascular recanalization in Buerger's disease in 20 consecutive cases. Ann Vasc Surg 2012;26(3):387–95.

103. Wu C, Li F, Niu G, et al. PET imaging of inflammation biomarkers. Theranostics 2013;3(7):448–66.

104. Casali M, Lauri C, Altini C, et al. State of the art of 18F-FDG PET/CT application in inflammation and infection: a guide for image acquisition and interpretation. Clin Transl Imaging 2021;1–41. https://doi.org/10.1007/s40336-021-00445-w.

105. Gormsen LC, Hess S. Challenging but clinically useful: fluorodeoxyglucose pet/computed tomography in inflammatory and infectious diseases. PET Clin 2020;15(2):xi–xii.

106. Nienhuis PH, van Praagh GD, Glaudemans AWJM, et al. A review on the value of imaging in differentiating between large vessel vasculitis and atherosclerosis. J Pers Med 2021;11(3). https://doi.org/10.3390/jpm11030236.

107. Arauz A, Hoyos L, Zenteno M, et al. Carotid plaque inflammation detected by 18F-fluorodeoxyglucose-positron emission tomography. Pilot study. Clin Neurol Neurosurg 2007;109(5):409–12.

108. van der Geest KSM, Treglia G, Glaudemans AWJM, et al. Diagnostic value of [18F]FDG-PET/CT for treatment monitoring in large vessel vasculitis: a systematic review and meta-analysis. Eur J Nucl Med Mol Imaging 2021. https://doi.org/10.1007/s00259-021-05362-8.

109. Pelletier-Galarneau M, Ruddy TD. PET/CT for diagnosis and management of large-vessel vasculitis. Curr Cardiol Rep 2019;21(5):34.

110. Fagart A, Machet T, Collet G, et al. FDG/PET-CT findings in a first series of 10 patients with polyarteritis nodosa. Rheumatology (Oxford) 2021. https://doi.org/10.1093/rheumatology/keab591.

111. Hackl G, Milosavljevic R, Belaj K, et al. The value of FDG-PET in the diagnosis of thromboangiitis obliterans–a case series. Clin Rheumatol 2015;34(4):739–44.

112. Seraj SM, Raynor WY, Revheim M-E, et al. Assessing the feasibility of NaF-PET/CT versus FDG-PET/CT to detect abdominal aortic calcification or inflammation in rheumatoid arthritis patients. Ann Nucl Med 2020;34(6):424–31.

113. Branchford BR, Carpenter SL. The role of inflammation in venous thromboembolism. Front Pediatr 2018;6:142.

114. Kaghazchi F, Borja AJ, Hancin EC, et al. Venous thromboembolism detected by FDG-PET/CT in cancer patients: a common, yet life-threatening observation. Am J Nucl Med Mol Imaging 2021;11(2):99–106.

115. Chen JX, Sudheendra D, Stavropoulos SW, et al. Role of catheter-directed thrombolysis in management of iliofemoral deep venous thrombosis. Radiographics 2016;36(5):1565–75.